Medicine and the Market

Related Titles in Health Policy and in Bioethics

Thomas H. Murray, consulting editor in bioethics

Medicine and the Market

Equity v. Choice

DANIEL CALLAHAN

ANGELA A. WASUNNA

The Hastings Center, Garrison, New York

The Johns Hopkins University Press

Baltimore

© 2006 The Johns Hopkins University Press
All rights reserved. Published 2006
Printed in the United States of America on acid-free paper
2   4   6   8   9   7   5   3   1

The Johns Hopkins University Press
2715 North Charles Street
Baltimore, Maryland 21218-4363
www.press.jhu.edu

Library of Congress Cataloging-in-Publication Data
Callahan, Daniel, 1930–
Medicine and the market : equity v. choice / Daniel Callahan, Angela A. Wasunna.
p. ; cm.
Includes bibliographical references and index.
ISBN 0-8018-8339-3 (hardcover : alk. paper)
1. Medical economics. 2. Medical care—Marketing. 3. Health services administration.
4. Medical ethics.
[DNLM: 1. Health Care Sector—ethics. 2. Health Care Reform—ethics.
3. Health Services Needs and Demand—ethics. W 74.1 C156m 2006]
I. Wasunna, Angela A., 1973–. II. Title.
RA410.53.C352 2006
362.1′068′8—dc22   2005023384

A catalog record for this book is available from the British Library.

For
Joab and Rose Wasunna
Dorothy Rice and Daniel M. Fox

Contents

Acknowledgments

If it takes a village to raise a child, as the saying goes, it takes almost that large a group to help someone write a book on medicine and the market. The topic is large, contentious, and international in scope. We were helped enormously by many people. We will begin with our research assistants—Mary McDonough, Juniper Lesnik, Rebecca Birnbaum, Michael Khair—and the staff of the Robert S. Morison Library at The Hastings Center. Gregory Kaebnick of The Hastings Center read the final draft and brought to it his considerable editing skills.

If that help was indispensable, the same can no less be said for the assistance of, and critical reading of various drafts by, a wide range of scholars from many countries: Migai Akech (Kenya), Ike O. Echeruo (Nigeria), Nuala Kenny (Canada), Ruud ter Meulen and Christi Nierse (the Netherlands), Eva Krizova (Czech Republic), Nicholas Pasini and Luciano Fasano (Italy), Hanspeter Kuhn (Switzerland), Kurt Fleschhauer and Ludger Honnefelder (Germany), Āke Bergmark and Christi Nierse (Sweden), Alan Cribb (United Kingdom), Herman Nys (Belgium), Miguel Kottow (Chile), and Khama Rogo and Chiaki Yamamoto (World Bank). Of particular importance was the wise guidance of Thomas Rice through the thicket of health care economics, from the beginning until the end of the project—the same Thomas Rice who is the son of Dorothy Rice (also a health economist), to whom, with others, we dedicate this book.

We also had the help of a special group of readers we brought together to go over an earlier draft of the book. They were, by turns, helpful, critical, cantankerous, prodding, and, best of all, often in disagreement with each other. It was a wonderful tutorial. Our thanks to Mark Pauly, William Hsaio, Richard S. Saltman, Meredith Turshen, and Thomas Rice. Alain Enthoven was exceedingly helpful with his insights as well.

Irene Crowe and the Pettus-Crowe Foundation supported our work on medicine and the market well before we began this book. Irene was an early believer in our project, and we were lucky to have her backing. Her assistance, and a grant from The Rockefeller, Tikvah, and Ira W. DeCamp Foundations, made possible some fine meetings in Prague, Cape Town, Santiago, and Tel Aviv and at Oxford University, as well as providing the financial resources necessary to write this book.

Medicine and the Market

Of Money, the Market, and Medicine

All of us seek health, the well-functioning of our mind and body, just as all of us recoil from pain and suffering. Yet the pursuit of health and the avoidance of suffering are a never-ending struggle. We are beset by a body programmed to decay and decline and by an external world that manages to bring harm to us from the outside, whether from accidents, plagues, viruses, deadly bacteria, or the depredations of our fellow citizens. Medicine and the health care systems of which it is a part are the main means of self-defense. These systems are in turn embedded in particular cultures with particular politics and particular sets of values. Each of them is also set within a world marked by the powerful impact of scientific progress, constantly reshaping the ways we understand life's possibilities, by shifting visions of the human good, and by long-standing debates about the best way to organize societies to pursue their collective welfare.

This book is about an important chapter of that larger story, focusing on the place of market theory and practice in medicine and health care. In recent decades health care reform has become a chronic problem in all parts of the world, sometimes mildly, sometimes harshly. While major changes may come slowly to health care systems (with some exceptions, as we will see), minor changes and endless tinkering with the details are almost annual events. Cutting through all these shifts are discussions, debates, and proposals about whether and how to deploy market practices to further health goals. Some countries seem far more prone than others to entertain and pursue market ideas, but hardly anywhere are those possibilities ignored. The seemingly con-

stant cost pressures on health care systems mean that there are repeated opportunities to renew old debates and to take another look.

We bring two perspectives to this tale, and no doubt some of the biases that
go with them. Callahan is American, long drawn to U.S. domestic health care
arguments and its attendant politics, and to an understanding of the unique,
almost idiosyncratic, fascination with the market that is a deep part of American culture. He is also a philosopher by training and thus drawn to questions of
the meaning of health and its place in human life, to the relief of suffering as an
ancient problem, and to the idea of, and difficulties with, medical progress as
one of the most cherished of modern values. Wasunna is a native of Kenya,
trained in international law and bioethics and, in recent years, caught up in the
ethical and social problems of HIV/AIDS and health care reform in developing
countries. She is also someone who has worked for years in the United States,
closely following the American arguments about restructuring of its health
care, wondering what, if anything, can be useful for her country. She has witnessed in Kenya, a developing country, the struggle to organize a more equitable health care system and to decide what role the market should play. The
international struggle over the price and provision of expensive antiretroviral
drugs for HIV disease, developed and produced by a profit-oriented pharmaceutical industry in developed countries, has been an inescapable part of that
larger struggle.

We mention our backgrounds for two reasons. One of them is to explain why
this book, which aims to be international in the scope of its analysis, uses
the American market debate as a point of departure, a foil against which to
assess the market arguments in other societies. The United States can fairly be
described as the heartland of market and health care arguments, experiments,
and passionate convictions for and against. The other reason is that, while an
American perspective will be brought in explicitly or implicitly on many occa-
sions, it no less offers a point of departure for thinking about the market in
developing countries. The United States provides evidence of some of the
problems and possibilities—call it a cautionary tale—that a bewitchment with
the market displays. Western Europe offers a different angle of insight, where
market practices are used but in a much more pragmatic, less ideological way
than in the United States.

In which direction will the developing countries go, in an American or a
European way, or some new way mainly of their own devising? They have a
number of different role models they can draw upon, but with of course one
fundamental difference: money and resources. The North American and Euro-

pean countries are rich in both, which better explains the good health of their populations than does the form of their health care. The developing countries start with no such advantage. Whatever they can learn from the developed countries will have to be applied in a very different setting and no doubt in different ways as well. How that all turns out will be determined not simply by ideas and theories of good health care, but by their general economic development and the kinds of political systems that take shape in the coming years.

THE MARKET: STEREOTYPES AND COMPLEXITIES

Like many people when they first come to the topic of "the market," we brought with us a number of stereotypes. For both of us, liberals by disposition, the notion of the market invoked suspicion and some hostility. Reminiscent of the ancient Manichean vision of the world as divided between the light and the dark, the good and the bad, to us the market bespoke crass commercialism, the commodification of important health needs and aspirations, a falling away from the ideal of health care that would be accessible and affordable to everyone. We cannot claim we totally overcame these stereotypes as our research progressed—and not all stereotypes are wholly false—but they surely underwent a change. The notion of "equity versus choice," reflected in the subtitle of this book, is itself inadequate, capturing one important political feature of the market debate but by no means sufficient to capture many other significant features.

Though starting on the equity side, we came to understand the attractions of the market as a possibly useful ingredient in health care reform, and in particular its understanding of human behavior and aspiration. There is a difference of great importance, for instance, between a view of the market that emphasizes its commercial uses, focused on economic growth and preference satisfaction, and one that focuses on its use as a more or less neutral behavioral and managerial tool to manage social institutions efficiently, including health care. Once we began to take account of that difference, we were led to recognize that, wisely handled, market ideas could well be helpful to the kind of health care we hope for (we say no more than that at this point)—health care that is affordable to all, sustainable in the long run, and respecting the culture of different societies.

The concept of the market, when played out in practice, is by no means clear and simple. A dictionary definition of the market is that it is "an exchange mechanism that brings together sellers and buyers of a product, factor of production, or financial security."[1] That formal definition is correct but not exactly revealing. A passage in a book on European health care, written by two distinguished analysts of that care (and something less than market enthusiasts), underscores the complexity and variety of market mechanisms:

> There is no single, simple concept of market that can be adopted for use in a health system. Rather, market-style mechanisms include a number of specific instruments such as consumer sovereignty (patient choice), negotiated contracts and open bidding. They can be adopted in markets organized on different principles: on price, on quality or on market share. Markets can, in turn, be introduced into different sectors of the health system: in health care funding, in one or more subsets of the production of health services . . . Competitive incentives can be brought to bear on the behaviour of physicians, nurses, support personnel or home care personnel. In practice, then, there is not one decision but a series of decisions to be made. Rather than a monolithic commitment to one of two abstractions—state or market—both Western and Eastern European health care systems confront a range of smaller decisions . . . it typically involves a multitude of approximations, if not compromises.[2]

If that quotation suggests the complexity inherent in any full analysis of "the market," the market-oriented economist Stuart M. Butler aptly reminds us that "markets develop and evolve in response to consumers' demands, and they do so in many different ways dependent in part on the framework of government rules affecting them."[3] The full story of the market in health care is one that is rich with variety and shadings (often confusingly so), a mix of success and failures, and as yet no definitive, easy-to-emulate guidelines on how to make it work well, much less to work well without doing harm to other important values. The same can of course be said of government-run or heavily regulated systems. Our aim is to take a look at that complexity, to survey a range of international initiatives to make use of market mechanisms, to see how the market has been integrated into different national health care systems, and, in the end, to offer some criteria for the use of the market in health care systems.

THE BACKGROUND TAPESTRY

To enter the realm of the market and health care is at once to observe a multicolored tapestry. It is made up of the interwoven strands of history, medical science, culture, politics, ethical and social values, and economic theory. It is beyond the scope of this book, and no doubt our capacities, to integrate fully these strands, to uncover all of the connecting threads, and to make sense of the entire pattern. But we will, when possible, attempt some integration, bringing the background tapestry to the foreground. Whether we succeed or fail in doing so, however, we want to lay out first of all what seem to us some of the more important background features. Taken alone or together, these have important roles in shaping the way the issues get laid out in public and professional debates. We single out four as especially noteworthy: the shifting and progress-driven goals of medicine and health care, which we take to be the most decisive force working to change health care; the interaction of history, culture, and politics; the work of health care economists and market advocates; and ethics and social values.

Shifting Goals of Medicine and Health Care: The Impact of Progress

In one sense, it may seem odd to speak of the "shifting goals of medicine and health care." People have always become sick and threatened with death from illness and disease, and they have always looked for relief. For at least a century, most societies have looked for ways to help provide the economic and medical means to pursue that relief. Two broad goals can be perceived in that individual and social effort: (1) the prevention of disease, now encompassing health-related behavior, and the protection and improvement of public health—which can be called the realm of population health; (2) the care of those who are sick and disabled, whether from the endogenous assault of disease or the exogenous accidents and vicissitudes of ordinary life—which can be called the realm of individual medicine and health care. In this second category, we can identify different kinds of health care services: for example, emergency care, primary care, acute care, chronic care, rehabilitative care, and nursing care.

Governments have taken an interest in both of these realms. There are many benefits of a healthy citizenry and many burdens of an unhealthy one, and many and variegated individual health needs. Medical and biological research, on the one hand, and health services research, on the other, have been pursued to improve outcomes in both realms. Because a great deal of health research is undertaken in the private sector, mainly for commercial purposes, the market has a central place, shaping the scope and direction of its research.

Though the description we have provided may be accurate enough, it is static. It does not well capture the dynamic and constant change brought about by medical progress and, even more perhaps, by medical progress that goes hand in hand with economic and social progress. Every one of the health care categories noted above is undergoing change and transformation: the general labels remain constant but the contents keep shifting. The dual goals of population and individual progress have led to a great increase in average life expectancy almost everywhere in the world, a shift of emphasis in developed countries from infectious to chronic disease, a gradual increase in the number and proportion of the elderly, and, in many parts of the world, a decrease in the proportion of children. In great part, the developing countries of the world have not benefited from the progress taken for granted in affluent countries. That terrible reality is all the more disturbing because it is by now well known what forms of medical research, public health measures, and improved health care delivery could radically ameliorate their dire health conditions.

We single out as most important the notion of medical progress, for three reasons. First, the market has been a potent force behind the medical progress in the commercial creation and production of medical goods of all kinds, drugs and devices. That progress has brought about great health benefits as well as great costs. Control of rising prices has been an important stimulus in the use of market mechanisms, whether the HMO (health maintenance organization) movement in the United States, the internal markets of the National Health Service in the United Kingdom, or assorted competitive and other tactics in Western Europe. A large portion of rising costs can be traced to the introduction of new technologies and the intensified use of old ones—estimated to account for 40 to 50 percent of American health care cost increases.[4] While there is a wide variation among countries in the use of high-technology machines and diagnostic devices, all have seen their steady increase, just as all have seen a steady rise in pharmaceutical prices.

Second, medical progress leads to a constant rise in the baseline of public expectations, of what counts as good health care, and a no less steady exacerbation of the old yet never settled idea of what counts as "medical necessity." Medical progress, as with most other forms of progress, is self-fueling: the more of it one gets, the more one wants. That progress breaks down any lingering fatalism about the inevitability of nature to do us in, seemingly open to any and all possibilities in the improvement of health. Just as the automobiles of 1960 no longer seem adequate—no air bags, poor environmental controls, more hazardous in accidents, and weak radios—so also the health care of 1960. The young and old expect to live longer and in better health than forty-five years ago, doctors have more ways of treating their illnesses, acute or chronic, mortality rates continue to decline in most parts of the world, and a whole range of new drugs and technologies have appeared on the scene.

Partly because of hype but mainly because of past success, the expectation is that the medicine of the next decade will be better than that of this decade, and so on with the medicine of the decades after that. Health care has a peculiar feature, at least in the developed countries: the greater the health progress, the more everyone wants to spend on it. The long-standing dream of eliminating, or at least radically diminishing, disease and forestalling death has received great encouragement from scientific progress—and yet, for all that progress, we still get sick and die, and only the most unbuttoned utopianism can envision something radically different in the future.

Third, efforts to understand the dynamics of improving health, and thus the main features of health progress—as distinguished from technical medical and scientific progress—have forced a valuable examination of just what exactly enhances health, individually and collectively, and in what ways. Assorted research has focused, for instance, on the role of medical research in improved health, on the place of socioeconomic determinants of health status (education, jobs, income, for instance), on the availability of good health care, drugs, and medical technologies, and on health-related behavior (smoking, a lack of exercise). While the heaviest emphasis of medical research has been on biologically related causes of poor health, American studies have pinpointed poor behavioral patterns as the primary cause of about 50 percent of deaths. Education levels are a good predictor of health status for most people, while the availability of advanced technology (among other things) is important for the life expectancy of those over age eighty. A series of well-known studies in the United Kingdom found a clear correlation between good health and occupational status, even for those with identical access to health care.[5]

If the previous few paragraphs adequately summarize some of the conventional ways of looking at medical and health progress, we want to offer an additional category, between what might be termed an infinity and a finite model, or vision, of progress. The infinity model has at its heart the conviction, even if usually unstated, that medical progress, as with scientific progress more generally, should be open-ended, always seeking—whatever the present level of health—even better health, committed to unending new biological knowledge and constant technological innovation. At its outer fringes this aspiration gradually blurs the boundaries between ordinary good health and enhanced human health—between, for instance, a now-average life expectancy and a much longer life (if aging itself is construed as a disease), or between a statistically normal child and one with enhanced physical and mental characteristics.

A finite model, by contrast (fitfully and erratically still present), would emphasize quality of life over length of life, accept illness, aging, and death as a permanent part of the human condition, stress population rather than individual health—and, in particular, would be skeptical of expressed preferences and desires as always the best indicators of what is good for us. Our conviction is that the infinity model of progress is in serious tension with the long-term financial sustainability of health care systems. Infinite goals cannot be financed with finite resources.

Even apart from open utopianism, the tacit logic and trajectory of contemporary research have no end in sight but the conquest of all disease (thought possible by some, for instance, as the long-term outcome of the Human Genome Project, mapping the human genome) and, as thought by the more venturesome, of death itself. "Death," William Haseltine, an important biotechnology scientist and entrepreneur, has said, "is nothing but a series of preventable diseases."[6] That kind of hyperbole can easily be dismissed, but then one can ask: just what lethal diseases is the National Institutes of Health prepared to ignore, to simply let be, as a cause of death? None that we can discern.

The phrase "medical necessity" came into use some years ago in an effort to specify a minimally necessary and adequate level of health care. There is no debate about the necessity of surgery for a ruptured appendix, but plenty of squabbling about Viagra as a necessity for aging males, with or without some clear medical pathology. And those are the easier cases. A whole host of new technologies are appearing that promise to improve health—such as new heart technologies (implantable artificial hearts) or expanded use of older ones (such as implantable cardioverter-defibrillators), or new cancer drugs that will not cure the disease but will turn it into a manageable chronic disease—with high costs and mixed benefits. Is an expensive drug that adds just a few months of life a "medical necessity" or a luxury item in a rich country? And are even those technologies that work well at moderate cost a necessity in comparison with the much wider good that might be done if the money was spent on diseases of childhood or drug subsidies for poor countries? Looked at in that light, the notion of medical necessity seems to disappear into a twilight zone, a mix of available money, cultural preferences, medical biases, and public information.

Inevitably, the market and medical progress will have an influence in determining "medical necessity." The phrase sounds like an empirical concept, something easily quantified and described. On the contrary, we believe it to be a function of available technologies, cultural values, and variable attitudes toward sickness and death. The history of medicine is filled with examples of new drugs and technologies functioning to change popular and professional thinking about what counts as a disease or a health care problem. A Czech geriatrician explained to one of us in the early 1990s that "Alzheimer's is not a problem in our country—people get old and forgetful; that's a problem of life, not medicine."[7] A decade later Alzheimer's had been acknowledged and is now as routinely dealt with in the Czech Republic—strikingly helped along by money from Pfizer, attempting to find a market for its drug Aricept. Neither baldness nor erectile dysfunction in aging men nor a less-than-desirable nose shape was considered a medical problem—until medicine found a way to do something about them.

Balancing Government and the Market: History, Culture, and Politics

While an interest in the market and health care can be traced back several decades, it took on a new energy in the 1970s, when cost pressures began to appear in a number of countries. By the 1980s, with the Thatcher and Reagan eras and gathering storms in the Eastern European countries, market ideas and advocacy began to circulate with growing force, particularly in the United States and the United Kingdom, soon to be picked up by the World Bank and its focus on developing countries. A parallel market stream, but with considerably less ideological flavor, was also developing in Western Europe, heavily influenced by globalization and competitive economic forces and by the need for financial sustainability of their health care systems.

At the center of this trend were debates over the role of government in health care. The more ideologically oriented market proponents could argue, by the early 1990s, that the downfall of the Communist countries, with their command economies, sent out a message about government in general: the need to loosen its grip, to turn more to the private sector, and to make use of the efficiencies that the market could bring. That was a lesson, many held, that health care systems needed to learn as well. While it is unclear to what extent these more general currents affected Western Europe, the 1980s saw a rise in market experiments and initiatives in those countries. Yet though such initiatives could be found almost everywhere in the face of economic recessions in

Europe—and worries about the future of the welfare state—they were limited by the force of strong and traditional communitarian convictions, summed up in the word *solidarity*. The World Bank, for its part, more affected by market ideology, saw it as the key lever for economic development in developing countries—and in their health care systems as well.

The abiding question everywhere, however, was how to find the right balance in health care between some government (or public control) role, which hardly anyone rejected, however much they disagreed on its extent, and the place of a private sector, evoking similar disagreement. Agreement on what might count as the "right" balance was thus elusive, a function of history, tradition, politics, and the flux of economic growth and economic recession.

Health Service Analysis

Economic analysis of health care is a major academic and professional field. A book of this kind could not be written at all without making use of the research and studies coming out of it. Yet as outsiders to the field, we did not find it altogether easy to reconcile the various arguments among health care economists or to find a wholly satisfactory way to characterize their work. We will replay a number of those arguments as this book moves along, but here we address only the nature of their work.

Two streams seem apparent, though with many connecting tributaries. The first, and most common in the academic field, might be termed the instrumentalist viewpoint, coming out of the tradition of welfare economics. Its characteristic mark is to treat "the market" as a set of tools and concepts of practical use in organizing various kinds of distribution systems, including health care. Its style is cool and analytical, committed to gaining solid quantitative data in the assessment of health care systems. Efficiency—the most effective means of achieving a chosen end in the provision of care—is perhaps its highest value. It steers clear of larger political and ethical debates and, at least so it seems to us, treats the issue of equitable access to care with a certain ambivalence. Some economists seem comfortable in dealing with matters of justice and equity (particularly in Europe). Others, especially in the United States, often label their judgments on such matters as "personal," or "value laden," not the outcome of economic theory.

The other perspective, which we will call the political viewpoint, embodies a combination of some important economists, such as Friedrich Hayek and Milton Friedman, together with a large and heterogeneous group of lay followers. In essence, their argument is that the market is the key to the spread and success of democracy, prosperity, and human freedom; it is more than an instrumental tool. Though its scope is not always clearly defined, the term *choice* is a leading value, the essence of economic and social freedom: among other things, the choice of a doctor and the choice by a doctor about how he or she wants to practice medicine, the choice of a health care system, and a personal choice about how much to pay for health care. This perspective has been taken up with vigor, and considerable influence, by the *Wall Street Journal, Forbes,* and the *Economist,* by the George W. Bush administration, and by a number of research institutions (the American Enterprise Institute, the Heritage Foundation, the Hoover Institution, and the Cato Institute, among the most prominent); it has both an academic and political following. If China can be seen at the moment as the great counterexample of the necessary relationship between the market and democracy, those with the political vision believe it is precisely the growing power of market activities in that country that will undermine its authoritarian regime. The political viewpoint, however, by no means ignores some mainline ideas from health care economics (it is simply at one end of the spectrum), believing the market brings invigorating competition, greater consumer-patient choice, and a reduction of top-down government power and influence.

Ethics and Social Values

If there have been long drawn-out struggles among health care economists on the appropriate place of the market in health care, and if those struggles have overlapped some more political and ideological battles about the civic virtues of market thought, there have also been some furious ethical and social debates as well. We generalize at some risk here, but three confrontations are worth noting. Perhaps one of the oldest is the long-standing Roman Catholic opposition to market ideas, even though there is a recent effort by some to find a theological grounding for the market. In nineteenth-century Europe, the social encyclicals of Pope Leo XIII, together with other Catholic influences, had an important role in establishing sick funds and planting the roots of universal health care.

That development emerged in the context of an otherwise conservative Church, hostile to modernism and suspicious of democracy, but whose often progressive social thought was usually embraced by autocratic regimes. If the Church did not like the modern world at all, it also did not like the industrial capitalism that was a part of it. The Church set its face against the market, against secular thought, and against the exploitation of labor. It remained a powerful force in European society for many decades, at the same time making many enemies on the right and left. In the United States, there is still considerable Catholic suspicion about the market, particularly among theologians, and they are joined by Protestant liberals, still with a strong tradition from an earlier time of the Social Gospel movement. Evangelical Protestant Christians are drawn to the Republican Party and to market ideas. In contemporary Europe, by contrast, where the influence of religion is weak and the general forces of the market strong (even if not quite as much as in the United States), a weaker individualism and a continuing dedication to a central role for public financing or oversight in ensuring welfare coverage of all kinds has led to a limited role for the market in health care.

Second, in the United States, the Democratic Party has for many decades been seen as an opponent of an untrammeled market and an advocate of a central role for government in the provision of social welfare. At least until the middle of the twentieth century, American physicians were a notably conservative group, opposed to government interference in their medical practice and hostile to universal health care. Efforts to introduce universal health have always come from Democrats, led by President Harry Truman just after World War II, Senator Edward Kennedy in the 1970s (though with a Republican ally in Senator Jacob Javits), and President Bill Clinton in the 1990s. Republican critics, harsh in their attacks on "big government" and "socialized medicine," resisted those efforts, almost always looking for market alternatives for health care reform. George W. Bush's success in pushing through a pharmaceutical plan as part of Medicare was in part a response to widespread political pressure, but also in part a major move toward the market in some of the plan's key provisions. The result received much criticism from Democrats for those market gestures, and no less from conservative Republicans for its expansion of the government reach.

The third and last grouping we will mention consists, in a more generic way, of some deep and enduring ethical and political tensions. Is there, as the United Nations has proclaimed, a right to health care? Put another way, what obligations do we have to others, as our fellow citizens and human beings, to come to their aid when they are sick and threatened with death? If there is a right to health care, is there an obligation on national governments to recognize and implement it? If so, does that obligation extend to all citizens regardless of income, or only to those who are unable to afford it? Since health care can involve people with different values and preferences, different ways of life, how extensive should our individual choice be in selecting our physician, the kind of health care plan we want, the type of care we desire, and the way that care should be paid for? Medical care as a profit-making enterprise, seen by some as a fundamental contradiction to its altruistic nature, poses a fundamental question: can profit be sought without harm to medicine's traditional patient-centered values?

We would note that, by our focus on the market debate, we will not give a great deal of attention to the important matter of the promotion and maintenance of health, which encompasses public health policies as well as the socioeconomic determinants of health. Moreover, when we refer to equity in health care, or equitable access to care, we will primarily be referring to access to organized medical care, of a kind and quality that is compatible with a nation's resources, affordable to everyone (which can allow some tiered variations in care, if not extreme in their variation). We will not deal directly with another set of important issues, those of health inequalities (which can exist in otherwise decent health care systems) or inequities (which can also occur in such systems), though we will frequently allude to them.

Market proponents are prone to want the scope of choice wide and capacious: liberty is a high, dominant value. Those wary of the market worry more about the fair distribution of health benefits, the protection of the poor, and financial security in the face of health care costs than about freedom of choice. The great struggle, over centuries now, between justice and liberty is played out again and again in market debates, just as it is played out in the larger sphere of national and international politics. Health care in the developing countries puts all of these problems in sharp relief, particularly in light of the AIDS debate.

Even if one agrees that there is a right to health care, and some obligation of government to ensure it, what obligations do rich countries have to poor countries? For those of us in the rich countries, people in the poor countries are surely our fellow human beings, but not our neighbors, not part of our own national communities.[8] Empathy and solidarity can be harder to come by. Market proponents, invoking neither rights nor solidarity, look to free trade, a vigorous domestic market in all sectors, and democratic societies to bring to poor countries the wealth needed to provide decent health care. The World Bank, as we will see later, has more or less forced developing countries to accept market practices for their economies in general and their health care systems in particular. Beyond that, the willingness of developed countries to help the developing countries through charitable aid programs has been erratic, with the European countries showing far more generosity than the United States. Nonetheless, the needs of those with HIV disease, tuberculosis, and any of a long list of deadly tropical diseases far exceed the amount of health resources that have been given to them. Once again, though different than at the national level, basic moral questions about the role of the market versus that of government, and the obligations of governments and international agencies, come to the fore.

A STILL UNFOLDING TALE

The story we want to lay out in this book rests on those background issues, and in many cases they will directly emerge. Our aim is to capture the dynamics and movement of the international debate about the proper, or sensible, or appropriate role of the market in health care. We begin, in chapter 1, with a broad survey of the development of market theory since Adam Smith in the eighteenth century and how, much later, market ideas and practices began to be applied to health care, sometimes zealously pushed and sometimes no less zealously resisted. We then turn, in chapter 2, to a comparison of health care in the United States and Canada, the former famous (or infamous, as the case may be) as the heartland of market approbation and the latter as a country that has embraced the market in most of its economy but not in health care. From there we move to Western Europe (chapter 3), comprised of a number of countries that have, for many decades now, worked to ensure full access to decent health care for all of their citizens, but where the market has, in varying degrees, been accepted as a way of supporting their commitment to good access.

Following that chapter we move on to the developing countries (chapter 4), where there are a wide variety of health care systems, little public money to pay for health care, and a fitful, erratic use of the market—stimulated by the World Bank—to help populations burdened by diseases and medical conditions long controlled in more affluent countries. With those country surveys behind us, we then examine the pharmaceutical industry (chapter 5), a major influence on all health care systems, a symbol of for-profit entrepreneurial medicine of the most vivid kind, and an industry that has long proclaimed the power of the free market as the source of energy, innovation, and international health benefits.

We conclude by attempting, in chapter 6, to synthesize the available evidence on the effectiveness of the most important market practices throughout the world. What actually happens when various individual market practices are used, such as competition, and what happens to health care systems when they decide to embrace, or not embrace, the market as a key feature of those systems? Finally, chapter 7 encapsulates our findings and offers some criteria for the introduction of market practices in health care systems.

We readily confess that we are proponents of universal, equitable-access, government-run or -supervised health care systems—and more so now than when we began our research. But we also readily acknowledge that the market may have some useful contributions to make if carefully managed and regulated, what we call the "second-best" solution. We more than suspect that the story we have tried to tell has many chapters left to be explored, that the present flux will be a permanent part of that story, and that the relationship between medicine and the market will, to a greater or lesser extent, always be a part of that story as well. In the end, that relationship turns on some old and enduring questions of individual and common good, and answers to them do not for long stand still.

CHAPTER ONE

From Adam Smith to HMOs

The Origins of Medicine and the Market

Consider two classic texts, one from the fifth century BC, the other from the eighteenth century AD. In his *Republic,* Plato writes that "the physician, as such, studies only the patient's interest, not his own . . . The business of the physician, in the strict sense, is not to make money for himself, but to exercise his power over the patients' body . . . All that he says and does will be done with a view to what is good and proper for the subject for whom he practices his art."[1] The more modern and familiar text is Adam Smith's 1776 book *The Wealth of Nations,* in which he writes: "It is not from the benevolence of the butcher, the brewer, or the baker, that we expect our dinner, but from their regard for their own interest. We address ourselves, not to their humanity, but to their self-love and never talk to them of our own necessities but to their advantages. Nobody but a beggar chuses to depend chiefly upon the benevolence of his fellow-citizens."[2]

A nicer, apparently more telling contrast between an animating commitment of medicine, altruistic at its core, and the animating principle of the market, self-interest, could hardly be imagined. Is that the whole story? Not quite. The doctor, Plato notes, in the words of a commentator, "is in one way a businessman," even though he does not act for his own advantages, only for that of his patient (picking up on the phrase "in the strict sense").[3] The fact that a physician takes money in return for his medical expertise does not, as such, turn him into a merely self-interested merchant; still, he is a merchant. The market and money have never been absent from medicine.

Yet if they have never been absent, there is a more interesting question:

why did medicine gradually make the move from a simple one-on-one economic relationship, doctor and patient, to an economically massive enterprise, that of the provision of health care, now of the highest importance in every country? A number of phases appear. They begin with the progress of medical knowledge and its successful clinical application, slowly in the seventeenth and eighteenth centuries and much more rapidly by the late nineteenth and into the twentieth centuries. In parallel with that development, the market as an idea and social reality gradually took on a life of its own, controversial but inexorable.

The two currents eventually converged into a massive and steadily growing economic juggernaut that invited market interest, both for its profit potential and for its organizational possibilities. The often raucous debates in most societies about the market, about the role of government in managing national economies, and about the place of welfare programs, including health care, have become daily fare. And no less so within medicine and health care systems. Again and again as the twentieth century moved along, the issues raised by Adam Smith played themselves out in medical research and in health care reform: the relationship of government and the market, the impact of the market on the culture and practice of medicine, and the way human nature, in its quest for health and its fear of sickness, is best understood.

If the altruism cited by Plato as the animating drive of the physician is not the full story of medicine, neither is the self-interest of the merchant, or his place in Adam Smith's thought, the full story of the market. *The Theory of Moral Sentiments,* published in 1759, reveals a fundamental aspect of Smith's thought, emphasizing the centrality of empathy in human relationships and the shaping of a decent society. Human beings are by nature dependent on each other. The dignity of the individual, at the core of Smith's thought, was always to be respected and a morally necessary part of market relationships. Yet benevolence, empathy, and respect for dignity could not by themselves sustain a commercial society.

Smith's claim, as the historian Jerry Z. Muller has aptly put it, "is that an economic system cannot be *based* on benevolence, which is a limited sentiment not easily extended beyond those one knows."[4] The great challenge, Smith believed, was to understand how to develop the potential social benefits of our propensity to self-love and self-interest. The market provides a way of increasing wealth while, at the same time, fostering social cooperation and valuable moral traits. Among those traits are discipline, delay of gratification, self-command, and prudence.

Would we object to a physician who displayed those traits, especially if undergirded by empathy and sensitive fellow feeling? Hardly, but we might hesitate in our judgment if the intention of such a physician is simply and only to make a good living. Not a few ambitious young people in the United States have chosen medicine as a career because of its financial reward, and then chosen a subspecialty because it offered even greater rewards. It is hard to know how Smith would have judged such a person, but the often misunderstood part of his notion of an "invisible hand" is that a distinction can be drawn between a person's intention in acting in a particular way and the actual results of such behavior. Dependent upon the institutional conditions of such behavior, the individual's "self interest may lead to socially valuable results."[5] Should I really care if my doctor is in it only for the money as long as he respects my dignity, treats me with empathy, answers my phone calls promptly, and provides me with high-quality medical care?

The moral premise behind Plato's description of the ethically responsible physician is that, while the physician must be some kind of merchant, selling his skills, his highest aim must, to be true to his profession, be altruistic. Though Smith does not take up the conduct of the physician, the implication of his willingness to separate moral intentions and social results is that the collective impact of self-interested (but prudent) physicians could result in as good medical care as those motivated by altruism. Our later examinations of market practices—and what actually happened to physicians' behavior within the market—will of necessity have to return to this implicit claim and Smith's notion of the invisible hand. Would a medicine that openly presented the doctor as a merchant, offering in a competitive marketplace services chosen by savvy patients labeled as consumers, be a tolerable medicine? And particularly if the services were of a high quality?

For now those last questions will be left hanging. Whatever the answer, it is important to understand that Smith believed it both necessary and possible to turn individual self-interest, the psychological reality behind the market, in the direction of the common good. In a parallel view, Plato believed that the physician who sold his services—since like the rest of us he must eat—could do so without harming the altruistic core of medicine.

Smith had other things to say of indirect importance to medicine and the market, and they should not be overlooked. While contemporary market advocates often present themselves as opponents of big government, this was not true of Smith. "Government in a civilized country is much more expensive than in a barbarous one," he wrote, and he expected that it would grow with the development of commercial society.[6] Nor was he an opponent of some features of what we would call the welfare state. The laboring man "whose whole life is spent in performing a few simple operations . . . has no occasion to exert his understanding . . . [and] in every improved and civilized society this is the state into which the laboring poor . . . must necessarily fall, unless government take some pains to prevent it."[7] While he was famous for his support of a free market for corn, Smith was prepared to have the government develop public projects to provide ways for helping the poor to pay for that corn. Concerning the poor he wrote, "No society can surely be flourishing and happy, of which the far greater parts of the members are poor and miserable."[8] Equity requires, he wrote, that those who help produce that which is needed by everyone should themselves be "tolerably well fed, clothed and lodged."[9] A contemporary reader could plausibly add "and with access to good health care."

By 1800, Adam Smith had been turned into the modern hero of commerce, a position he still holds but one that does not do justice to the complexity of his thinking.[10] Like Bernard Mandeville in his ironic 1723 book *The Fable of the Bees,* Smith saw self-interest as a primary human drive. But he did not think it necessarily led only to luxury and vanity, though he agreed they are dangerous. They can also, if properly managed, help generate a decent society.[11] It is not a stretch to contend that Smith's philosophy can be understood to be what Stephen Darwall has called "sympathetic liberalism," embodying a liberal theory of social justice and equal individual dignity as the basis of a free market.[12]

Smith's effort to develop both a theory of a virtue ethics and a libertarian market theory has a particular importance for this book. When claims are made about the value of market principles for medicine and the health care system that provides it, we should inquire into the implicit models of human nature and of government that lie behind them. Smith offers a way of joining those two dimensions of human life, attempting to integrate self-interest and the sympathetic virtues with a view of government that can serve as a check to the self's more rapacious side. That kind of aim poses a challenge to opponents of the market, who must show that such a commitment necessarily entails harm to medicine's traditional altruism. It is no less a challenge to many market proponents, who must show that the ideology of the market and its characteristic practices can be safely deployed to maintain that altruism.

Any sharp contrast between the altruistic aims of medicine and the self-interest focus of Adam Smith's work, in any case, immediately collapses in the face of a closer examination of each one. Nonetheless it seems true that in the eighteenth and early nineteenth centuries medicine was not, unlike many other commodities such as corn, seen as a subject for organized market application. As the debate on the role of the market developed in the nineteenth century, medicine still remained in the hands of solo practitioners (what we now call "fee-for-service" medicine). Despite the effort of organized American medicine to eliminate the competition of quacks and to establish the hegemony of physicians in the organization and practice of medicine in the late nineteenth and early twentieth centuries, medicine went its own way and the larger market debate another.

What was to bring them increasingly together in the twentieth century? Why did many in medicine come to think of their skills as a profitable commodity, ripe for market tactics—but remain anxious to hold on to the individual doctor's value as a purveyor of his skills to individual patients? And why, on the other hand, did market proponents, indifferent to medicine and health care in the eighteenth and nineteenth centuries, begin to see them as fruit to be picked in an expanding market vineyard in the twentieth century?

THE TRANSFORMATION OF MEDICINE AND HEALTH CARE

Though money was always involved in the interplay of doctors and patients, there was no serious interaction between medicine and the market in any organized sense in the United States (or elsewhere for that matter) until the second half of the nineteenth century. There was, for one thing, no open trade in medical care as was the case with other commodities such as food, cloth, and machines. Medicine was not thought of as a commodity at all, but as a service, though doctors did on occasion compete for patients, and sometimes on the basis of price. The quality of the doctor's care mattered the most, often reflected in his fees. The doctor-patient relationship was essentially contractual, the doctor giving patients what they wanted in return for a fee. The relative ineffectiveness of medicine made it an unlikely target for market theorizing. Doctors could do relatively little to cure and control disease, to rehabilitate the injured, or to solve mundane medical needs. Medicine was thus not a necessity of life, as it has become today. Nor was it organized enough to make it attractive to financial speculators.

Yet as far back as the end of the eighteenth century, the ground began being laid for a radical change in the nature and economic status of medicine, as well as for the emergence of organized national health care systems. Four features of the change seem particularly important, each intensifying the other:

a new vision of medical possibilities, a decline in mortality and morbidity, an enthusiastic embrace of medical research, and the emergence of a market for medical care.

A New Vision of Medical Possibilities

While Francis Bacon and René Descartes in the sixteenth and seventeenth centuries had raised the possibility of using science to conquer the infirmities of the body, it is hard to beat Benjamin Franklin's optimism: "It is impossible to imagine," he wrote to the distinguished British scientist Joseph Priestley, "the height to which may be carried, in a thousand years, the power of man over matter . . . all diseases may be prevented or cured, not excepting that of old age, and our lives lengthen at pleasure even beyond the ante-diluvium standard."[13] The famous American physician Benjamin Rush was hardly less effusive. The American Revolution had itself "opened the doors to the temple of nature . . . [making possible] a knowledge of antidotes to those diseases that are supposed to be incurable."[14]

There were no medical breakthroughs in that Enlightenment era to lend credibility to such claims. Yet there was an Enlightenment faith that science held the key to most of the riddles of life, including an understanding of nature's way of ravaging the body. We call particular attention to Franklin's statement that "all diseases may be prevented or cured." It was an influential position and a foundational statement of our notion of an "infinity" model of medicine, that of unlimited frontiers, seeking not simply the amelioration of the human physical condition but its ultimate mastery. Benjamin Franklin can hardly be considered a spokesman for contemporary medicine, but his language captures well its main scientific themes: an uncommon optimism about the future, a great faith in science, and a deep belief that medicine can, someday, radically change the human condition.

This utopian theme emerged again and again in the United States. A physician writing in the *Journal of the American Medical Association* in 1914 said that "in fifty years science will have practically eliminated all forms of disease."[15] After World War II, as the National Institutes of Health was growing and flourishing, the tradition of unlimited optimism remained powerful, reflected in the annual congressional appropriation hearings for the regularly expanded NIH budget. Again and again it was said that great breakthroughs were on the horizon, with each new discovery opening the way to even greater ones.

Richard Nixon's declaration of the war on cancer in 1970 reflected this theme, as did the Human Genome Project, initiated in 1990, and the excitement about stem cell research as the new millennium dawned further embellished it.

A Decline in Mortality and Morbidity

If there was in the eighteenth century little foundation for the optimism of a Franklin or Rush, that reality gradually began changing in the nineteenth century. From 1800 to 2000, average life expectancy in the United States moved from thirty-five to sixty-eight years. What came to be called the "health transition" (meaning the long-term reduction of mortality) moved after 1800 through various phases and stemmed from a variety of causes. It came to be associated with the "demographic transition," the movement from high mortality and fertility to low, and in the words of the demographer James C. Riley, "the health transition has not yet stopped . . . It is an ongoing thing that we manipulate and manage with great variation in skill."[16]

A 1953 United Nations study broke down the health transition into three phases: the emergence, before 1850, of a higher standard of living (better nutrition, housing, and clothing); important sanitary projects between 1850 and 1900; and after 1900 a mix of medicine, economic developments, and public health.[17] An important study by Thomas McKeown in 1976 shifted his own earlier emphasis on public health and medical advances, stressing instead a rising standard of living, particularly nutrition, and, even more broadly, modernization. The last of these, encompassing development of political, legal, and economic institutions, was apparently seen by McKeown as a "prerequisite for mortality decline."[18]

The epidemiological transition—the shift of mortality from infectious to chronic and degenerative disease—was influentially described by Abdel Omran in the early 1970s and, though criticized and amended, has remained illuminating.[19] With an emphasis on disease, four stages can be described: (1) between 1670 and 1750 there was a decline in major plagues; (2) between 1750 and 1890, a drop in communicable disease, such as scarlet fever, smallpox, diphtheria, and whooping cough; (3) in the late 1800s, a drop in respiratory disease and infant mortality, and by 1939 a decline in tuberculosis, chronic bronchitis, and infant mortality (less than 5% of infants by 1939); (4) and after 1900, the shift from communicable to noncommunicable diseases, which saw a rapid shift in deaths from infancy to late adulthood. That last phase began the era, which remains our own, of heart and circulatory disease, cancer, and

respiratory diseases as the leading killers.[20] This pattern, characteristic of
North America and Western Europe, has not necessarily been the same in other,
poorer parts of the world, which can exhibit diseases that still kill children and
young adults, but also those degenerative diseases that take the lives of the
elderly.

By 2000, most people living in developed countries could expect to live
beyond the age of sixty-five (75%–80%), and the infant mortality rate, earlier
over 100 per thousand, had dropped to 6 to 7 per thousand. Maternal mortality
has all but disappeared. While hardly absent, the threat of death in childhood
or adulthood has radically diminished. Our children, far fewer in number per
family, have an even better chance of making it to old age than we do. The
vision of Bacon, Descartes, Franklin, and Rush has come to look, if not a sure
thing, at least strikingly plausible. By 2000, the ancient fatalism in the face of
nature had begun to fade, and good health as a realizable hope came to the fore.

The Embrace of Medical Research

That hope gained considerable help from the health transition (with its mix
of causes), but needed still more to seize its full possibilities. That help came
by the mid to late nineteenth century, with a formal and organized effort to
embrace medical research, primarily in the medical schools and the pharmaceutical industry. There had, of course, always been some medical research—
think only of Leonardo da Vinci's splendid anatomical drawings—but the difference is suggested by the phrase "formal and organized." The British and
French carried out medical research in the eighteenth and early nineteenth
centuries, but it was the Germans, and the international pharmaceutical industry, that created the great leap in research in the second half of the nineteenth
century.[21]

The Germans were the leaders in both respects, educational and commercial. Their universities and medical schools, with substantial government support, gave a prominent place to research, serving as a stimulus and model for
other countries, particularly the United States. After a slow start, American
medical schools worked hard by the end of the century to give research an
important place, even competing with each other to gain noted researchers and
helping to subsidize research journals, notably the *Journal of Experimental
Medicine.* Research was seen as important not just for medical progress but
also for the prestige of the schools.

The combination of the fresh research initiatives by the turn of the century and a growing interest in science and medicine more generally was a stimulus to the media, which began to popularize and report on scientific news. These developments caught the eye of some of the United States' wealthiest philanthropists, and in particular John D. Rockefeller. In 1901 he established the country's first independent research organization, the Rockefeller Institute for Medical Research (eventually renamed the Rockefeller University). By 1928 he had contributed $28 million to the institute. Rockefeller was assisted by a Protestant minister, Frederick T. Gates, also a savvy businessman. "Medical Research," Gates wrote, will "educate the human conscience in new directions and point at new duties."[22] That was an interesting and prescient insight into some of the larger social ramifications of medical research and a large step in what we have called its "infinity" thrust.

Despite occasional suspicious glances directed toward the philanthropic backing of medical research as a capitalist, not altruistic, move, there is little support for that accusation. The same cannot be said for the pharmaceutical industry, which early on displayed its characteristic mix of research and marketing. The German industry led the way. By combining a scientifically oriented system of higher education, well-trained scientists, and partnership among industry, government, and higher education, the German drug companies led the way in research and the marketing of its products. That model was soon emulated in the United States and other Western countries. By pioneering the use of alkaloid chemistry to extract useful compounds, the development of synthetic dyes from coal tar, and the formal use of research to develop new drugs, the pharmaceutical industry set the stage for the still greater advances in the twentieth century, right up to the emergence of the biotechnology industry in the 1970s. The fact of a patent system that allowed a monopolistic control of the industry's products did not hurt that development.

Given this international background, the stimulus of the medical schools, and the prestige accorded medical research by the philanthropies, the American government, slow to get involved in medical (though not agricultural) research, came to see the light. The inauspicious beginning of the National Institutes of Health in 1937 gave way to an enormous boost after World War II, stimulated by the broad scientific advances the war generated and by the medical progress it fostered, from surgery to drugs. Thereafter, with steadily rising congressional enthusiasm, and with the help of some zealous and politically skilled laypersons (Mary Lasker and Florence Mahoney most notably), the NIH budget rose each year. Gradually, the present research pattern emerged, with the NIH doing the basic research and the pharmaceutical (and device) industry doing the "translational" work to turn that research into marketable products. Because of this division of labor, the government lays the foundation for clinical applications, but industry carries them out. The industry, that is, gets to use publicly funded basic research, aimed at the public interest, to advance its own private, commercial interests.

The Emergence of a Medical Market

While there was, during the nineteenth and early twentieth centuries, already a fragmented market in medicine, it was disorganized and ad hoc. These were proprietary hospitals and medical schools, but their life span was increasingly short in the twentieth century. In 1900, proprietary hospitals constituted 64 percent of the hospitals in the United States, a percentage that had declined to 18 percent by 1940.[23] The opposition of the medical profession to such hospitals was largely responsible for this shift, in great part because it found that community and other nonprofit hospitals could provide the needed capital for hospitals, a steady stream of patients, and a good income through their professional fees. The proprietary medical schools, a source of much of the quackery that the profession was working to overcome—in part to establish its own monopoly—were swept away by the early-twentieth-century reforms in medical education.

Yet even if there is considerable evidence for the market-like activities in the nineteenth and twentieth centuries, it is hard to detect any theory or ideology of the market in operation. "The market" was not invoked as an animating idea, even though it was being put into practice. As we describe in the next section, there was a constant debate after Adam Smith about the role and the place of the market in society, but remarkably little application of that interest to medicine and health care. While the American Medical Association displayed considerable hostility to any government role in the provision of health care, that was not because it was caught up in the larger argument about the market that could be found among intellectuals and political theorists. At most, the AMA was willing to tolerate the low-level market practices of proprietary hospitals and medical schools, but soon came to jettison them as well, willing to settle for a simple fee-for-service medicine and a few small-group practices (but in general opposing prepaid group practices).

No particular historical moment, or health care personage, emerges that might be identified as that moment when an important question occurred among those thinking about the management, problems, and future of health care: if the market is an important engine of efficiency, choice, and innovation in the overall running of society, why could it not bring those same virtues to medicine and health care? But it is worth speculating that only after the government in the post–World War II era became the most important actor in the health care system did the market idea begin to make inroads, adding prestige and massive amounts of money to the enterprise.

A number of developments signaled that move. The 1947 Hill-Burton Act stimulated the building of hospitals. The rapid development of the NIH in the 1950s and 1960s was an enormous stimulus to nonprofit and for-profit research. The Medicare and Medicaid Acts of 1965 established massive programs of health care for the old and the poor. And the 1980 Bayh-Dole Act, allowing government-supported researchers to patent their findings, became a major incentive for universities to enhance, and sell, their research capabilities.

Yet two specters were emerging as well, the one undeniable, the other potent but highly controversial. The undeniable specter was that of rising health care costs. It was beginning to be noticed in the 1960s, but not taken with full seriousness until the 1970s, signaled by President Nixon's effort to find ways of controlling costs, and heightened still further by Presidents Carter's intensification of those efforts. While there was, and still is, debate on the main drivers of costs, market proponents saw an opportunity: if patients were made more conscious of, and responsible for, the costs of their health care, if there was more competition among health care providers, and if there were fewer government regulations and red tape, that would make a great difference as well. The main point, however, denied by few, was that rising costs posed a serious challenge that, one way or the other, had to be dealt with. If the market proposals were contentious, the fact of a problem was not. It was by then well recognized that third-party insurance, mainly provided by employers, masked the true cost of health care from its recipients and insulated patients from feeling the impact of rising costs.

Far more provocative was the market-inspired argument that government regulation had become too much a part of American health care, just as it had become too large a part of American society in just about every other area. The rising cost and regulatory scope of Medicare and Medicaid were cited as two prominent examples, but assorted government regulations of hospitals and medical practice were also part of a long list of complaints. If at first the complaints were a minor theme in the years after World War II, easily pushed aside during the 1960s, as one expansive program after another was enacted, market advocates and political conservatives began to be heard in the Nixon era and gained an increasingly strong role in subsequent years.

While this story will be unfolded further as our book moves along, some conclusions about the entrance of organized and aggressive market thinking by the 1970s and 1980s can be proposed. In the case of medicine—which in a fee-for-service doctor-patient relationship had always had a basic market transaction at its core—it would take the development of the health care system, as a steadily more costly and complicated enterprise, to bring in market practices in more ambitious ways. The changing ideology of health, stimulated by the reigning infinity ideology, steady medical progress and great health success, and the dawning possibility of satisfying demands beyond mere ordinary good health, made a great difference as well. Though drug costs were no more than 5 percent of health care spending in the 1970s, the pharmaceutical industry in particular capitalized on this constellation of forces. By emphasizing research, endless progress, and ever-expanding patient choice, it skillfully used the market as a means and glorified it as an end.[24]

THE EXPANDING MARKET DEBATE

The history of the market debate following the work of Adam Smith is rich and suggestive about the nature of commercial societies and their various social institutions.[25] But, with the exception of twentieth-century arguments about the welfare state (and then usually only indirectly), there was remarkably little application until recent years of the larger motifs of that debate to medicine and health care. Though health economists became interested in market practices in the 1930s, and much more intensively in the 1980s, that was not because, as with the historical market discussion, it was stimulated by some key theorists, but because that more general discussion came eventually to permeate all major institutions.

We want to attempt now to pick out some of the larger themes of that long historical debate and to make explicit where they seem suggestive for our contemporary health care situation. Toward that end, we will make use of three categories, the potential effect of markets and market thought on doctors, on patients, and on health care systems. These three categories encompass the two dominant issues that have been part of the general market debate for two hundred years, that of the effect of markets on cultural values, and that of the relationship between the market and government.

The Potential Impact of Markets on Doctors as
Healers and Merchants

In the debates that followed in the wake of Adam Smith's work and the rise of industrialism, the impact of the market on traditional values and cultural institutions was one of the most important. "Which human type is promoted by capitalism?" was one question.[26] We think it fair to say that the pervasive culture of the market in the United States tends to promote the idea of the physician as merchant. The doctor's skills are taken to be valuable in themselves and, all the better, profitable to sell. While internists, geriatricians, and pediatricians can (and should) mutter about their more affluent subspecialty colleagues, those with special technical skills and expensive technologies to deploy them, it is not considered wrong to make lots of money. The large number of physicians who have become wealthy entrepreneurs, or executives in health care corporations (nonprofit as well as for-profit), is hardly frowned upon either. The line between the physician as altruist and the physician "as something of a businessman" can get fine indeed in as commercial a society as the United States.

Yet it is not for nothing that the romantic figure of the nineteenth- and early-twentieth-century physician, working as a solo practitioner, making his lonely house calls by horse at night or in bad weather, remains a powerful memory. The famous nineteenth-century William Fields painting of a doctor kneeling at the home bedside of a sick child (*The Doctor*) captures that image perfectly. But if that is a less dominant image now than a hundred years ago, it well may be because the kind of romantic conservatism promoted by the organized medicine—but accompanied by some hard-core economic interests—of the late nineteenth and first half of the twentieth century has long ago passed. This kind of romanticism about market-stimulated activities was challenged in the eighteenth century by the German intellectual and government official Justus Möser. While he countenanced a limited role for the market in economic life, he saw its expansion as a threat to the existing institutional order and to traditional and social and cultural values.[27]

One can easily catch a strong flavor of this kind of cultural impact—often eroding even though never overcoming the altruistic tradition—in the ideology of the prewar AMA, with its glorification of the solo practitioner, its opposition to new-fangled group practices, and its utter rejection of "socialized medicine." Despite his reservations about the market, had Möser been an early twentieth-century physician, he might well have become a president of the AMA. For he wrote that government bureaucracy was mostly an "arrogant interference in human reason, destructive of private property and violations of freedom."[28]

Other thinkers accepted the market and its logic within the commercial sphere, but objected to an assumption that its values should be applied to other areas of life, particularly politics and culture. Medicine would, it might be guessed, be one of those places the market ought not to go. Edmund Burke, a supporter of the market and commercialism, became famous nonetheless for stressing the importance of tradition, habit, and custom. That emphasis might well have led him, in our day, to hold on to other older traditions of medicine. In particular, he held that a commercial society rested on a noncommercial base. The notion that society could be reduced to a social contract was a mistake. Our most important obligations and relationships, Burke wrote, are not contractual—and there is reason to think that this view would apply to the doctor-patient relationship as well.[29]

As did Burke and Adam Smith, Georg Hegel, a German professor of philosophy, believed strongly that a person's good cannot be defined by his or her preferences. Adam Smith understood the process of becoming moral to be a social process, and Hegel extended that insight to an argument that our social and political institutions are related to what we should become as persons, and that what kind of person we will be is partly shaped by historical institutions.[30] We might ask, in that vein, what kind of person should the doctor be and what should be the role of the institution of medicine—its goals, mores, and traditions? Medicine, in particular, has historically stressed the importance of the senior, seasoned physician as the role model for medical students and residents. But is one doctor, a senior ophthalmologist who advertised on New York radio in 2003 that he had done thirty thousand laser procedures on the eye, a good role model? At the least he is, it is not unfair to say, "something of a businessman," along with many other entrepreneurial physicians who establish medical businesses, whether investing in scanning devices as auxiliary services or developing "boutique" medical practices at a high cost.

Markets and Patients

It is reasonable to speculate that Burke and Hegel would have rejected any claim that the doctor-patient relationship can be reduced to the contractual model, a joining of buyers and sellers for mutually self-interested aims—or consumers and providers, as they are now often called in health care. The complexity of the relationship, the uncertainty of many medical outcomes, and the vulnerability of patients make that an inappropriate model. Yet even if their relationship is not that of fee-for-service, which is surely a contractual one, but is instead mediated through a third party (such as an HMO [health mainte-nance organization] or an insurance policy), it is partly a contract. Where it ought to differ, and must in great part importantly differ, is well brought out by an insight from Hegel's ethics. The role of social institutions, he held, is peda-gogical, helping to direct our desires and to shape our preferences. That insight would seem particularly appropriate in the case of the patient. Our health preferences, whatever they might spontaneously be, are not necessarily a good guide to better health. There we typically, and not unreasonably, turn to the doctor and the medical culture he or she represents to learn what medical knowledge has to teach us about our health.

The psychiatrist and law professor Jay Katz has written brilliantly on the idea of the doctor as educator.[31] That idea is not a model hostile to the freedom of patients to accept or reject the education, but it can offer a helpful way for the patient to knowledgeably screen the growing number of direct-to-consumer advertisements and other market blandishments designed to sway people's judgment. It was Hegel who noted, as Smith did not, that the market does not just satisfy wants; it also creates them. One of the most important contempo-rary tasks of doctors—and behind them the institution of medicine—is to help us know the difference between medical needs and medical desires. But this means that medicine itself must be ever busy with self-examination, trying to discern when it is unduly influenced by the cultures in which it is embedded, when its patients are so influenced, and how medicine can, amidst such pres-sures, remain true to its core values.

Hegel is particularly instructive on the distinction between needs and de-sires in a way pertinent to a theme of this book, that of the infinity model of medical aims, which sets limitless goals and stimulates a constant transforma-tion of wants into needs. Because the commercial market creates wants, es-chewing any notion of adequacy, those wants know no principled boundaries. To be sure, the price of health care can set boundaries, but they are usually treated as temporary obstacles, capable of being overcome by better manage-ment and cost-lowering research. Nothing should long be allowed to stand in the way of endless progress. Hegel called this way of thinking a "bad infinity," an idea foreshadowed by Aristotle's notion of *pleonexia,* that of a quest for acquisitions without end—and even more than the quest for material goods. In much the same vein, our present health can never be good enough, if only because good health will always be temporary, and medical progress will constantly redefine what good health means.[32]

The wise doctor, it might be said, is one who knows how to find a good balance between helping patients achieve better health while educating them on the limits of medicine to bring any final human perfection. As the social scientist Daniel Bell noted, since the earliest days of capitalism there has been a tension between finite ideas, stressing prudence, self-discipline, and a control of wants, and an infinite, Faustian idea captured in the notion of science as "the endless frontier," with, as its goal, the complete transformation of nature. "The ascetic element," Bell observed, "and with it one kind of moral legitimation of capitalist behavior, has virtually disappeared . . . The notion of common ends was dissolved into individual preferences."[33] This movement is the ultimate danger that the inroads of market ideas can pose for medicine, rejecting any unitary concept of health tied to any coherent view of human nature and its flourishing. Medicine would then be reduced to the management and satisfaction of health desires, whatever they are and whatever their validity, and however little they may have to do with the historical goals of medicine.

Government and the Market

If the impact of the market on culture and politics has been a perennial topic of debate for two hundred years, hardly less important has been the effort to discern a good relationship between government and the market. On this latter issue, there have actually been two threads, often intertwining but still separable: the role of government in monitoring and regulating the market in commercial matters, and the place of the market within or parallel to government efforts to deal with welfare problems, whether poverty or health. As it happens, of course, most health care systems show a mixture of both threads, ranging from the United Kingdom, with its National Health Service (NHS) at one end of the spectrum, where government runs the entire system, and the United States at the other end, with a strong for-profit sector, often contracted with by government to run health and welfare programs.

Behind the ascendant prominence and influence of market ideas and practices in the 1970s, and even more vigorously in the 1980s, lies another era. The 1920s and 1930s saw economic distress on a widespread scale, and market failure and depression as the fate of many otherwise affluent countries. The general reaction, signaled by the work of John Maynard Keynes, was the advent of what have been called "mixed economies," with a heavy role for government and a toleration, only, for market ideas (despite the prominence of market-industrialized societies). While World War II helped revive many flagging economies, most notably in the United States, the need for postwar reconstruction in Europe, and the continuing needs for strong welfare programs, provided the impetus for strong centralized governments. As one set of commentators has put it, " 'government knowledge'—the collective intelligence of decision-makers at the center—was regarded as superior to 'market knowledge'—the dispersed intelligence of private decision-makers in the marketplace."[34] The British nationalization of many private services and the founding of the British NHS in 1947, and Lyndon Johnson's Great Society programs, including Medicare and Medicaid in 1965, nicely symbolize that era.

That era came to an end in the 1980s. The stage was set for this change in the United Kingdom in the 1970s, when Keith Joseph, a politician and intellectual gadfly, stimulated an interest in market ideas, notably those of Adam Smith and Friedrich Hayek, and then caught the eye of Margaret Thatcher. When the Conservatives won the 1979 general election and Thatcher became prime minister, she undertook a systematic, and initially most unpopular, campaign to put market ideas into practice. Privatization of government-owned enterprises, including the state-run electric power monopoly, British Coal, and British Air, was a striking result. Remarkably untouched, however, was the National Health Service, uncommonly popular and seemingly untouchable (even up to the present).

The United Kingdom was the European flagship nation for market practices. Thereafter a number of countries, though hardly all by any means, set out in a similar direction. The reflections of Friedrich Hayek were particularly influential. The main contention of his 1944 book *The Road to Serfdom* was twofold, "that the rise of fascism and nazism was not a reaction against the socialist trends of the preceding era but a necessary outcome of those tendencies," and that "the guarded transformation of a rigidly hierarchical system . . . where man gained the opportunity of knowing and choosing between different forms of life, is closely associated with the life of commerce."[35] The market and democracy are natural allies, each necessary for the other.

To make his case, Hayek had to downplay the ancient notion of a "common good" and comparable concepts. "The welfare of a people, like the happiness of a man," he wrote, "depends on a great many things that can be provided in an infinite variety of combinations . . . the rules by which our common moral code consists have progressively become fewer and more general in character." His main objection was to "directing all economic activity according to a single plan."[36] Yet there remains some ambiguity about his view of ethics. He sounds, for that matter, very close to John Rawls, who held that no free society should be guided by some overarching conception of the human good (though Rawls was far more interested in justice than was Hayek). Democratic pluralism requires rules of justice and fairness, but not a monolithic view of human ends. Even so, Hayek and Rawls sound much closer than most would expect.

We mention that last point because it touches two matters central to this book. One of them is whether there is, in the historical tradition of medicine, at least an implicit view of the human good and the place and meaning of health in that good. And, if so, ought it to be cherished and cultivated, or modified or rejected as medical progress and human values change? A precise answer to these questions cannot be extracted from that tradition, but an inexact answer can be proposed. It is that humans strive for wholeness of mind and body (a Greek legacy) and a capacity to function well in different aspects of individual and social life. That goal is as modern as it is ancient. Yet the preservation of health should not itself be a goal of life. It is a crucial means, however, and when possible it should be protected and cultivated.

Can we then say of medicine and health care what Hayek says of economic systems, that the human needs and aspirations, and the scientific possibilities of the medical future, are diverse, raising "innumerable questions . . . but to which existing morals have no answer and where there exists no agreed upon view on what ought to be done"?[37] While there is no doubt that considerable diversity exists on the proper ends of medicine and health care, there remains the bedrock of illness, pain, suffering, and death—and, we think, considerable agreement on the need to deal with them, even if they are not, in some communal way, always the worst of human evils.

Hayek was by no means an opponent of many elements of what we now think of as the welfare state, including government support of health care. Like Adam Smith (and most other economists), he appears to make a distinction between market freedom in the economic sphere, requiring a minimizing of a state's interference, and the provision of a minimal level of security for its citizens, which can require that interference or some compensatory government assistance. He distinguishes between "security against physical privation, the security of a given minimum of sustenance for all . . . and the security of a given standard of life." "There is no reason," he concludes, "why in a society which has reached the general level of health which ours has attained the first kind of security should not be guaranteed to all without endangering general freedom."[38] Of course, the idea of a "given minimum of sustenance for all" invokes the long-debated ideal of a guaranteed level of care to meet "medical necessity." That issue is at once political, determining the scope of government support for health care, and substantive, defining the meaning of *necessity* in the context of the shifting goals, possibilities, and aspirations of medical progress. Since the market creates wants as well as responding to needs, that flux will inevitably influence what comes to be meant by *necessity*.

Milton Friedman, notably in *Capitalism and Freedom,* follows Hayek in emphasizing the intrinsic relationship between the market and democracy. Though he is more ambivalent about the notion of a "given minimum of sustenance for all," to use Hayek's phrase, he does appear to support programs against poverty as long as they are focused on the poor, not on special classes of citizens or occupational groups. His views on health care are notable for suggesting the development of "medical teams" analogous to what we would now call group practices or HMOs, and which he likened to "department stores of medicine." Such stores, selling their services, will have strong market incentives for reliability and quality. Over time, "consumers would get to know their reputations."[39]

Friedman would not do away with individual medical practice, but said he was only trying to show that there are many more ways of organizing health care than have so far been used. Writing as he was in 1962, he turned out to be prophetic about some directions in health care. Most strikingly, health care in the United States is increasingly treated as a commodity like any other and, for many, medicine is seen as perfectly suitable for the commercial marketplace. Though she does not cite him, Regina Herzlinger, of the Harvard Business School, shows the influence of Friedman's way of thinking in her book *Market-Driven Health Care.* She treats medicine uncompromisingly as an ordinary commodity and says of patients, "don't call them patients." They are consumers, and indeed they are increasingly becoming revolutionaries: "the consumer revolutionaries want their health care system to provide them with the same kind of convenience and mastery they've found with Home Depot, Consumer Reports, and NordicTrack, so that their health status and costs will improve still further."[40] Herzlinger is a regular contributor to the op-ed page of the *Wall Street Journal* (though rarely cited in the professional health economics literature).

THE CONVERGENCE OF MEDICAL CHANGE AND
MARKET PRACTICE

The English political scientist Michael Moran rejects the view that the need for cost containment or the force of ideology can adequately account for the convergence of the market and health care. Instead, he argues that health care became part of a broader industrial politics in developed countries. That politics has been intent on advancing national competitiveness and technological progress, and fueled as well by greater lay involvement in health care, emphasizing choice and political power. "The rise of market ideology" in health care, he wrote, "has occurred because it can be appropriated by a range of different interests. In this lies both its strength and its weakness: it promises different things to different people, but not all promises can be reconciled."[41]

We cite Moran's judgment, even though it is a bit too abstract and reductionistic to be wholly persuasive. A more complete picture of the way market thought and health care came together has to include a concern with cost containment and a general frustration with the difficulty of managing large health care systems. The collapse of Communism and its command economy brought into sharp focus the future role of government in health care no less than in everything else. Market thought made a great political leap in the 1980s and 1990s. Health care had become an obvious arena to test its applications and implications. The "reform" of health care—whatever the culture, whatever the reigning system—became an international movement. Market advocates were quick to jump at the opening that movement offered.

Market thought and theory have, over their history, not been indifferent to the cultural effects of market practices. But as Jerry Muller has emphasized, market conservatives have never been well able to reconcile the commitment to market freedom and their recognition that the market can be, and has been, a solvent for many important cultural values, including some that market proponents themselves value. In Hayek's case, Muller writes, "his antipathy to the notion that government exists to protect any particular culture . . . led him to ignore the need for a shared ethos, however limited—what Hegel has called *Sittlichkeit* . . . Hayek's opposition to the use of government to enshrine any single culture led him to deny that there might be any shared cultural standard for the sake of which the market might be restrained. As a result, he had no way to evaluate the negative effects of the market or to suggest a principled reason to try to remedy them."[42]

The books of Regina Herzlinger and the ideas of Milton Friedman suggest some of the "negative effects" on health care theory that a too-libertarian view of the market carries with it. Nonetheless, that much said, it seems reasonably clear that there are streams of thought in the history of market thinking, beginning with Adam Smith, that leave open the possibility of a market orientation sensitive to the altruistic tradition of medicine and prepared to grant the importance of a government role in providing a health safety net and other social services. The hard question is whether government can support them vigorously in practice.

The Nobel laureate Amartya Sen, known for his commitment to social justice but no enemy of the market, has written that "we have good reasons to buy and sell, to exchange, and to seek lives that can flourish on the basis of transactions. To deny that freedom in general would be a major failing of a society."[43] Our question remains: how far, and in what ways, can the market go in that direction without doing harm to the moral values of medicine, most notably the primacy of patient welfare and professional integrity? The important historical figures we have surveyed did not take up that question, though most were aware of and troubled by the general threat that market values pose to all traditional institutions and values.

ECONOMISTS AND PHYSICIANS: TWO MARKET STRUGGLES

By the 1980s, a vigorous international debate was underway about the market and health care. Sides were chosen, politics came into play, and both the developed and developing countries saw a great push to determine what the market had to offer for health care reform. In this section, we look at two areas of contention, each encompassing a different set of actors, each aware of the other but bringing its own special interests to the fray: health care economists and market advocates (not always the same), and physicians (worried about medical values and physician integrity).

Before developing our analysis, it is time to define our terms, necessary to make certain the reader understands how we will be using the language of the market; different academics and pundits, it turns out, sometimes understand "the market" in different ways, or with very different emphases. We were struck early in our research by how rare it is for most health economists to specify exactly what they mean by "the market," as if when writing for each other they can assume some common understanding; but then they can become quite technical when making necessary distinctions about market practices. We could not help noticing also that the strongest critics of the market assume everyone knows what they are talking about as well, a kind of monster that anyone can see if they just open their eyes. Nuance about different market practices is not often pursued.

The traditional technical definition of the market, that it is a system of exchange of wages and goods based solely on supply and demand and free of government interference, is not very helpful. No nation has a purely market-dominated health care system, just as no country has a purely government-run system. The main debates are almost always about specific market mechanisms, the use of this or that market technique, or mixture of techniques, to bring about some desired individual or system outcome. Market mechanisms can be used when the ultimate aim, the famous bottom line, is financial profit. But market mechanisms can also be used within nonprofit systems, seeking to influence doctors or patients to act in ways that foster their altruistic aims in a financially viable way. As two seasoned international observers have contended, "there is no single, simple concept of market that can be used in a health care system."[44]

The Italian health care economist Maurizio Ferrera has, nonetheless, nicely summarized some leading features of market methods. They include, among other things, a managerial rather than bureaucratic style in the organization of services, the promotion of cost-conscious behavior by the "consumers" of health care, and the stimulation of competition and other characteristic market-type interactions between purchasers and providers.[45] To this list we would add a choice of health plans, even though this is a common feature of many government-run or managed systems.

For our part we want to distinguish between two types of market mechanisms. There are those that aim for major changes in health care systems. These include the privatization of major parts of a system, moving them out of government hands altogether, sharply reducing the government role, or attempting to bring competition into as many parts of a system as possible. Then there are those mechanisms whose aim is, for the sake of greater efficiency, quality, or cost management, to influence individual and institutional behavior without changing the underlying health care system. At the individual level, deductibles and copayments are a common way of attempting to influence patients' behavior, just as financial incentives and disincentives can attempt to influence physicians' behavior. In Europe it is common to speak of "quasi-markets" (or "social" or "internal" markets), which one commentator has defined as "markets where provision is left to a competitive market, but the state provides the finance for, and in some cases also acts as the purchaser of, health care."[46]

Health Economists

In the United States, the field of health economics began to take shape in the 1930s with research on health care institutions, technology, and policy, but then took a great leap during the 1960s, stimulated by the theoretical and econometric work of Kenneth Arrow, Martin Feldstein, Selma Mushkin, and Gary Becker.[47] Kenneth Arrow's 1963 paper "Uncertainty and the Welfare Economics of Medical Care" was of particular importance for subsequent debates on the place of the market in health care.[48] In brief, he argued that health care could not well fit with conventional models of perfect markets. Such care is marked, he said, by irregular and unpredictable demand, uncertainty of outcomes, inadequate information, and erratic supply conditions. Inevitably in those circumstances there can be no perfect market, and thus a need for non-market interventions and control. Put another way, health care is inherently subject to market failure (an inefficient allocation of scarce resources).

For us, the most interesting feature of the subsequent debates among health economists, and those from other disciplines that entered the fray, was whether and to what extent various market ideas and mechanisms could effectively be used in health care in the absence of a perfect market. With the exception of a relatively small handful whose hostility to the market has remained strong and persistent, such as the articulate Canadian Robert Evans, most health economists have been prepared to consider the use of market mechanisms. A sympathy for markets has been a traditional feature of mainline economics. Even where there has been skepticism, the possibility of using market practices to make health care systems more efficient, more innovative, more open to patient choice—and perhaps even more equitable—has been a strong lure. As more than one commentator has asked, in the face of inefficiency, public discontent, and seemingly unmanageable costs, where else might we better look for some solutions?[49] The collapse of the Communist systems in the late 1980s was simply one more strong push in that direction.

Yet for all their academic prestige, their adeptness in the use of quantitative data, and their prevalence in the policy arena, there has been a perennial lamentation by many leaders in health economics that their work has not been taken with sufficient seriousness. One of the most distinguished economists, Victor R. Fuchs, a former president of the American Economic Association, presented the results of a survey of his economist colleagues that he conducted in 1995, not long after the failure of the 1993–1994 push of the Clinton administration for universal health care. It showed a great diversity of views and little consensus on health care reform. "My principal conclusion," he wrote, "is that value differences among economists, as well as among all Americans, are a major barrier to effective policy-making."[50]

Fuchs noted that the Nobel laureate George Stigler had said, in his 1964 presidential address to the American Economic Association, that economics was "at the threshold of its golden age," because "the age of quantification is now full upon us," and would thus be far more useful for policy purposes than theory unsupported by empirical evidence. But Fuchs said that, despite the massive outpouring of empirical studies in the years that followed, they did not "narrow the range of partisan disputes and make a significant contribution to the reconciliation of partisan differences."[51]

In answer to the question of why there is so little agreement among American economists on policy-value questions, Fuchs speculates that "most health policy decisions have significant implications for freedom, efficiency, justice, and security. Health economists (like other Americans) probably desire all these goals, but (again like other Americans) they probably differ in the values they attach to them, or in the way they define them."[52] Moreover, he notes, even when there is considerable agreement among economists on empirical issues, it is poorly communicated to legislators and the public.

We cite the judgment of Victor Fuchs because it helps us make sense of some important features of the medicine and market debate. As outsiders and non-economists, we have been struck by a combination of considerable convergence on some broad policy issues and unremitting trench warfare on the technical details. Our reading of these struggles is that there are two key groups contending over the economics of health care. One of them, the mainstream, might be termed rationalistic and instrumental. While issues of equity are not ignored, or political passions wholly put aside, they hardly stand out—they are more between the lines than visible on the surface. The other group is those we call the politicals, a coalition of some economists and many more laypersons—politicians, pundits, and some political scientists—who wear their values on their sleeves: smaller government, the inherent connection between democracy and the market, the importance of competition, and the sovereignty of personal choice.

Instrumentalists and Politicals

The important questions for the economics mainstream are instrumental: means not ends are dominant—what works and doesn't work. If a health system decides to embrace copayments for drugs, for instance, aiming to make patients more sensitive to costs and thus to help control an unnecessary overuse of drugs and to contain costs, what will be the likely results? Will patients use fewer drugs, will system costs be held down, and will there be any harm to patients' health? We liken that mode of reasoning to an elaborate kind of chess game: if tactic x is used for the sake of greater efficiency, then what are the likely consequences, a, b, or c? And if, say, a is chosen, how might it affect, in turn, the present policy y, which may still have some important benefits? Should x simply replace y, even if the hazards are great, or should x be tinkered with in a way that makes it compatible with y?

While theory is not beside the point with this mode of reasoning, empirical evidence about possible policy results is golden—and yet debates about the meaning of the evidence are often present. As Robert Evans has said of arguments for and against private insurance, "God and the devil are both in the details." "Instrumentalists," as Evans calls them, advocate "particular structures or policies because they expect certain consequences to follow."[53]

Instrumentalists, characteristically, do not take the fashioning of health care goals as their domain. The other domain is politics and values, outside the scope of their professional skills. The historian Evan Melhado concludes his analysis of this tradition in health economics, which he calls the "economizing model," by saying that "its answers will likely serve the goal of economic rationality, but will not sustain the passion that would be needed to support improvements of benefits and expansion of entitlements."[54] We should add, however, that many mainstream economists are supportive of universal health care and decent access to such care. But they are often also careful to specify these as their values and not an expression of their professional expertise at work, which is limited to economic theory and the value-free collection of relevant data (though their putative value-free nature has been repeatedly questioned).

Little such nuance marks the work of those Evans has called "the fundamentalists," those who hold "particular forms of economic organization to be good per se."[55] He does not mention any health economists who fall into this category, and we would prefer to use the term "the politicals," those who fit Evans's general description but with a twist: they are market advocates who generally are less than anxious about market failure and other market liabilities, and have a clear set of political ends that shape their choice of instrumental means. They share many common features: they are prone to be antigovernment, at least in the sense of wanting a minimal government role in health care; they want maximum consumer choice and do not hesitate to think of patients as consumers; they believe that the health market generates technological innovation, which has both medical and economic value; and, for them, freedom is clearly a more important value than equity.[56]

Milton Friedman would be the commanding economist in their eyes but, on the whole, the politicals do an end run around conventional health economics. Their larger goal, going back to Hayek, is to promote the marriage of the market and democracy, each of which needs the other in pursuit of the ultimate value, freedom. This is no doubt what gives them their political strength, embraced by the Republican right, the editorial pages of the *Wall Street Journal,* and many conservative media commentators. The fact that even many market-oriented economists do not take them seriously because of their failure to grapple seriously with the technical problems of a health care market is beside the point. If Fuchs is right that disagreement among economists is one reason they are not taken more seriously in shaping public policy, then it is irrelevant that serious economists disagree with the politicals; with bigger game in mind, that is not the group the politicals aim to influence. Legislators, pundits, media editorialists, and politically conservative party leaders are a more important audience.

BALANCING MARKET AND GOVERNMENT

Yet there is at least one important point of consensus among health economists, even including most of "the politicals" (even if not something the latter group stresses): that the basic economic and political issue is to find a good balance between the market and government. There will never be, nor should there be, a health care system that is organized along purely market lines, even if that is a libertarian's dream; and there will no longer be health care systems so thoroughly organized from the top down that there is no room for market practices. Most economists stress that the balance to be achieved will and must reflect the culture, politics, and history of different countries, making it hard to propose any binding international principles or planning schemes. "It all depends" might be defined as the working basis among most health economists for reform efforts.

There is a further complication, which any outsider who surveys the health economics literature cannot fail to note. There is an admirable attention to detail, nuanced arguments, and empirical data, with impressive mathematical equations common enough. And along with that professional elegance, there is often a mind-numbing complexity, full of technical squabbles with fellow economists, and conclusions either too ambiguous, or too dependent upon controversial assumptions or politically implausible scenarios, to be of great help to policymakers. (Our own fields, philosophy and law, have been subject to the same criticisms, so we too live in a glass house.) In her fine collection of essays, *Markets and Health Care,* Wendy Ranade notes one source of the complexity: "All health care systems are a mixture of public and private elements: the rise of the market in health care involves an incremental shift and the selected application of various market 'tools' or instruments to different parts of the health system, rather than a wholesale move from one kind of system to another."[57] While this judgment appears true for developed countries, it is not the case for many countries in economic transition and newly industrialized.

An instrumentalist approach to health care, embedded in a discipline striving to be value-free in its technical work and suspicious of the passionate rhetoric of the visionary or reformer, might be said to be ideal for an incrementalist approach. As John Appleby notes in the Ranade volume, it may seem a paradox that there is at once a strong consensus among economists, going back to Kenneth Arrow, "that health care is generally an unsuitable commodity to be traded in a market," but that there is nonetheless "a surprising attraction to market-based solutions to health care problems." But if it is understood that "market *tools* can be applied to *parts* of health care systems and do not have to be all-encompassing," then one can see why "the recourse to market-based solutions to perceived problems in health care systems has been piecemeal rather than total."[58] But, of course, this piecemeal thrust invites piecemeal counter-thrusts, constant problems of integrating the new pieces into a reigning system, and what can be termed slippery-slope anxieties: "but if we do that, even if reasonable, we open the door to eventual harms of a serious kind," an often persuasive kind of argument even in the absence of any decisive evidence that the slope will be slippery.

Three major efforts to use market tools and ideas to reform American health care show the pitfalls of trying to do what, at first blush, seems perfectly reasonable: a proposal by Mark Pauly and three market-oriented colleagues of a plan for "responsible national health insurance"; the work of Alain Enthoven in developing the concept of "managed competition"; and the Clinton Health Security plan.[59] All of these plans shared some important common threads: that some form of universal care is necessary, that there should not be an excessive government role, and that a competitive market should be built into some parts of the plan.

For Pauly and his colleagues, the key was to require people to obtain health insurance based on a competitive choice among policies and tailored to their financial situation and their particular needs and desires, and open to government assistance to pay for such policies when necessary. It incorporated the idea of a minimum benefit level and refundable tax credits reflecting different income levels and risk categories. The marketing of different competing insurance policies would serve the need for choice and efficiency, while the government support would serve the need for equity. The essence of the Enthoven approach was to mandate employer payroll contributions to health insurance premiums (to serve equity), and the development of competitive HMOs (to serve competition and efficiency). The latter specification called for the regulation of the terms of health insurance and the establishment of "health purchasing alliances" to allow small businesses to purchase insurance at affordable costs. The plan also called for a limit on tax deductions for employer-provided health benefits. The Clinton plan incorporated many of the features of the Enthoven approach, but picked up also on a California plan that brought in a more elaborate system of purchasing alliances and more government regulation.

While there has been much discussion over the years why none of these plans succeeded in winning over Congress, it seems fair at least to say this: the Pauly plan was too market-dependent, the Enthoven approach aroused hostility among those who felt it did not guarantee true universality of coverage, and the Clinton plan appeared too complex and heavily dependent on centralized government control. But all three plans were complex, perfect targets for various political and business interest groups and the play of clashing ideologies, and full of enough detail to allow academic critics to inflict upon them the ancient Chinese idea of death by a thousand cuts. Interestingly, the Enthoven approach found a warmer reception in the United Kingdom and the Netherlands, and was influential in devising the "internal markets" of the British National Health Service (a nice example of using market practices for nonprofit aims).

We conclude this discussion with a look at an interesting exchange in 1997 between two distinguished economists, Mark Pauly and Thomas Rice, both admirably thoughtful and careful thinkers. Pauly is someone who has worked since the early 1970s to advance market ideas and strategies in health care, while Rice has a strong record of supporting universal health care and a strong role for government (or, as Europeans might prefer to put it, publicly operated systems). Rice has noted and emphasized what many others could hardly fail to notice: the government-controlled European and Canadian health care systems, though full of problems at the margins, have delivered health care outcomes as good as or better than the United States in ways efficient enough to spend much less per capita on health care along the way.

Rice begins the exchange by trying to show that economic theory does not automatically support the superiority of the market in health care. "If one accepts the viewpoint that economic theory does not demonstrate the superiority of market forces in health," he writes, "the obvious corollary is that all important questions must be answered empirically . . . Market forces may indeed have a prominent place in health care organization and delivery . . . but economic theory does not show them to be necessarily a superior approach to health care policy."[60]

Pauly responds by arguing that even those who embrace the competitive model as the best route for reforming health care "do not base that conviction on the belief that economic theory shows the market to be superior to government regulation . . . theory tells us that, at best, the ideal market can tie an ideal government, not that it can do better." We should, he contends, be talking about "imperfect markets versus imperfect government."[61] That seems to us a sensible response, and Rice in effect responded to that contention by publishing an important book, *The Economics of Health Care Reconsidered*. In its first edition, he offered a criticism of fifteen assumptions about market competition, none of which, he showed, is well fulfilled in health care. Then, in the second edition, he balances the ledger by examining the strengths and weaknesses of government in health care.[62]

Our main point in highlighting this exchange has been to take note of an implicit agreement among American health care economists (it seems to us) that market theory as such does not provide the answer to the best relationship between medicine and the market. Yet we might add that, if (1) theory applied wholesale solves few problems, and if (2) only empirical studies will resolve many of the problems, then we are left with some questions. One of them is whether it is a mistake to simply look at present systems of health care and ask whether various market practices might improve their efficiency and their equity—that is, a strategy of putting aside the question about the basic values a health system should manifest, accepting those as a given, and simply tinkering with its means.

Alternatively, might it be more valuable to follow Richard B. Saltman's recommendation that the best way of dealing with the market-government balance is by simply positing that universal access to necessary health care is "a central organizing principle of a good society. From this normatively defined starting point, a market becomes an instrument of social policy, rather than a religious belief system."[63] There is something eminently sensible about Saltman's recommendation, and it has been the starting point for almost every European nation and Canada. Its obvious drawback as a method is that market proponents could agree on the importance of a normative starting point (and have in fact done so). But they specify choice, freedom, and competition as that point as well, not equity and universal care, and with the market also simply an "instrument of social policy," but subordinated to a very different overarching good. For the politicals, choice wins out in the struggle with equity

When one leaves the disciplinary world of health economists, standing just outside as we do, some observations come to mind, not so much about what kinds of problems they deal with, but about what is characteristically missing: a passion for equity, concern about the effects of the market on the culture of medicine, and an interest in what we have termed the "infinity" model of progress. It is surely not the case that the problem of equitable access to health care is absent from their work. Victor Fuchs, as a leader of an earlier generation of economists, and Thomas Rice, as a younger one, have, along with many others, supported universal health care.

But the more characteristic flavor is a subordination of equity to efficiency, in keeping with the technical bias of economics. As for the "infinity" model, there has been a continuing interest in the impact of technological innovation on health care costs, but counterbalanced by a recent group of health care economists who argue that the economic benefits of medical research are so great that its generation of such "externalities" as rising health care costs is put into the shadows.[64] How is efficiency, much less equity, to be pursued if a rise in costs, often to unaffordable levels, has become inherent in health care because of the combination of technological progress, aging societies, and rising public demand? The market obviously beckons as an attractive safety valve for hard-pressed government programs. That question becomes all the more insistent as more and more technologies are seen as medically worth the money, however expensive they might be, passing cost-benefit analysis barriers with

ease for the care of individuals—but adding enormously to the aggregate social cost of medical care while having a small effect on overall population
health (e.g., kidney dialysis or open heart surgery for those in their eighties
and nineties).

THE MARKET AND MEDICAL CULTURE:
COMMERCE AND INTEGRITY

While we will return to those issues again, we want to close this chapter by
looking at the matter of the culture of medicine. As we noted earlier, the long-
running general debate on the place of markets in society, going back to Adam
Smith, has been dominated by two large themes: the relationship between the
market and government, and the effect of markets on professional and national
cultures. The health economists have given considerable attention to the former issue but very little to the latter, other than indirectly. In the broader
debate, we may recall, even many recent market proponents have been prepared to concede that markets can be harsh solvents of traditional values and
practices, the note struck by the title of Irving Kristol's book *Two Cheers for
Capitalism*.[65] Health care economists have not, by and large, taken up this issue
in looking at the impact of the market on health care. Many American physicians, however, have reacted negatively to the rise of market thought and a
growing commercialization of medicine, and do so even as many of their colleagues enthusiastically embrace it.

The middle of the 1990s provides a convenient entry point to observe this
phenomenon. In the aftermath of the failure of the Clinton health plan, the
HMO movement accelerated, and soon a majority of Americans were enrolled
in one HMO plan or another, with a sharp rise in for-profit plans. By the
mid-1990s the HMOs had simultaneously managed to hold down the hitherto
strong rise each year in health care costs, one of their primary aims, while
alienating many laypeople and doctors in the process. Efficiency worked, but
for many the result was not pleasing. "The market," one typical article noted,
lamenting the loss of the medical virtues defended by the AMA for over 150
years, "has done what it was asked to do, controlling costs, [but] . . . the market has shown little interest in preserving the sanctity of the doctor-patient
relationship."[66]

The steady stream of articles in the leading medical journals laid their heaviest emphasis on the employment by HMOs of various market practices. They
included, most notably, price competition, assorted cost-control measures, the

use of financial incentives to manage physician behavior, a heavy-handed denial of types of care wanted by doctors and patients, and, perhaps worst of
all (so it was charged), MBAs rather than MDs deciding about what counted
as appropriate care. Over against those practices were the core values of medicine, which one article called the "6 Cs": choice, competence, communication,
compassion, continuity (of care), and (no) conflict of interest.[67] Patients' trust,
a critical ingredient of the doctor-patient relationship, was being eroded, subverted by doctors either forced to compromise their ethical principles by
bottom-line-oriented administrators or lured to do so by enticing entrepreneurial possibilities that embodied gross conflict of interest.[68]

"Investor-owned care," two prominent medical critics said, ". . . embodies a
new value system that severs the communal roots and Samaritan traditions of
hospitals, makes doctors and nurses the instruments of investors, and views
patients as commodities."[69] A sentence from the writings of Milton Friedman
(though he was not speaking specifically of health care) was frequently cited as
emblematic of the market virus sweeping through American medicine: "Few
trends could so undermine the very foundations of our free society as the
acceptance by corporate officials of a social responsibility other than to make
as much money for their stockholders as possible."[70]

Dr. Arnold S. Relman, in the 1990s the editor of the *New England Journal of
Medicine,* was one of the most persistent critics of the market, not hesitating to
use the bully pulpit of that journal to inveigh against it. Writing in the *Atlantic
Monthly,* he noted that not only did the Hippocratic Oath enjoin physicians to
serve only "the benefit of the sick," but Moses Maimonides, a thirteenth-
century physician of great and continuing renown, said that "a thirst for profit"
or "ambition for renown" should not be allowed to interfere with the doctor's
professional duties. As did many other physician critics of the market, Relman
drew a sharp distinction between medical practice and commerce, but noted
that the physicians were being drawn into the nexus of the "medical-industrial
complex." They were increasingly using advertising, marketing, and public relations techniques to attract patients, and their professional societies
viewed competition among physicians "as a necessary, even beneficial, feature
of the new medical marketplace."[71] Relman's successor as editor of the journal,
Jerome P. Kassirer, continued in the Relman tradition, as signaled by the title of
a 1997 editorial, "Our Endangered Integrity: It Can Only Get Worse."[72]

Nearly a decade earlier, however, the witty and admired health care economist Uwe Reinhardt had criticized Relman (in a published exchange between
the two) and other market critics for their sanctimonious view of physicians.[73]

Reinhardt was by no means a market enthusiast, but he felt that physicians had long been captured by economic incentives of their own making. Relman had particularly objected to Reinhardt's description of physicians as differing in no significant way from other "purveyors of goods and services."

Reinhardt did not retreat from that description, observing that "piece-rate compensation is the sine qua non of high quality medical care." "No one," he said, "could leave a doctor's office without dealing with the cashier on the way out," and "physicians, like everyone else, like to locate in pleasant areas where there is money to be had." He added that the AMA had determined through an internal legal analysis of its Principles of Medical Ethics that a physician could "arbitrarily refuse to accept any person as a patient, even though no other physician is available . . . [and has] a perfect right to refuse patients who are not insured or on welfare." He concluded that "one would be hard put to distinguish organized American medicine from the trade association of any other group of purveyors of goods and services."[74] Reinhardt's assault was not easy to evade, even though in response Relman stressed the ideals of medicine, agreeing that they have hardly always been lived up to. He was prepared to agree as well that far too many physicians behave more like businesspersons than altruistic doctors.

What kind of ethical and professional rules ought to guide physicians in their commercial activities, including the devising of rules that would altogether ban some of them? A number of initiatives were undertaken and proposals offered. Noting that some federal and professional agencies were looking at various aspects of physician commercialism, Linda Emanuel of the AMA wrote that "these projects are responding to the need for accountability on professional medical standards," but she argued that new standards were not necessarily needed. "More to the point," she said in response to some proposals advanced by a prominent business professor (John McArthur) and a no less prominent physician (Francis D. Moore), both from Harvard, is to "redirect existing structures to suit the specific standard-setting needs of current commercialism."[75] At the same time, a number of studies were undertaken to determine in what ways physicians were caught in the web of commercialism, with a particular interest in the use of financial incentives to affect physician behavior.[76]

We conclude this brief survey with two observations. While considerable attention was, and still is, paid to what McArthur and Moore referred to as the "culture of commerce" and its difference from the "culture of medicine," there is another, even more encompassing and potent culture that should be identified as influential. We call it "the culture of money and affluence." Beginning in the 1980s most prominently, and plainly visible in the Reagan years, the idea of affluence and prosperity caught on in a furious way. For one thing, the long-standing claim that the market led to a more prosperous society was seemingly verified in a most dramatic way by the collapse of Communism, which failed so dismally to bring about prosperity for countries behind the iron curtain. Self-interest as a deep market principle was finally being given its day in the sun, with Ronald Reagan and Margaret Thatcher leading the way. For another, the idea that there is nothing wrong with a desire to make money and to in-dulge in the pleasures of affluence (or, even better, real wealth) was increas-ingly visible in domains where it once evoked only hostility or suspicion.

Amateur sports all but disappeared, for example, and it became acceptable for once disdainful academic scientists to make money, good money, in the commercial sector. Universities began competitively vying for academic stars with higher and higher salaries and sweeter perks. Offices were opened to make money from faculty research, and biomedical researchers were encour-aged to come up with profitable ideas. That was the spirit of the times, bound to penetrate medicine, whether in seeking good money for physicians' "piece work" (to use Uwe Reinhardt's term) or looking for investment possibilities to enhance their regular income. The fact that a medical education was expen-sive, leading to heavy debts, that it was hard and long, leading to a desire to catch up later on the other pleasures of life (including money), and that the professional societies, while concerned, were not condemnatory of money and the market—all provided a further rationale for the making of money, if any was needed.

Our second observation is that the HMO movement has undergone many changes since the mid-1990s, many calling into question its use of market practices—not because they were ineffective, which they were not, but because they generated a great patient and physician backlash. Their help in control-ling costs, which had stimulated great optimism that perhaps the ultimate key to cost control had been found, shortly came to an end. By the end of the 1990s annual costs were once again on the rise, and by the early years of the new millennium were back into the 10 to 20 percent range.

Part of the reason for the mixed record of HMOs was that the critics had been heard (and probably too much so). As a result of legislative mandate or compet-itive pressures or patients' and physicians' complaints, many practices designed to control costs were dropped or modified. Those practices included oversight and report-card keeping on physicians' prescribing practices, rules about the use of primary care physicians as gatekeepers or their elimination altogether, too heavy a use of evidence-based medicine as a rationale (whether reasonable or not) for the denial of various therapies, and requirements that doctors gain permission for expensive procedures. As with most so-called competitive practices, which the HMOs were forced into, the emphasis is almost always competition as a way of holding down costs. But the other side of that coin is that competition can just as easily drive up costs. The reason is almost self-evident: you often cannot well compete for customers by offering fewer desired services or amenities in a market such as health care, where people want better not worse care.

The development and maturing of HMOs, even though they failed, at least politically, can well be seen as a pertinent experiment in what a universal health care system might have to look like. To be economically feasible, it would probably have to work with global budgets, that is, an overall government-determined annual health care budget with a cap on expenditures. It would have to find ways to control physicians' behavior and technology expenditures, on the supply side, and patients' expectations, on the demand side; and it would have to do unpleasant things of that kind by one form or another of explicit rationing. It would surely have to make use of copayments and deductibles. In sum, to be viable and economically sustainable, any universal health care system would have to do just about everything that brought such opprobrium on HMOs in the 1990s.

If universal care advocacy took the direction of competitive HMOs and insurance policies, they would have a politically adventurous time dealing with an American public. That public, as the 1990s' HMO debate showed, wants fine health care benefits with no bureaucratic cost-control measures to limit that care. Americans are the most market-loving people on earth, but the minute the market gets in the way of what they want, they can be just as enraged as they would be with any scheme to adopt a government-run "socialist" system, which would also have to say no to them on more than one occasion. Markets have their own way to say no to our unconstrained desires, and so do government-run systems. And since there are not that many ways of saying no to people who want what they want—free, democratic people—market-based and government-based health care will be fraternal twins, with a strong family resemblance. Neither will do well with what we consider the most daunting problem: how to cope with the infinity model of health progress, one result of which is to keep everyone dissatisfied with the status quo, however high the level of health.

We move next to the first of what can be called our case studies, studies of the way the market debate has developed and market practices have been deployed (or restrained) in a number of countries, developed and developing. We begin with a comparison of Canada and the United States, two countries that are remarkably similar in many ways on the surface but went in radically different directions in the provision of health care a little more than forty years ago. The comparison shows the great difference that culture and history make in response to market ideas, and the way different political systems can decisively affect the outcomes of market debates.

CHAPTER TWO

A Tale of Two Cultures

Canada and the United States

Who wants to live next to a giant, even if for the most part a friendly one who speaks your language, offers you movies, TV sitcoms, automobiles, and, to top it off, a huge market for your exports? But that same giant brings with it a culture capable of swamping yours. It has a history of hostility to government, an individualism that at times seems opposed to the very idea of human inter-dependence, an unparalleled love of the market, and a health care system that, for all of its objectionable qualities, has just enough intriguing experiments and fancy technologies to catch even the resistant eye.

For its part, the giant does not reciprocate that last compliment. It has vaguely heard of its northern neighbor's health care system, but mainly from some old rumors that the doctors don't like it, that patients on waiting lists often die, and that desperate Canadians come in great numbers to the United States for their health care. Hardly anyone takes the trouble to check out those rumors, and in any case the Canadian system doesn't count as a model, fatally flawed by its dependence on government financing.

Canadians are far less uninterested in their neighbor and its health care system. On the contrary, they worry about becoming "Americanized," facing a culture overwhelming in its sheer size and economic force and ignorantly indifferent to Canadian strengths, not the least of which is a notably successful health care system. A comparison of Canada and the United States in their response to market ideas and practices offers as fine an example as one could ask for of the way in which two countries apparently so much alike can go in opposite directions. That difference is the product of history broadly taken, a different starting point some two centuries ago. But there is a history more narrowly taken, what Carolyn Hughes Tuohy has called the "accidental logics" of the development of health care in the two countries that, at critical junctures, led them down divergent paths.[1] That broader history is one marked by the growth of the United States as a world power, fueled by an intense commercial drive ("the business of the American people is business," as President Calvin Coolidge once said), by a love of innovation and technological prowess, by a breakdown of community in many places, and by an embrace of the market that has now reached into nearly every sphere of American life, from athletics at one end of the alphabet to universities at the other.

That broader history has been marked in Canada by a more reserved development, sharing many of the American traits, but in a quieter way, eager for business success, ready to accept the market in most spheres but not (for the most part) in health care, attracted to technological prowess, yet holding on to the idea of community and solidarity in the provision of welfare for its citizens. The narrower history of Canadian health care reflects those influences but, in its embrace of universal health care, diverged in an important way from traits and trends that were often enough otherwise similar between Canada and the United States. It is that narrower story of the two countries that we want to tell here, focusing on debates about the market, but which is usefully set as an introduction within the context of the broader story.

THE EARLY CANADIAN BACKGROUND

Many Americans are hardly aware that Canada is a younger nation by a century, coming into existence as a coherent state in 1867 with the establishment of the Canadian Confederation, uniting Ontario and Quebec, and gradually adding other provinces in the years to come. If it first had to throw off the influence of the French, who early colonized much of the country, it had later to deal with the British. But in the latter case the bond with Great Britain was to endure and, even if Canadians desired their independence, which finally came about in 1982, they maintain to this day a friendly postcolonial relationship with the mother country. The seeds of that bond were in part planted by British loyalists who fled to Canada during the American Revolution, and fertilized by a steady stream of British migrants.

If the United States can be seen as a child of the Enlightenment, Canada was a child of the monarchy. The British immigrants and loyalists brought with them a different set of values from those of the liberal, individualistic, and populist American settlers. As the American sociologist Seymour Martin Lipset put it in his fine comparative study of Canada and the United States, "Canada has been and is a more class-aware, elitist, law-abiding, static, collectivity-oriented, particularistic (group oriented) society than the United States."[2] Canadian writer Frank Underhill put the difference more sharply: "Our forefathers made the great refusal in 1776 when they declined to join the revolting American colonies . . . [and] they made it once more in 1867 when the separate British colonies joined to set up a new nationality in order to preempt [American] expansionism."[3]

Yet as the earlier struggle with the French influence indicates—carried on into the present by the sporadic threat of secession by the province of Quebec, and by the country's liberal immigration policies—Canada is a richly multicultural society. It thus has all of the strengths and stresses that go with attempts to mix people of different histories and ethnic cultures. All the more remarkable, then, has been the kind of unity expressed in its universal health care system, surviving many challenges and cutting across party lines, winning an enduring public support.

Prior to World War I and well into the early 1960s, Canadian and American health care developed along similar lines, marked by a fee-for-service medicine, a gradual growth of health insurance plans, efforts to establish the legitimacy and authority of medicine, and a resistance among physicians to the interference of, or regulation by, government. Yet with some exceptions, there was a difference: though Canadian physicians for many decades were hostile to health insurance and particularly government-run health care, that resistance gave way more rapidly than in the United States. The twenty-three-day strike of Saskatchewan doctors in 1962 against that province's Medicare plan might be seen as the last serious gasp of Canadian physicians' resistance.[4] When it became obvious in the aftermath of World War I that the poor health of its draftees could be traced to inferior health care, a movement to bring insurance into the system was surprisingly successful, not fought with the enduring force American physicians brought to that development; and that Canadian movement set in motion the impetus for national universal care.

As early as 1911, Canadian physicians resisted the introduction of health insurance, worried about cold bureaucracy replacing charity and a government exploitation of the medical profession. The Canadian Medical Association nonetheless gave some support to the idea, provided that it would help increase physicians' income and with fees set by them. By 1917, the president of the CMA warned doctors that "mercenary reasons" should not be invoked to oppose insurance, and in 1919 Mackenzie King, who was to become prime minister, made health insurance part of Liberal Party policy.[5] Thereafter, with the Great Depression as a stimulus to the development of a wide range of social services as a political right and without means testing, health insurance was steadily pursued. The way was not always smooth. A comprehensive health care bill passed the British Columbia legislature in the mid-1930s, but it was resisted by the province's College of Physicians and Surgeons, who voted against it 613-22. That vote led to its indefinite postponement as law and, finally, political abandonment.[6]

The CMA eventually came to see public financing as an antidote, not a threat, to the economic troubles of the profession. Unlike the United States and Britain, "the most vocal supporters of health insurance were prominent members of the Canadian Medical Profession. It was always a qualified support and enthusiasm varied inversely with the economic condition of the profession."[7] Led by Alberta and Saskatchewan, insurance plans were put in place after World War II, and by the mid-1950s two-thirds of the population had some hospital and physician insurance. But it was not until 1966, with the Medical Care Insurance Act (Medicare), which had a 50:50 patient cost-sharing feature, and 1984, when the Canada Health Act removed that limitation, that full-scale equal-access coverage was established.

THE EARLY AMERICAN BACKGROUND

That has not been the American story. While it is a contentious subject among some American historians, Joyce Appleby has persuasively made the case that the first post-revolution generation established what became an enduring American identity, that of a nation that democratized politics and created a "liberal, commercial, or capitalist society of unparalleled scope and social influence, but also constructed the peculiar national identity of autonomous and enterprising individuals."[8] It was, Appleby argues, Thomas Jefferson and the Jeffersonian Republicans who were most responsible for that development, that same Jefferson who was a representative of the small farmers, hostile to a centralized government, and a forthright individualist in his ideological leanings. His lavish style of life, the source of lifelong debts, indicated a man who was not averse to a life of affluence and high taste. Some decades later, Alexis de Tocqueville caught the flavor of this kind of American: "It is strange to see with what feverish ardor the Americans pursue their own welfare . . . He is so hasty in grasping all within his reach, that one would suppose he was constantly afraid of not living long enough to enjoy them."[9]

In his research on early American medicine, the medical historian George Rosen was quickly able to pick up the lasting influence of a national market outlook and the individualism that went with it. Physicians in the mid-nineteenth century, he wrote, shared the social values of American society: "the individual should be free of government interference and given full scope for initiative, self-assertion, and the development of self-interest . . . After all, the United States was a free society, in which competition was the life blood not only of trade but of the professions as well."[10] Even so, by that time American physicians, prepared to accept competition as part of their professional life, wanted it on their own terms. Part of that acceptance meant establishing their social authority, controlling or eliminating those who would be part of the competition, and finding ways to make use of government while not being dominated by it.

Increasingly, as Paul Starr puts it in *The Social Transformation of American Medicine,* American physicians had to find ways to use their growing authority in order to turn it "into high income, autonomy, and the rewards of privilege and to gain control over both the market for its services and the various hierarchies that govern medical practice, financing and policy."[11] They did not have an easy time of it at first. Their efforts to control medical education, licensing laws, and professional associations ran into considerable public opposition. Licensing laws, in particular, were often struck down in a backlash against a medicine that was too often grossly ineffective and marked by visible quackery. Even so, after 1850 and into the 1930s, physicians' authority was consolidated by a return to licensing laws, by reform of medical schools, by a successful campaign to defeat quack competitors, and by the growing impact of a medical research and clinical progress that for the first time in American history offered real benefits to patients.

Among those victories was also a rebuff of attempts to establish health insurance, group practice, and physicians in the employ of various industrial companies. The United States at the beginning of the twentieth century was decentralized, with a weak federal government and hostile to any ideas that might deprive the practitioner of control of his (and rarely her) practice. The term *socialized medicine* began to be heard—particularly applied to the notion of compulsory health insurance—a term that remained potent well into the end of that century and can still be heard on occasion today. The forces and virtues

of the market were directly pitted against just about any and all reform efforts—
other than those that would consolidate the power and control of physicians
over American health care, their clinical judgment, and their income. Even
doctors a bit too generous in providing charitable care were seen as a threat to
the high value of competition.

Not until the 1930s did what Paul Starr describes as the "triumph of accommodation" begin to emerge, opening the way for health insurance of some
consequence and a gradual move of solo practice medicine into a corporate
medicine, one that saw the emergence of a massive hospital industry, the Blue
Cross–Blue Shield programs, and prepaid group practices. This effort lagged
behind the Canadians, but it gradually came. The American Medical Association (AMA) was a bit premature when, in 1907, it proposed business training
for physicians, but it saw where the future was going—physicians with MBAs
are, needless to say, no longer a rarity.[12]

If in an important sense American medicine did mirror the market ethos of
the society in which it existed, an important qualification is in order, reflecting
a professional ethic going back to Plato and Hippocrates: physicians had important moral duties toward their patients. Doctors still made house calls,
usually without a surcharge, and at any time of night. If some surgeons wanted
cash first for their operations, many general practitioners, as they were then
called, were willing enough to extend credit to their patients, not to harass
them for payment, and, if worse came to worst, simply write off their bills.
Mutterings about patients who defaulted on their debts were common, but the
pro bono tradition was often strong enough to avoid the harshest kind of retri-
bution, that of refusing further care to patients who had not paid their bills.
Doctors in the pre–World War II era made a good living, putting them usually
in the upper middle class, but nothing like the kind of living that the Medicare
era made possible beginning in the 1960s.

If there was a softening of the market drive at the doctor-patient level in the
name of charity, moreover, it was also visible at the higher level of medical politics. What George Rosen noted and Karl Polanyi characterized as the "double
movement," affirming the value of the market while at the same time working to
limit its harmful effects, could be seen as well in medicine. As Rosen observed,
"Both the ethics and medical theory enshrined and legitimated the primacy of
the relationship between the physician and the family he treated and thus
created formal constraints preventing the worse excesses of competition."[13]

Thus while economic liberalism worked against any market restraints, what

Polanyi called "social protectionism" attempted to curb the effects of the market on traditional institutions. As Starr puts it, "professionalism, charity, and government intervention were efforts to modify the action of the market, without abolishing it entirely."[14] Similarly, medicine's opposition to corporate medicine, with profit as its goal rather than patient care, came from the same source. It was, in short, acceptable for the individual practitioner to treat *his* practice as a market-driven, competitive profession, but not acceptable for that same practitioner to put himself in the service of corporations with profit as *their* principal motive. The distinction may seem a fine one, but it was to surface again in the 1980s and 1990s when physicians came to depend on for-profit health maintenance organizations (HMOs) for their livelihood.

But even noting that qualification, there was a transition from what has been called "guild free choice," dominant in the late nineteenth and early twentieth centuries, to "market free choice." It was forced along by a 1979 Fair Trade Commission ruling that the market practices of the AMA were a "restraint of trade," and thus no longer acceptable. The essence of "guild free choice" had been to forbid price competition among physicians and to control the kinds of economic arrangements or innovations physicians could make.[15]

The net result, as the medical historian Nancy Tomes notes, was that "the social transformation of American medicine was bankrolled chiefly by paying patients."[16] That transformation was helped along as well by an increased public perception of medicine as a luxury good and a parallel development of what became the distinctive twentieth-century consumer culture. Ironically, as Tomes observes, in various efforts to strengthen consumer protection with health-related goods, "pro-market arguments rooted in the need for consumer protection and 'getting one's money worth' appeared more effective than those couched in the language of social justice and citizen entitlements."[17]

THE POSTWAR YEARS AND THE TRANSITION TO THE PRESENT
Canada: Postwar Reforms

If there were many similarities between American and Canadian physicians in the early history of each country—notably, a desire to maintain professional independence and an initial resistance to health insurance—the years after World War II saw the beginning of a real divergence. The Canadian chronology, worth looking at first, lays out a relatively clean and straight line from fee-for-service medicine through the 1950s to the Canada Health Act (CHA) of 1984. The latter established a government-run program that set in place five principles, cited again and again as the hallmark of the Canadian system: universality, accessibility, comprehensiveness, portability, and public administration.

1947: Tommy Douglas, premier of Saskatchewan (1944–1961) introduces universal hospital insurance in Saskatchewan.

1957: The federal government passes the Hospital Insurance and Diagnostic Services Act, providing for a 50:50 cost sharing with provinces that have universal health care.

1964: A Royal Commission Report (the Hall Commission) recommends publicly funded universal insurance for physician care.

1966: The Medical Care Insurance Act (Medicare) is enacted, with 50:50 patient cost-sharing for physician services.

1977: The federal government abandons its 50:50 cost-sharing formula.

1984: The Canada Health Act establishes the five principles cited above, prohibits user fees (copayments) and third-party insurance; physicians can "opt out" but, if they do, cannot get back in.

1990s: Cost and management crisis arises; widespread budget cuts.

2000–2002: Three reform reports are published; a reaffirmation of the Medicare program, additional money to be put into the federal part of the system, but lingering anxieties about the future.

2003: The Ministers' Health Care Renewal Accord increases federal transfer funds to the provinces.

2004: Additional federal funds are provided in response to widespread criticism of the health care system.[18]

For the story we want to tell about its early history, four features are worth laying out: the gradual shift in the attitudes of Canadian doctors to universal health care; the important role of provincial initiatives in changing the federal perspective and policy; the fortuitous economic and cultural background features; and the general Canadian approach to welfare services of all kinds.

Changes in the attitude of physicians to the idea, first, of health insurance and, second, of a universal, government-financed system were crucial in the development of the Canadian Medicare program, but they did not initially come along peacefully. Far from becoming a model for Canadian doctors, the emergence of the British National Health Service (NHS) in 1947 was for many British doctors a dispiriting experience. Many of them voted with their feet by migrating to Canada, joining unhappy Canadian doctors in opposing universal health care. Joining that chorus were nasty portrayals of the British NHS sent across the border by the American Medical Association. The 1962 strike by Saskatchewan doctors, reacting against the province's Medical Insurance Act, was a dramatic signal of the vehemence of their opposition (with one in five of the province's physicians those who had fled the NHS).

But the Saskatchewan rebellion was up against a larger force. As two commentators put it, "The doctors had everything going for them—money, authority, prestige—everything except public opinion. Right from its inception, Medicare would prove to be a favourite of the people."[19] That was probably understandable. In 1961, 30 percent of Canadians had no health insurance at all. Even so, the profession remained adamant. With the full support of the AMA and speaking against the work of the Royal Commission, the CMA saw a government-run system as a "measure of civil conscription . . . contrary to our democratic philosophy."[20] Its complaint did not carry the day. The shift in elite physician opinion turned out to be crucial in removing the last obstacles to universal coverage.[21] The physicians were in the end willing to trade off some entrepreneurial and economic control in order to hold on to clinical decision-making.[22]

As the Saskatchewan initiative suggests, it was the leadership of the Canadian provinces that was of great importance as well in leading up to the 1966 Medicare Act.[23] Ontario's support in the 1950s of a variety of welfare ventures, but especially the devising of a federal-provincial health insurance program, was an encouragement to other provinces and opened still another path for universal care, that of a creative and close federal-provincial relationship.[24] The prosperity and rising incomes of the 1960s were also a great help, with strong political support for welfare programs of all kinds.[25] If Canada did not quite have the political slogan of a "Great Society," as did the United States during the Lyndon Johnson years, it had the same substance. But in the case of Canadian health care that substance received the fortuitous support of a changing medical profession and the warmer federal-provincial relationship.[26]

It was a perfect instance of the "accidental logics" noted by Carolyn Hughes Tuohy. Everything fortuitously came together for those eager for universal care. It was no less a moment of great defeat for its ideological opponents. As one writer notes, "Both the insurance industry and organized medicine framed the issues in terms of free enterprise versus 'socialized medicine' . . . the medical profession would lose its professional autonomy and the public its freedom of choice."[27] As it turned out, doctors did not lose their autonomy and, in most respects, the public did not lose its freedom of choice.

The United States: Postwar Years, Postwar Frustrations

The American story for the years after World War II and into the present era was far more complicated. It was marked by a gradual expansion of health insurance (mainly employer-provided), a repeated failure to enact a universal health care program, and an increasingly complicated for-profit sector. The latter was marked in particular in the 1990s by a spurt of for-profit HMOs, the sale of many nonprofit hospitals to for-profit organizations, and the use of business techniques and models for health care organizations. As we did with the Canadian developments, we lay out a chronology of important market-related developments pertinent to the themes of this book:

1943: A bill that would have reorganized social insurance and introduced a national medical and hospital insurance plan (the Wagner-Murray bill) was not supported by the Roosevelt administration and failed to get as far as congressional hearings.

1942–1947: The creation of Kaiser Permanente (California), the Group Health Plan (Seattle), and the Health Insurance Program (New York) was the origin of prepaid group practice plans, later called HMOs.

1945: Another bill introduced in Congress (the Wagner, Murray, and Dingell bill), supported by President Truman to provide a moderate form of universal health care, also failed, in great part because of vehement opposition of organized medicine.

1946: The Hill-Burton Act passes, supporting hospital construction.

1965: The Medicare program (for the elderly) and the Medicaid program (for the poor) are established during the Lyndon Johnson administration.

1971: Initiative is taken by President Richard Nixon to support and subsidize HMOs, characterized as a "new national health strategy."

1975–1993: Heavy emphasis is placed on cost control; rising number of uninsured.

1994: President Clinton's Health Security bill, providing for universal care through managed competition, is defeated.

2003: A pharmaceutical benefit plan is adopted as part of the Medicare program—at the same time as the George W. Bush administration begins talking about cutbacks in Medicare and increased privatization of part of it.

This chronology does not tell a happy story. The number of uninsured has risen steadily over the decades, reaching forty-six million people by 2005. Employers have gradually cut back on health benefits, and cost inflation has been running from 10 to 12 percent a year (but with a slight decline in 2003). Liberals seeking universal health care have failed time and again to gain it, yet strong market proponents can boast of few striking gains either, with the Bush Medicare pharmaceutical program a significant exception. Those seeking a strategically clever mix of market and government to achieve universal coverage have yet to find a way that will work to bring together disparate interests and ideological foes. The postwar years show a trajectory that has satisfied hardly anyone.

While the Reagan years gave a large boost to a market ideology, the postwar momentum was already moving in that direction. With the end of the war against fascism, the beginning of the cold war against Communism immediately took its place, emphasizing the dangers of socialism (usually confused with Communism), including "socialized medicine," and extolling the virtues of capitalism. The advent of employer-based health insurance during the war, introduced as a tax-free fringe benefit in the face of restrictive wage and price controls, was the beginning of an important development. It meant that the majority of Americans who were not clearly poor or old, but simply employed, could count on decent health care coverage—but at the same time excluding the working poor and those employed by small businesses unable to provide health insurance to their employees. That combination would, together with other factors, provide just one more obstacle to universal health care by the 1990s: with a strong majority of people reasonably well insured, there was a public unwillingness to risk their own benefits by any radical change in the de facto system.

If the AMA can hardly be blamed for everything that happened in recent years, it had a major role in the postwar years in opposing many types of reforms, but particularly universal health care managed by the government. As noted, it even helped Canadian physicians in their opposition to such care. While the AMA gradually softened its stance, accepting various forms of group practice and corporate medicine, it did so much more slowly than the Canadian physicians. Moreover, as Tuohy has noted, Canadian physicians have had a tradition of "red toryism," which she has described as "an ideology that emphasizes the social responsibilities and obligations of those who hold privileged positions in society."[28]

A well-placed group of Canadian physicians with just that ideology proved decisive in bringing Canada its present health care system. In the United States, by contrast, the combination of medical and business opposition, particularly from the insurance industry (the latter continuing into the 1990s and the Clinton health care debate), was exceedingly powerful. The former aimed to hold on to its economic and clinical power while the latter aimed to avoid, in the case of the insurance industry, a loss of business. Other industries were wary of the possibility of a government attempt to have them pick up the bill for expanded health coverage (as well as being ideologically opposed to a government-run program). Canadian business posed no comparable obstacle.

Ideology and Incrementalism in the United States

While it is often thought that interest-group politics were the dominant force in the American health care struggle over the years, ideology has been even more important in the United States than in Europe.[29] In Europe, for that matter, the leading countries could fight against Communism but at the same time put in place strong welfare programs, and altogether avoid letting universal care be labeled as "socialist." That label would in any case have had little negative resonance in postwar Europe, with its many strong socialist and left-wing parties.

A strong welfare tradition, going back to a number of authoritarian governments, beginning with Germany in the late nineteenth century, showed in any event that good health care programs could grow in various soils, liberal or conservative, democratic or authoritarian. While Bismarck's Germany and Castro's Cuba have little in common, both believed that government has a key role in the health and economic welfare of its citizens. The Germany of that era—we note as an aside—was the parent of the modern pharmaceutical industry by virtue of its pioneering and profitable mixture of scientific and marketing skills.

Two American events are worth greater attention for our purpose: the emergence of incrementalism as the dominant model of health care movement (and some would say progress) in recent years, and the Clinton health care debate of the mid-1990s. The repeated failure of national health insurance efforts from the 1930s through the 1990s, aiming at wholesale change in the system, stimulated incrementalism as the fall-back position. Its strategy was to nibble away at the problem of universality bit by bit, hoping eventually to have full access for all. The Medicare proposal, and eventually government program, provides an interesting twentieth-century case study of the wisdom and practicality of incrementalism—which failed as a first step to universal care.

In the 1960s, with many calls for large-scale reform in the air, supported by public opinion polls, and with President Lyndon Johnson's election and his Great Society, the time seemed ripe to introduce important new health care programs that would nicely open the way for further programs, eventually culminating in universal care. With the elderly at that time the poorest age group in American society, and with much agitation for their better care, the Medicare program seemed not only to offer a fine response to the elderly problem but to serve as a forerunner for a more comprehensive plan; and the addition of the Medicaid program at the same time seemed to open that gate still further.

The future did not turn out that way. The rising costs of Medicare and Medicaid, the fact of continued efforts toward universal care that got nowhere in the 1970s, and, in that same decade, the development of new interest-group coalitions with competing agendas took much of the luster off incrementalism. For a time the idea more or less disappeared, not to be heard much about until its reappearance in the new millennium. But that most recent shift has turned out to have two faces, pointing in opposite directions.

From the liberal side, with no serious prospect for universal care in the offing, incrementalism in the 1990s seemed the most prudent course, focusing in particular on the effort to provide pharmaceutical coverage of some kind under the Medicare program. From the pro-market conservative side, that same pharmaceutical debate offered the possibility of incrementally moving the Medicare program in a privatizing direction. Conservative House Republicans threatened not to vote for the $400 billion drug benefit package (a figure lower than later estimates) unless it could control costs and promote competition between the standard Medicare program and private health plans. The fact that strong congressional figures of the same stripe revealed a desire at the end of 2003 to find ways to cut back Medicare expenditures in general, and to promote even more privatization of the whole program, signaled a move in the same direction. Incrementalism, it turns out, is a game that two can play.

Yet if incrementalism has now returned, on the right as well as the left, there was in the mid-1990s one further effort to create a universal health care system, that of the ill-fated Clinton Health Security bill. Paul Starr uses the term *accommodation* to describe the gradual shift of the American medical establishment from its early opposition to any and all forms of corporatism to a final, though not necessarily enthusiastic, acceptance. The word *accommodation* can also be applied to the Clinton effort, but of a different kind. It was an attempt to accommodate the strong voices in favor of market strategies, the need to control costs, the worries in the business communities about those costs, and the long-standing, but constantly dashed, hope for universal care. Clinton had made that last hope part of his election campaign.

The decisive failure of that effort within two years has been attributed to many causes—political ineptitude, excessive detail, weak congressional support—but the feature worth looking at from the perspective of this book is the attempted marriage of health care and the market. If there were many who wished for a single-payer plan—an extension, for instance, of the Medicare program to all citizens—President Clinton as well as most other observers felt that to be a hopeless option.

Instead, in the idea of "managed competition," he and his advisors felt they had found a way to get the best of two worlds, a universal health care plan that would cover everyone but in a way that embodied the central market concept of competition. Government's role would be the "managed" part, with the market supplying the kind of competition needed to control costs and maximize efficiency. As noted in the previous chapter, it was Alain Enthoven who developed the theory of managed competition (which he had brought earlier to the British National Health Service in the form of an "internal market"). It was later taken up by the Jackson Hole Group, an influential group of market supporters, by the Washington Business Group on Health, supported by large corporations, and by a number of insurance companies and managed care organizations. But by the time Enthoven's ideas had been mulled over and debated by those with other ideas, what found its way into the Clinton bill incorporated a number of deviations from Enthoven's original conception, which itself had changed a bit over the years.[30]

The net result of what at first seemed a good combination of the market and universality turned out to be exceedingly unstable, picked apart by market proponents and universal-care advocates alike. Big business failed to support the bill, small business came to oppose it, and a wide assortment of other organizations and interest groups brought forth many objections to this or that feature of the bill. Republicans, highly partisan at a time when Democrats controlled the Congress and the presidency, were intent on defeating Clinton's efforts one way or the other. Many of Enthoven's allies and groups sympathetic to his views, along with Enthoven himself, objected to the idea of a cap on national health care expenditures, an important part of Clinton's plan, and came to have doubts about an employer mandate, requiring business to pick up much of the bill for the universal care.

Worse still perhaps, as the Clinton bill ran into trouble, a number of alternative proposals were advanced, and from every part of the political spectrum. None of them succeeded either. The myriad objections from the right and left to the Clinton bill reflected what has sometimes been described as the "hyper-pluralism" of the American health care scene. What the Clinton bill mostly failed to surmount was the politically motivated but deeply rooted hostility toward government. It was there from the beginning, in early American history, but stoked to a new frenzy in the Reagan years by an increasingly partisan Republican Party that aimed to reduce the size and impact of government (always referred to as "big government"). Despite public opinion surveys indicating support for some kind of major reform, the strong role to be played by government was fatal. Perhaps most significant for the future, the 1992–1994 debate spawned a large number of new interest groups, none friendly to government and most of them certain to oppose any future universal health care program that requires central control, even of a decentralized, regional-control kind.

CANADA: THE PRESENT SCENE

The passage of the 1984 Canada Health Act brought universal health care to the country. It put in place a health care system that was dedicated to the five principles cited earlier—universality, accessibility, comprehensiveness, portability, and public administration—and prohibited copayments and parallel private insurance. For patients it allowed a choice of physicians, and for physicians it allowed freedom of practice (choice of location, type of practice, professional self-governance). The price of care is set by fee schedules determined by the provincial medical societies. If a physician is to remain in the system, he or she must accept the set fee. "Extra billing" of patients, earlier accepted, was eliminated and, with it, physician entrepreneurialism.

While physicians grumbled about the fee schedules, often complaining that their provincial medical associations did not bargain well enough in their behalf, the period between 1984 and the mid-1990s was notably successful. The CHA worked well. If it did not provide a model that American medicine and American legislators would consider following, it did allow many Canadian commentators and health policy experts to crow about its superiority to its big neighbor to the south. The combination of physician leadership, public opinion, and a culture that embraced a full welfare state brought the present Canadian system to life and, for a time, it seemed to have a bright and secure future.

The main features of the Canadian system can be summed up (though hardly in full) as: publicly funded and privately delivered care, patient and physician choice, no private health care provision for services covered by the provincial health plans, resistance to two-tier medicine and discouragement of privatization, federal-provincial transfer payments, and provincial responsibility for health care but with many conditions set by the federal government. There are limits on beds and technology, less technology than in the United States, waiting lists, a failure to include pharmaceuticals and home care fully in the system—and significantly lower per capita health care costs than in the United States as well as a higher life expectancy.

In 1998, the public share of spending for doctors was 98.7 percent, for hospitals 91.1 percent, for capital expenditures 81.8 percent—but only 31.0 percent for drugs and 10.5 percent for other health professionals. Those proportions reflect the early history of universal health care, when medical and hospital costs were high and the emphasis was placed on catastrophic costs. The result, as Terence Sullivan and Patricia Baranak note, "is that the continued emphasis on public payment for medical and hospital care no longer offers the same comprehensive protection for Canadians from financial risk as it did in the past."[31]

At least through the early 1990s, public opinion was highly favorable toward the system. There would be considerable agreement with the judgment rendered some years later by two well-placed commentators that three elements of the system are unique, fundamental, and worth preserving: (1) the fact that Medicare is a subsidy and resource transfer program, meeting the needs of all and ensuring a comparable level of care in each province; (2) the simplicity of the program, keeping administrative costs to a minimum by virtue of a single public-payment system; and (3) its ability to control costs because of the bargaining power of a single payer.[32]

Emerging Troubles

But if those were, after 1984, the basic ingredients of the system and much praised and supported in Canada, there was trouble ahead. By the 1990s, a combination of federal and provincial deficits, complaints about mismanagement, and a rapidly rising proportion of the gross domestic product (GDP) going to health care (up to 10% by 1992, second only to the United States) led to a number of sharp budget cuts. Saskatchewan, the province that had been the Canadian pioneer for Medicare, was particularly hard hit by financial troubles, closing some fifty-two rural hospitals. Alberta went the same way, with huge Medicare cuts. By the mid-1990s, every province but British Columbia had sharply reduced its health budget.

All of those troubles were exacerbated by federal cuts in the amounts transferred to the provinces. For some eight years, from 1990 to 1998, there was an erosion of quality in the system (a decline in doctors, hospital beds, and investment in new technologies) and a decline in expenditures. Not until the end of the 1990s was there an upturn, both in the financial health of the country in general and in health care expenditures. Despite the problems of those years, Canadians continued to prize their system, resisting the idea of a strengthened private sector. "Canadians," two commentators summing up public opinion said, "rejected the notion . . . that the private sector could deliver health care more fairly or efficiently. The drift in public opinion toward individualism took an abrupt halt when the conversation turned to health . . . Canadians lost confidence in the government's ability to manage the health care system, but they remained resolute in their belief in a collective approach."[33] At the same time, they note, patients were becoming more demanding, reflecting the rise of a consumer movement but one still set within the lines established in 1984; it is a consumer movement, it seems, that does not hanker for an expanded private health care sector.

Nonetheless, if there was an economic pickup by the end of the 1990s, and no sign that Canadians were prepared to abandon the basic system, considerable uneasiness remained. There was, for one thing, the ever-growing fear that Canadian health care (not to mention the entire society) would be "Americanized," a note struck again and again in the literature on Canadian health care, popular and professional.[34] American ideas were seen as dangerous, not only because they challenged the Canadian way, but also because they came across the border so easily—a border where the majority of Canadians live within fifty miles of the United States, a border breached daily by the media, which brought news about the United States and much of its TV entertainment; it is a slow-acting virus.

A consequence of this worry has been a spate of articles over the years about the superiority of the Canadian system and a steady flow of articles touting the system. An active practitioner of this effort has been the prominent British Columbia health care economist Robert Evans. The flavor of that pride is well caught by his comment in 1999, when the Canadian system was just pulling out of its troubles, that Canadians "are among the healthiest people in the world, and we are becoming healthier . . . on the standard measures of life expectancy and infant mortality, we outperform the United States."[35] All of that is true, but we want to note that he seems to have felt it necessary to say that time and time again, as if Canadians needed renewed inoculations against Americanism and arrogant Americans needed renewed reminders of the failures of their system.

Yet if Canadians have endlessly worried about Americanization and see its footprints everywhere—a latter-day Big Foot—at least one analyst of Canadian values has forcefully argued, with provocative data, that far from converging, the cultures of the two societies are going in opposite directions. The trend in the United States, he argues (based on public opinion surveys in both countries), has been that "for several decades now Americans have been dismantling FDR's New Deal, while Canada has been struggling to make its public programs sustainable and to expand the rights and freedoms of its citizens."[36] If that judgment comes across as a shade too chauvinistic, it seems valid, given the recent weakening of American welfare programs (which began in the Clinton administration), the George W. Bush administration's desire to insinuate more private sector choices into the (U.S.) Medicare program, and, on another cultural front, the legalization of gay marriage in Canada well before the United States.

We call attention to the anxiety about Americanization and the constantly reinforced strain of national pride in Canadian health care because they now coexist with considerable uneasiness about the actual state of that care. It is as if, when Canadians look south across the border they swell with pride, but when they look within they shrink back, seeing many problems and feeling much uncertainty about the future. While the health care system regained some stability by the end of the 1990s, the complaints did not stop, the uneasiness if anything increased, and important federal and provincial reports were commissioned.[37]

Waiting Lists

The complaints as the new millennium began took in just about every feature of Canadian health care. At the top were the waiting lists and waiting times, which always seemed to get longer. On the one hand, they are not inconsistent with universal care and equal access—*eventually* almost everyone will get what they need, just not right away. On the other, when there are fixed budgets and budget caps, and control of expensive technologies, waiting lists are an inevitable result; and they are a source of unhappiness whenever they appear. That is just what has happened in Canada, exacerbated by occasional but well-pub-licized cases of deaths that resulted from too long a wait for needed care. A *New York Times* survey in 2003 found significant increases in waiting times in Canada between 1993 and 2003 in orthopedic surgery (a median wait of 32 weeks), ophthalmology (27 weeks), neurosurgery (17 weeks), and gynecology (17 weeks).[38] (Waiting lists are hardly unknown in the United States.)

While waiting lists provide good fare for the media, their actual health impact may not be as great as many imagine: they are an important inconve-nience, sometimes harmful to health, but perhaps not nearly so crucial as other problems. Among the latter are a shortage of nurses, estimated to be as high as twenty-five thousand; a shortage of doctors, particularly in rural areas; com-plaints by both doctors and nurses of overwork and inadequate pay; a shortage of such diagnostic technologies as CT (computed tomography) scanners and MRI (magnetic resonance imaging) unit, and underequipped hospitals. A doc-tors' strike, not seen for many years, reappeared in January 2001 in New Bruns-wick because of lower physician wages in that province (and belying the claim of provincial equality).[39] The Conference Board of Canada, in a 2003 assess-ment of Canada in general, titled its section on health "Dispelling the Myth—Canada Is Not a Top Performer."[40] It went on to point out that Canada finishes ninth among twelve OECD (Organization for Economic Cooperation and De-velopment) countries on some basic health indicators—even though, in terms of perceived health status, Canadians were number one, with 88 percent of Canadians reporting good health, considerably above the average of 73 percent for the other countries.

Three important reports, in 2001 and 2002, addressed most of these prob-lems, though in different ways—but each, one way or another, taking up the question of an appropriate future balance between public and private sector health care. A 2001 report from Alberta, known as the Mazankowski report after its chair, former Conservative deputy prime minister Don Mazankowski, came out strongly for a much stronger private sector role, continuing a tradi-tion of market sympathy for some years in that province. While stressing that "no one should be denied access to essential health care services because they are unable to pay," it went on to say that "it is time to open up the system, take the shackles off, allow health authorities to try new ideas, encouraging compe-tition and choice, and see what works and what doesn't."[41] With language reminiscent of Regina Herzlinger, the report frankly says of patients, "let's call them 'customers.' "[42] Its clear target was the federal monopoly on health care financing and the straitjacket of federal domination. A 2002 report by the Canadian Senate (the Kirby report, named after Senator Michael Kirby) called for expanding coverage of drugs, post-acute home care, and palliative home care, and different modes of taxation for care. It also wanted the way open for more private initiatives such as medical savings accounts and copayments.[43]

The most important report, at least in terms of its federal backing, was the one issued by the Premier's Advisory Council on Health, chaired by Roy J. Romanow, a former premier of Saskatchewan.[44] In keeping with the traditions of Saskatchewan, a province considered the cradle of the national Medicare program, the council flatly rejected an expanded role for the private sector, reaffirmed the core values of equity, fairness, and solidarity, and called for a massive increase in federal health contributions to the provinces.

As for increasing the role of the for-profit sector, or introducing market practices, the Romanow report had not a good word to say. One by one it took on various market ideas and one by one rejected them. It no less decisively rejected a widespread view that the present system is economically unsustainable, a source of much Canadian concern, even if it might be classified as the free-floating kind, not based on any clear evidence about the future. "The Commission," the report stated, "is strongly of the view that a properly funded public system can continue to provide the high quality services to which Canadians have become accustomed."[45] The Romanow report was an uncompromising document, its optimism rejecting widespread anxieties about the future, and its all-out attack on the use of market mechanisms was a sharp rebuff to a rising call for their use.

The report suggested, in fact, that even some private provisions should be eliminated (by increased public funding of diagnostic devices, for instance, now a growth area for the private sector). Just give us more money—some $15 billion (Canadian)—was the message to the federal government. The report was not without its critics. Those from the left felt it had not adequately addressed such problems, for instance, as underfunded, stressed hospitals, and from the right that the market was hardly given a nod as a way out of the financial difficulties of the public system.

The Market at Bay—but Agitating

Despite the many difficulties facing the Canadian health care system, market proponents have so far made little progress. Stephen Harper, of the conservative opposition Canadian Council, said of the Romanow report (with more hope than evidence) that "this is the last gasp of 1960s ideology. We have enough watchdogs and bureaucracies."[46] The National Citizens' Coalition and the Atlantic Institute for Market Studies have similarly pressed market ideas, but without much success. These ideas include increased public-private partnerships, parallel private insurance for hospital and physician care, and medical savings accounts, for instance. In general, as in other countries, the main motivations behind market proposals are the increased financial pressure on the public program together with increased demand and expectations. There is also the familiar refrain that the market will bring greater efficiency, reduced utilization, and increased freedom of choice. Far from fearing Americanization, many Canadian market proponents look with favor on the American system with its strong private role. But they have not made much progress with those arguments: the spirit of the 1960s remains strong.

If it seems fair to say that the market is being held at bay in Canada—in 2002 the proportion of private sector spending reversed a long trend in the other direction by actually decreasing, from 29.8 to 27.4 percent, with public sector spending going from 70.2 to 72.6 percent—the reforms put in place after the three reports cited above may not be sufficient to avert a troubled future. The main reform was the Ministers' Health Care Renewal Accord of 2003. That accord resulted from a meeting of the provincial and federal governments and put in place an increase of federal transfer funds of $30.9 billion over a five-year period, a number of special initiatives including a special fund for diagnostic and medical equipment, and a Health Council to monitor the results of the accord. But it did nothing to eliminate the provision of private services within the framework of public financing, thus failing to act on that recommendation by the Romanow report.

On the face of it, this array of reforms seems strong and responsive to many of the complaints about Canadian health care. But Allan Detsky and David Naylor, two of Canada's most respected health care analysts, point out that public opinion surveys show a sharp decline in satisfaction with the system, noting that in 2001 some 59 percent of Canadians believed that the system requires some fundamental changes, and 18 percent that a complete rebuilding is in order.[47] These analysts are doubtful that the Renewal Accord is strong enough in its reforms to allay public and physician anxiety about the future of the system.

While there is no good evidence to suggest that the core principles of the system will be rejected, there is sufficient restlessness and uneasiness to suggest that the future may be difficult. Market supporters, so far unsuccessful in any significant way, are standing by in the wings waiting for their moment to come. Detsky and Naylor conclude their analysis by writing: "We foresee continued turbulence as provinces pursue overdue reforms of their regional programs, as the federal government seeks to hold provinces to account for new funding, and as a growing proportion of Canadians lose patience with health care systems that they perceive as no longer delivering reasonable access to core services."[48] Janice MacKinnon, finance minister in the government of Roy Romanow from 1991 to 2001, is hardly more optimistic. She notes that "health care costs are increasing at a faster rate than the revenue of any government, and other critical priorities are being underfunded in the scramble to cover those costs." "Health care," she says, "may be the Canadians' highest priority but not their only priority."[49]

Taking an even more pessimistic stance than the Romanow report and the Canadian Institute for Health Information, the Conference Board of Canada said, in a 2004 report, that the health care system is not sustainable in its present form.[50] The fact that its report was funded by the province of Alberta led some to question its pessimism, but its projection of future costs and burdens is plausible. If the market is now being held at bay in Canadian health care, there are many opportunities for market proponents to find soft spots to exploit.

An important opening was provided by the Canadian Supreme Court in June 2005. It ruled that Quebec's prohibition on private services covered by the public system violates the province's bill of rights. Whether similar prohibitions in other provinces will also be challenged is unclear, but the Quebec decision represented an important break with a long-standing feature of Canadian health care. Since most European countries allow private insurance, however, with no major threat to their public systems, a Canadian shift in other provinces need not unhinge the Canadian health care system.[51]

The narrow reelection of Prime Minister Paul Martin of the Liberal Party in 2004, but the loss of that party's majority, could spell trouble for the reform efforts earlier pushed by Martin, aiming to put into place many of the Romanow proposals. The continuingly fractious province of Alberta in 2004 issued a report, *Alberta Health First,* promoting privatization, with the premier threatening to take Alberta out of the Canada Health Act and go it alone. Prime Minister Martin, however, announced in September 2004 that the federal government would put an additional $14 billion into the system, aiming to deal with the most persistent complaints. For many of the system's critics, that was seen as a stop-gap, inadequate amount of money.

THE FUTURE OF AMERICAN HEALTH CARE:
LOOKING INTO THE FOG

If Canada has managed to hold on to its traditional health care values and organization, fending off market proponents, there is a nervousness about the future. Where is the United States? The only perfectly clear answer is that it is south of the border from Canada. Nothing else is evident. Its complex combination of public and private, undergoing constant change, and a political scene that has become increasingly partisan and more ideologically divided than in the past, at times nastily so, make a traditionally unclear future even more so at present.

We offer four generalizations we believe few observers would deny. The first is that there is no large-scale organized effort, or serious political leadership, to pursue universal health care, much less a government-run, or simply government-financed, single-payer system. The fact that public opinion polls have for many years indicated a public willingness to accept universal care seems almost irrelevant (a 2003 national public opinion poll showed support for a government-run universal care program by a margin of 62% to 32%).[52] The sticking point is that no one has a sure-fire idea of how to bring that about, and political support for the idea is scattered and uncoordinated.

The second generalization is that there is a serious problem with rising health care costs, a refrain heard for thirty years, but cutting more deeply now. It is reducing employer-provided benefits and putting pressure on government programs (particularly Medicaid at the state level), and its impact is now reaching into the middle class.[53] The third is that a major contributor to rising costs in the United States is that of technology—between 40 and 50 percent of increased health care costs, whether new technologies or more intensively used old ones. They are constantly fed into the health care system by the drug and device industries, and almost always welcomed by physicians and health care consumers, expecting and demanding constant progress, a perpetual playing out of the infinity model of progress.

The fourth is that the organizational and historical culture of American health care, intensified by its current economic problems, opens a fertile field for the intensified introduction of market ideas and practices, however untested or found wanting in earlier incarnations. While it could of course be said that the current situation also opens the way for renewed pressure for universal care and a stronger government role, the obstacles to a move in that direction

seem at least balanced by forces intent on widening market strategies. Ironically, where it was the power of organized medicine in the nineteenth and
early twentieth centuries that was able to shape the agenda of American health
care, it was the effort of physicians to hang on to their "entrepreneurial discretion and clinical autonomy" that turned out, in the long run, to foster an entrepreneurialism that came to threaten, even overthrow, professional objectives
or collegial decision-making.[54] The influence of physicians has diminished but
not disappeared, now centered on payment policy, quality and clinical innovation, and medical education and training.[55]

The American health care system is obviously in trouble, at least in the eyes
of most observers. But what does the word *trouble* mean in this context? With
the exception of some minority groups, the health of Americans has never been
better: increased life expectancies, dropping mortality rates for all age groups,
declining disability for the elderly, and the rehabilitation or successful maintenance of many who would have been dead in earlier times. Yet forty-six million people are uninsured, and many more underinsured or temporarily uninsured. Between 1996 and 1999, some eighty-five million had no insurance at
some point.[56] Moreover, many countries have a better general level of health
than the United States despite the fact that the United States spends 15 percent
of its GDP on health care and by far the most per capita. As for minority groups,
it is not good for your health to be a black male or a native American in the
United States.

In trying to sort out the role of the market in recent years in the United
States, we want to look briefly at three events of special significance: the failure
of the HMO movement to control costs and the resultant trend to reduce benefits in employer-provided insurance, the emergence of corporate medicine,
and the 2003 Medicare pharmaceutical debate. The thread that runs through
these three events is the way each has embodied or espoused market practices
as a way of dealing with the troubles noted above.

Managed Care: An Economic Success and a Political Failure

Managed care (by which is usually meant health maintenance organizations) has been, in the apt words of James C. Robinson, "an economic success
and a political failure."[57] Its aim has been twofold: to provide integrated health
care services and to stifle increasing costs; and for a time it seemed to do just
that (but less so with integration than cost control). Since HMOs are, at least in
many places, competitive with each other, the hope and expectation was that

they would control costs, and from about 1993 to 1997 they seemed to do so. There was also a deeper agenda among many proponents of managed care: its success would demonstrate the value of market ideas. Gerald Burke wrote in 1996 that "Americans have embarked, by default, on a grand experiment in free-market medicine and that it may be a decade or more before we can fairly judge its successes and failures."[58] Alain Enthoven and Sarah Singer, writing in 1997, were buoyant: "Since the early 1990s, cost pressures have moderated significantly, and there is no explanation except competitive markets and managed care . . . market forces are the only practical means to contain costs while maintaining quality."[59]

Well, to paraphrase a cliché of that era, something happened on the way to the market. It was a failed experiment in cost containment, and if it worked for a time, it had little staying power. What went wrong? There seems to be no definitive explanation, but Robinson's description of managed care as a "political failure" is the most plausible. As Alain Enthoven, echoing Robinson, succinctly put it, "managed care has broken down under an onslaught from lawyers, politicians, consumers, and doctors."[60] Physicians' and patients' complaints, often ferocious, were directed at HMOs: angry and anguished cries about denied patient services, physicians angered at being forced to work with HMOs, the difficulty of access to specialists, requirements that physicians get permission for expensive procedures, and a lack of choice of plans for patients (usually the fault of employers who offered only one choice). These complaints got through, sometimes leading to legislative mandating of denied or restricted services ("drive-through baby deliveries"), and sometimes to increased competitive pressures (the need to keep up with the offered benefits of competitors).

But one message seemed clear enough: HMOs operate with spending caps, forced to budget their services in light of what insurers or employers will pay them—and that means rationing and limit-setting. Americans do not like that.[61] Nonetheless, if HMOs have been a failure in controlling costs, or proving the benefit of market competition, they have proved to be effective in delivering integrated care, far better than a fragmented fee-for-service medicine. Yet their troubles also show what any universal health care plan, particularly one forced to live within a fixed budget and with some reasonable caps on services and expenditures, would be up against—and could there be any other kind? The American public seems wedded to an infinity medicine, a medicine eager for unending technological innovation, a medicine that must always get better, and a medicine resistant to any financial or medical restraints, whether market- or government-imposed.

An important consequence of the failure of HMOs to control costs has been that employers are cutting back on benefits.[62] Since employers provide the bulk of care for those not covered by Medicare or Medicaid, their behavior has a widespread system effect, increasing the number of uninsured and leading to the use of various market tactics to manage their costs. On occasion it has also led to some negative judgments on employer-based health insurance altogether.[63] Employers have responded to cost pressures, in some cases by eliminating employee health benefits altogether (in small businesses), by decreasing benefits (most drastically by eliminating family coverage), and by forcing employees to pay more out of pocket through copayments and deductibles.

Employees are paying 40 percent more out of pocket than three years ago, and in 2003 two-thirds of employers increased the employee share and 79 percent said they planned to do so again in 2004. Union opposition has been strong, but only fitfully successful. The employer rationale, in addition to controlling costs, has been that a market-driven system can best address the inefficiencies and poor quality of American health care and increase employees' personal health responsibility by forcing them to directly confront the cost of their care.[64]

While in one sense the difficulties of managed care in living up to its early promise seemed to open the way for more "consumer-driven" health care, that movement may not have the force behind it that many expected to see.[65] Patients' complaints about HMOs, particularly restrictions on choice, surely reflected a climate of growing consumer force, but some recent developments suggest some hesitations. While there are different definitions, the essence of consumer-driven health care is to provide a greater choice of health plans, more personal control of medical spending, and to make consumers more conscious of the real cost of medical care. But a recent study of employers' attitudes toward such programs suggests some ambivalence on their part. They are uncertain about the effect of such programs on costs and quality and, most significantly perhaps, whether such programs will in fact be popular with employees (with some evidence that they will not be).[66] In conclusion to a comprehensive study of consumer-driven health care, Karen Davis, president of the Commonwealth Fund, says that the early evidence of its efficacy is inconclusive about its long-term value, but notes also that "if it is primarily a tool for shifting costs from employers to employees it will quickly be discarded."[67]

The Corporate Practice of Medicine

In his painstakingly detailed and tightly argued book *The Corporate Practice of Medicine,* the health economist James C. Robinson argues that the basic problem is the "conflicting pressure between expenditure-increasing technological change, on the one hand, and revenue-constraining resistance by taxpayers, employers, and individual purchasers on the other." That way of stating the basic problem (which can be repeated around the world) seems to us just right. Robinson, in a book published in 1999, but written earlier—during the palmy days of temporary cost containment—argues that the solution to this conflict is corporate medicine, which will embody the fact that "the principle and promise of organizational innovation is firmly established in the historical record and contemporary marketplace."[68]

By *corporate medicine* he means to draw on what he judges to be the great success of the American business corporation, when freed of excessive regulation (e.g., the airline industry, utilities, energy). These corporations, he argues, have been outstandingly innovative and deft in their competitive strategies, reducing costs, increasing efficiency, and improving quality. More specifically he means "the endeavor to bring together, not individual physicians into medical groups, but medical groups into larger health care systems . . . multiple markets, physician-hospital organizations that combine, and health plans that design multiple products . . . In the final analysis it is not incremental improvement in price and quality that counts, but . . . radical competition . . . that strikes not at the margins of the profits and outputs of the existing organizations but at their foundations and their very lives. This is the corporate practice of medicine."[69]

Another book of that era, *The For-Profit Healthcare Revolution,* focuses in particular on the creation of investor-owned hospitals, pioneered by, among others, Bill Frist, Jr., now majority leader of the U.S. Senate, and the creation of the Health Corporation of America. Along with others in the industry, that corporation bought up nonprofit or other for-profit hospitals so that, by the mid-1900s, thirteen hundred hospitals were investor-owned, 20 percent of the nation's hospitals. "Cost pressures," the authors note, and "competition has never been more fierce."[70] After charting the emergence and growth of for-profit hospitals and some other aspects of for-profit health care, they conclude their book by asking "who best manages the economic resources that pay for our healthcare services . . . In the final analysis, the individual market will determine the most effective structure."[71] That last sentence was surely the spirit of the times. What then happened? Costs have not been controlled, and hospital costs in 2002 overtook pharmaceutical costs as the major source of increasing health care costs. Where there was pressure in the 1990s to reduce the number of hospital beds—a major cost item—by 2003 there was once again talk of a shortage of those beds.[72]

Should we be surprised that corporate medicine, a source of much profit and much financial churning, has not dealt with the cost problem? The economist Victor Fuchs, writing in that era, noted that, while it was too early to reach final conclusions on the outcome of massive mergers, acquisitions, and consolidations of health care organizations, "the historical evidence is that the history of mergers in the American economy in general suggests that many of the larger mergers and acquisitions in health care will prove to have little social value. Studies of mergers in other industries have not shown widespread cost reductions or improvements in profitability, on average."[73] And so it has turned out in the health care industry. No less deleterious, at least in the hospital industry, is that competition from for-profit hospitals has forced the nonprofits to copy their "undesirable behavior."[74]

REFORM PROPOSALS

As noted above, there is no well-organized drive for, or political support of, universal health care, and the $700 billion expected cost of the new Medicare pharmaceutical benefit package (and a growing budget deficit in general) is not likely to encourage any further major reform efforts in the immediate future. Nonetheless, there are a number of ideas for reform available. Most, but not all, have an expanded role for the market. In that context, however, a significant finding of the Community Tracking Study, surveying households, physicians, local health system leaders, employers, and insurers, found deep skepticism about the ability of market-based reforms to produce urgently needed improvements in the efficacy and quality of the nation's health care system.[75] That may not be good news for those looking for an expanded market role. We briefly describe five proposed ideas for reform, beginning with a proposal for a single-payer national health insurance plan.

A National Health Insurance, Single-Payer Plan

This plan has been put forth by a group of physicians. It would be a government-run system, financed by direct taxes. Its aim would be to cover "every American for all medically necessary services, including long-term care, mental health and dental services, and prescription drugs and supplies." In addition to dismissing just about every claim ever made in favor of market practice—defined contribution plans, tax subsidies and vouchers for the poor, and mandated employer-coverage voucher plans—it forthrightly declares that the "pursuit of corporate profit and personal fortune have no place in care-giving. They create enormous waste and too often warp clinical decision making."[76] But, that much said, the details are not spelled out. It is not clear whether this plan would require government-salaried health care workers, low-paid physicians, a federal pharmaceutical and device-manufacturing program, and federalized nursing homes, hospitals, and clinics, and whether it would elimi-nate copayments and deductibles. A contemplation of the political and cultural history of American health care would lead to even further questions.

A "Medicare for All" Bill

This bill, formally called the United States National Health Insurance Act (HR 676), was introduced into the House of Representatives by John Conyers, a Democratic congressman from Michigan.[77] It would expand the current Medi-care program to include all U.S. residents, creating a "publicly financed, pri-vately delivered health care program" that aims to "ensure that all Americans, guaranteed by law, will have access to the highest quality and cost effective health care services regardless of one's employment, income, or health care status." Notably—as with the Canadian system—private health insurers would be prohibited from selling coverage "that duplicates the benefits of the USNHI program," but the plan would allow private coverage for benefits not covered by the program. The program would set reimbursement rates for physicians and other health care providers, and negotiate prescription drug prices. Unlike the physicians' plan noted above, far more details are provided, including a proposed funding of $1.8 trillion per year (compared with the present $1.7 tril-lion for U.S. health care costs). As with the physicians' proposal, it turns its back on market practices, with no apparent aim to politically sweeten its pro-posal to appeal to market proponents.

An American Medical Association Proposal

This proposal, advanced in 2004, moves strongly in a market direction. It would include tax credits for the purchase of individual health insurance policies and a strengthening of individual and group health insurance markets. It aims to empower individuals to choose their health plans and to give patients and their physicians greater control over their health choices. Insurers would be stimulated to respond more to the "demands of individual consumers and be more cautious about increasing premiums." The AMA looks to the development of new insurance markets through legislative and regulatory changes, "to foster a wider array of high-quality affordable plans." "Consumer choice"— choice of plan and choice of physicians and other health care professionals—is the cornerstone of the AMA's proposal to expand coverage. The AMA would limit the role of government, avoiding a "one-size fits all approach to coverage."[78] The emphasis of this proposal is on expanding coverage, not on providing universal health care (though it seems to believe that its tax credit plan would push in that direction), and it offers no estimate on how great that expansion would be. It is a remarkably market-oriented proposal, showing that the supposedly old-time resistance of the AMA to government-dominated plans is still alive and kicking.

Managed Competition Redux

Alain Enthoven, the leading proponent of managed competition during the Clinton push for universal care, but not of the final version that was put forward, has come back with a revised proposal. Its idea is "for the employer to increase competition by offering employees a wide choice of carriers and plan designs, a responsible choice (employees fully responsible for premium differences, individual choice, informed choice, and multiple choices of delivery systems)." The Federal Employees Health Benefit Program and the California Public Employees Retirement Systems provide successful models, he argues. The managed competition model encourages cost-reducing innovation, opens the market to selective networks, and creates effective market forces. "Exchanges" would be crucial, bringing together numerous employers and employees who "can meet with numerous carriers and offer choices." Business leadership would be needed, together with tax benefits, tax exclusion for participating employers, and a regulatory body "to be sure that exchanges actually promote competition and expand the competitive market."[79]

In a later article, Enthoven wrote that "it is late, probably too late, to avert the inexorable progression to 'Medicare for All,'" but he was quick to add that the Medicare model will not deliver efficient health care systems: "A properly structured model, based on existing demonstrated successes, could."[80]

Enthoven's phrase "inexorable progression" is interesting. We have not noted any "inexorable progression" and wonder if that is a sound prediction or a voice of defeat from someone who has worked tirelessly, but without success, for a market-oriented managed competition plan.

A Voucher Plan

A prominent physician and ethicist, Ezekiel Emanuel, and a distinguished economist, Victor Fuchs, have proposed a voucher plan. "Every family or individual," they write, "would be given a voucher to purchase a policy that covered basic services . . . People who want more services . . . could pay a premium over the voucher." An ear-marked tax would pay for the vouchers, with the level of the tax a function of public willingness to peg the tax to the level of public demand for health care. The strategy behind this proposal is that "Democrats have long favored the notion of universality, while Republicans have instinctively favored vouchers and have longed for the demise of Medicare and Medicaid."[81] Just how this proposal will deal with the basic unwillingness of taxpayers to pay more for health care in the first place, or deal with antigovernment sentiment (it will require government financing and regulation), or with pro-market proponents' desire to get rid of government control altogether is not explained (and, in their defense, it must be said that the authors did not have space to fill out the details).

While he does not present a plan for full-scale health reform, the market-oriented economist Stuart M. Butler echoes some common features of market-oriented reforms: a change in the tax treatment "to reduce the market-distorting bias that favors employer control of health coverage rather than consumer control of health dollars"; investment in information systems (a common idea on both sides of the ideological divide); alternative groups and intermediaries (e.g., churches, unions, ethnic groups) to act on behalf of consumers; and "regulatory steps to spur competition."[82] In contrast, the Harvard economist David M. Cutler argues that a universal health program, with the government forcing people to buy insurance (with the same range of choices now possible for federal employees) and working hard to remove inefficiencies and improving quality, could bring genuine reform. "Universal coverage," he notes (as well he might), "means a larger role for government than is the case now."[83]

Maybe one of these ideas will catch on. Emanuel and Fuchs speak of "a crisis [that] is at hand." But the United States has shown a remarkable talent to muddle through its "crises," a term heard every decade or so, and to resist any basic changes. Moreover, none of these ideas, so far as we can see, appears to offer a way of dealing with the disturbing findings from the work of the Dartmouth epidemiologist John E. Wennberg: wide and often inexplicable medical practice variations in different parts of the country in hospital beds and admissions, use of technology, and treatment of disease. Most revealingly, his studies have shown that more hospital beds or available technology do not necessarily lead to improved health outcomes.[84]

If Canada can be said to have a crisis, as many observers would say, it has one great advantage in dealing with it. In its five principles (in the CHA) and its history of universal care it has a good starting point. The United States, with its mixed public-private system, has no such bedrock, just a luxuriant jungle of competing interests and values that add up to no coherent whole. As noted in chapter 1, health economists usually say that it is not a matter of market *or* government, but of getting the right balance. True enough in some abstract way, but as the Medicare drug debate revealed, the pro-market people have a different notion of the right balance than the pro-government people.

THE MEDICARE DRUG BENEFIT DEBATE

This section can fittingly end with a discussion of the Medicare drug benefit debate, which came to a climax at the end of 2003. It ended with a drug benefit program that changed the nature of the Medicare program itself, making room for large government-paid incentives to jumpstart a major private sector role. The Medicare program, providing health care for the elderly, came into existence in 1965 at a time when 30 percent of the elderly had incomes below the federal poverty line. It embodied the idea of a social contract between seniors and society to be renewed from generation to generation, and it was the equivalent of a single-payer health care system, financed totally by the federal government (with some patient out-of-pocket provisions). It has been, by most accounts, enormously popular with the elderly, better able to control its costs than the private sector, and the beneficiary for a time of strong bipartisan support in Congress.

That bipartisan support was to dissolve in 1994–1995. As the political scientist Jonathan Oberlander has shrewdly noted, Medicare has become the battleground of the market versus government struggle.[85] That change began with the election of Republican majorities in both houses of Congress in 1994 and the later decision of Newt Gingrich in his conservative Contract with America to make reform of Medicare a targeted issue. The aim was clear enough: to give the private sector a greater role in the program, bringing the market into play as much as possible—more patient choice, more competition, less regulation, a reduced government role. As one market proponent noted at the time, while his side was not getting all it wanted, it was "moving the ball down the field."[86]

By 2003 that ball had moved very far indeed. Despite the fact that the Medicare+Choice program had not been a success, beginning with 8 percent of Medicare recipients in 1995, peaking at 16 percent in 1999–2000, and declining to 11 percent by 2003, that proved no discouragement to those pushing for an expanded market role. Moreover, the Bush administration made it known that it was prepared to cut back on the Medicare program later if the costs, including the new drug benefits, got too high. But the more immediate goal was, with the help of a Republican majority in both houses, the addition of a pharmaceutical benefit to the Medicare program. Such a benefit would close one of the most obvious gaps in the original program as well as offering the potentially great political prize of greater elderly support for the Republican Party. For its part, such a benefit was no less attractive to the Democrats and for the same political reasons. The question, as the debate on a bill opened, was who would win—and, in order to win, which side would be willing to make what compromises? From the start, however, it was clear to the Democrats that the Republicans would work to privatize as much of the drug benefit as possible, and no less clear that Democrats would have to accept some of that privatization if any bill was to get through.

There is no need here, much less space, to detail all of the changes in the program that came out of the debate (now widely publicized), which on balance saw the Bush administration get most of what it wanted. There were a number of market items included in the purported $400 billion budget: medical savings accounts, subsidies to begin in 2006 to support private plans competing with Medicare's traditional fee-for-service arrangement, a 28 percent tax exemption for corporations offering retirees drug benefits, and a reliance on insurance companies and private health plan to manage the new drug benefit. Most strikingly, the bill also prohibits the government from negotiating lower drug prices for those on Medicare, thus making it impossible to use the single most important power used by other governments to control drug costs. One need not be overly cynical to see the hand of the pharmaceutical industry behind that provision. The idea of price controls on drugs in the United States, standard fare in most developed countries, is about as low in their eyes as hell was in Dante's.

The Democrats, led by Senator Edward M. Kennedy, particularly protested that last provision, but there were many other objections as well. Forced to compromise to get a bill through, a large number voted for the bill, a bill that undermines many of the values that lay behind the original program. It was, as a *Wall Street Journal* story aptly put it, "a classic compromise: a Democratic benefit and a Republican delivery system."[87] That delivery system will, at least for the immediate future, be a bonanza for the health care industry, drug companies, and private insurers.

If the Democrats had to swallow a lot of distasteful features of the bill to get it through, there was also some surprising conservative opposition. Dick Armey, a Republican and the majority leader in the House from 1995 to 2002, wrote that "the conservative, free market base in America is rightly in revolt over this bill."[88] John Iglehart, the perceptive founding editor of *Health Affairs,* noted that, if conservative Republicans did not like the bill, neither did many Democrats, objecting in particular to the benefits it bestowed on drug companies and its threats to traditional Medicare.[89] No doubt President Bush was pleased to see the bill make it through Congress. An editorial in the *Wall Street Journal* said that "trillions of new dollars in spending . . . will only increase pressure for taxes to pay for it . . . Republicans may soon find themselves becoming the tax collectors for their own welfare state."[90] That may not have occurred to the president.

CANADA AND THE UNITED STATES: WHERE ARE THEY GOING?

A final word on the comparison of Canada and the United States. We characterized the present Canadian situation as "the market at bay," but noted persistent agitation on the issues and enough problems to help push it along. In light of President Bush's success in putting market practices in his drug benefit bill, it is tempting to characterize the American situation as "the market ascendant." If most of the reform proposals we sketched above open a wide door for market practices, the Community Tracking Study—with its finding of a decreasing ardor for market strategies—leaves a less clear picture. If Canada has its Medicare program as its bedrock from which to start any debate about an increased role for the market, even in the face of great cost pressures and other problems, the United States is now prone to react ambivalently to its cost problems, with some calling for a market push and others for a stronger government role.

In theory, American health care is market-prone, but in practice the record is considerably more mixed. Canada has a weak tradition of market advocacy for health care. The United States has a strong one. The outcome of the (U.S.) Medicare drug benefit debate, pushing the United States further down a market road already well traveled in the past, showed how much that strong difference matters, at least at the moment.

Yet the hint of an undercurrent of skepticism about the future suggests that the Bush victory may not serve as a predictor of future trends. Much will depend on the future of health care costs, still going up in comparison with general costs (even if moderating a bit in 2003 and 2004). Those increases are now affecting the whole system and reaching into the middle class. One in seven Americans had difficulty paying their medical bills, and 68 percent of those having such problems had health insurance. Of the twenty million families facing difficulties in paying their health care bills, 20 percent had incomes below the federal poverty line, while 22 percent were in the "low-income" category. Those latter figures are familiar, but the high percentage of the insured with problems in paying their health bills signals something new. It is beyond our wisdom, such as it is, to predict where all of this will go, and even the deity might beg off telling us what the American health care future will be. One of the few promising signs, perhaps reminicent of the Canadian history, is that a few states have taken initiatives to provide health care for all of their citizens. Their outcome remains uncertain.

If Canada and the United States show the great difference that culture and political systems make, the countries of Western Europe provide still further examples of their importance. Yet the development of universal care in Europe, though showing some features similar to its development in Canada, by no means followed an identical path. Its history is more deeply rooted and different in character, and the fact that so many countries with different languages, history, and culture embraced universal health care is noteworthy (think of the difference between Italy and Norway, France and Germany). In the next chapter, we look at the values that have sustained the commitment to universal care but, no less important, the variety of ways in which market practices have made their way in European health care.

CHAPTER THREE

The Endurance of Solidarity

Universal Health Care in
Western Europe and Elsewhere

One country, the United States, has never proclaimed a principle of affordable health care for all. Another country, Canada, was late getting there. Yet a large number of other countries have been there for a long time, riding out wars, depressions, political upheavals, and, in recent decades, the beckoning embrace of the market. The nations of Western Europe have been the heartland of universal health care. Technically, not all European countries have mandatory health care coverage (Germany, the Netherlands, Belgium, and Switzerland do not), but all aim for full coverage, one way or another, of all their citizens. Thus when we speak of universal coverage we will mean a system of health care that provides everyone with full access to adequate care, whether through direct taxation, mandatory employer-employee contributions, or affordable private insurance (or some combination of these). The experience of Europe in holding on to universality over the decades, gingerly incorporating some market practices into their health care systems, is thus an important part of the contemporary saga of medicine and the market.

The fact that almost every one of those systems is now struggling in various degrees to contain costs puts them at a critical historical juncture. Or is it this year's juncture? One can go back for three decades and find statements about a "crisis" in funding health care and the need for reform, but especially during the late 1980s and into much of the 1990s. The desire for health care reform in Europe as elsewhere is best likened to a chronic disease; the disease is not cured, just managed. Can the European countries hold on to universal health care—and its foundational value of solidarity—and can they embrace market practices without giving up some long-held moral and political commitments?

While various forms of health insurance in Europe go back many centuries, the birth of national health policies in Europe has been traditionally traced to Otto von Bismarck, the German chancellor from 1862 to 1890.[1] The first initiative came in 1881 from the German emperor William I, who at Bismarck's behest wrote a letter to the German parliament saying that those disabled by age and illness had a strong claim to care from the state. The result was an old-age insurance program adopted in 1889. Together with retirement and disability benefits already in place, a sickness insurance program enacted in 1883, and an 1884 workers' compensation program, the net result was a comprehensive system of income security (at a time when loss of income from sickness was considered far more important than the cost of medical care). The main method for implementing these programs was the development of "independent" social insurance funds, but in fact quasi-governmental in operation, heavily regulated by government, and typically dependent on mandatory payroll deductions.

Contrary to a long-standing belief, retirement benefits under Bismarck began at age seventy, not sixty-five (though changed many years later to the latter figure). More important, the motives behind Bismarck's program were not, as many today might assume, liberal in their thrust. The main aim was to promote the well-being of the work force and thus to maximize efficiency—and thereby to inoculate his country against more radical socialist alternatives. As would happen later with similar health care developments in Europe, the early welfare state development was heavily influenced by Catholic social thought, and usually put in place by authoritarian, conservative, and paternalistic governments.

While the Bismarckian tradition, relying on private sickness funds, can be seen as the primary stimulus to European health care programs, it was eventually complemented by a shift in the post–World War II era to tax-based systems in a number of countries (e.g., the British National Health Service), giving the government a more direct hand in financing and managing each country's system. Yet even the social health insurance systems are under tight government regulation and supervision. (See table 3.1 for a breakdown of tax-based and social health insurance systems.)

Various theories have been proposed to account for the rise of the welfare state and the health care systems that have been an important element of it: as

TABLE 3.1
Social Health Insurance (SHI) and Tax-Based Systems

	Predominantly SHI-based	Predominantly tax-based	Year of major legislative change from SHI to tax-based
Market Rejectors			
Canada		X	–
Denmark		X	1972*
France	X		
Italy		X	1978
Sweden		X	1970*
United Kingdom		X	1946
Market Accommodators			
Australia	X		
Belgium	X		
Germany (until 1990)	X		
Israel	X		
Netherlands	X		
Switzerland	X		
Second Thoughts			
Czech Republic		X	–
New Zealand		X	–

Source: Adapted from Richard B. Saltman and Hans F. W. Dubois, "The Historical and Social Base of Social Health Insurance Systems," in *Social Health Insurance Systems in Western Europe,* ed. Richard B. Saltman, Reinhard Busse, and Josep Figueras (Maidenhead, UK: Open University Press, 2004), 26.
*SHI never played a significant role, but the year indicated marks, arguably, a break point where the central state took increased financial responsibility to provide more extended coverage and the role of the tax-based system was increased largely.

part of the logic of industrialism, when traditional sources of social security such as the family and the church began to lose their force; to save capitalism from an uprising of the masses; and as a consequence of the spread of democracy, putting voter pressure on politicians for social benefits. We will not attempt to pass judgments on these theories. What needs to be noted is that the notion that comprehensive welfare programs are inherently "socialist," a deeply embedded American and politically conservative idea, does not reflect their origins or their later histories, supported by the left and right.

If the nineteenth century saw only a slow growth of the idea of health insurance in Canada and the United States, by the end of that century it was widespread in Europe, even if not in as comprehensive a form as with the Bismarck program. Behind much of this development was the idea of "social citizenship": social rights are granted on the basis of citizenship, not market performance. A citizen's place and productivity in the workplace are put to one side in favor of a universal standard of entitlement, based entirely on their individual value and their place as citizens, on nationality and nothing else.

THE MEANING OF SOLIDARITY

At the heart of the European model is the concept of solidarity, a communal or communitarian moral premise for the provision of health care, not the more individualistic notion of rights (though they seem to be invoked more frequently these days and are the characteristic language of most international statements on health care). Solidarity has been there from the beginning and animates the European idea of health care to this day. It encompasses the mutual responsibility of citizens for the health care of each other, equitable access to care, and it assumes that, in the face of illness and the threat of death, we are bound together by common needs that require a community response.

The principle of solidarity can rightly be treated as a moral and political paradigm, a statement of the ideals of solidarity, not necessarily its actual practice. As we try to show in what follows, it is the effort to remain true to those ideals in the face of a variety of economic obstacles that has been a prime vehicle for the entry of market practices. We do not mean to state a paradox here. We only want to underscore a point about European health care systems: there have been three sources of attraction to the market—for the sake of greater efficiency within health care systems that want to hold tightly to solidarity values; as a way of containing costs; and to express an ideological drive toward greater consumer choice and self-determination. For the most part, the first and second motives have been the most significant, but the third is on the rise in many places.

Nonetheless, in continuing support of solidarity even as market debates break out and various market practices are adopted, it is important to note how many of the countries cite various international documents and covenants to justify their commitment to that principle. One of the most prominent is the *International Covenant on Economic, Social and Cultural Rights* of the United Nations, adopted in 1966 and put in force in 1976. Article 12 includes "the right of everyone to the enjoyment of the highest attainable standard of physical and mental health."[2]

This is an ambiguous statement, suggesting that everyone has the right to whatever is medically possible, now or in the future. Even though it is a shade less ambitious than the 1947 World Health Organization (WHO) definition of health—which defined health as "a state of complete physical, mental and social well-being and not merely the absence of disease and infirmity"—by omitting any reference to the availability of resources to achieve that high goal, the 1966 aspiration provides a grounding document for what we have referred to as the "infinity" model of medicine, that of an open-ended commitment to progress.[3] Whether the European countries or any others can afford health care systems that are so ambitious in their aspirations, or can do so without being forced to call upon the market to bail them out when the costs can no longer be borne, is an issue we will explore further.

A SELECTIVE COUNTRY SURVEY

Before continuing with generalizations about European health care (by which we principally mean Western Europe), we turn to a summary of the relationship between the market and health care in a number of selected countries. Our aim is to capture the nature of the market debate, the extent of market practices, and the way the market and solidarity values are integrated. Since we will be looking at a wide range of countries, it is not feasible to provide a history, or a full description, of the health care system in each country (as we could more easily do with the United States and Canada). Instead, we will use a shorthand description of their main features. We describe countries as either in the Bismarckian tradition, that of independent and private sickness funds overseen and coordinated by the state and financed by mandated contributions of employers and employees; or in the Beveridge tradition, where government provides health care services that are paid for by direct taxation (typically known as "single-payer" systems). Alan Jacobs has usefully reminded us that, while a convergence toward market practices in Europe can be widely discerned as a part of general health care reform, there have been great differences in the goals and content of the strategies employed. Those differences are brought about by ideological differences among ruling parties or coalitions, by different political institutions, and by the preexisting health care structures.[4]

We want to make use of some categories of our own as a way of helping us to capture and describe the market debates in various countries. While claiming no great precision for these categories other than as a rough sorting device, we thus group countries under the following headings:

Market rejectors. Countries in this category have a history of rejecting large-scale market practices and continue to do so even in the face of economic pressure—even though all of them accept some limited role for the market. They include, for instance, in Europe, Denmark, Ireland, Italy, Sweden, the United Kingdom, and France as a borderline case; and Canada, Cuba, and Tanzania.

Market acceptors. These are countries where there is a relatively great willingness, even eagerness, to put in place market ideas and mechanisms as part
of their health care systems. With varying degrees of intensity, these countries
have back-up, safety-net government programs, but there is a proclivity toward
private sector market practices rather than government-dominated programs.
Under this category we include Argentina, Brazil, Chile, the United States,
and Vietnam. A few countries, notably India and China, go one step further
than simply embracing the market as organized and state-regulated policy.
They may be characterized as *laissez-faire countries,* where the market is allowed to flourish in an unimpeded and unregulated way with few if any safety-
net features.

Market accommodators. In this category we put countries that, while wanting to hold on to solidarity values and universal access, have worked to find a
role for some market practices and on the whole have a favorable, though
cautious, attitude toward them. Among such countries are, in Europe, Belgium, Germany, the Netherlands, and Switzerland; and Australia and Israel.

Second-thought countries. We can think of no better term for a few countries
that took a sharp turn toward the market at one time, became disillusioned
with the results, and moved back to a strong solidarity model. Two examples
will be offered: the Czech Republic and New Zealand.

Coerced marketers (pertinent to the next chapter). These are countries, all in
the developing world, that put in place various market practices under pressure from the World Bank: Ghana, Kenya, Malawi, Zambia, and Zimbabwe.

A few qualifications are in order. Every country in the world has some
degree of market practices, just as every country has some kind of government
program for at least some categories of its population. Every country, that is,
shows a mix of public and private, for-profit and nonprofit activities. Our
aim with the above categories is to interpret where countries seem to fall on
a government–market continuum, not only in order to understand present
patterns but also to get some sense of where those patterns might move in
the future.

In what follows, we focus on a few countries in particular, then move on to a
more general analysis, bringing in the example of other countries along the
way. We have included among the few countries some that are not European
but have been greatly influenced by Western European values and have had
similar debates (New Zealand and the Czech Republic).

We start with some countries that can be called "market rejectors." In each case, they are examples of countries where there is some small degree of private insurance, some minor experiments in market practices, and some slight degree of pressure, political and ideological, to extend the scope of market practices—but in no case any significant loss of commitment to universal care and equitable access. It is not possible, we believe, to find a country in Western Europe that can be presently described as a market acceptor.

MARKET REJECTORS
The United Kingdom

The British National Health Service (NHS) was founded in 1948 and, to this day, stands as the model of a "single-payer" system financed heavily by taxation and run by the government—the homeland of the Beveridge system.[5] Some 84 percent of all health care expenditures are supported by general taxation, with no more than 10 percent of the population carrying additional private insurance (and which relieves them of none of the taxes for the NHS). Most of the private expenditures are for various out-of-pocket payments for services that are, in some part, provided by the NHS but not wholly paid for by taxes (e.g., dentistry and optical services, drug copayments). In most cases the out-of-pocket payments are income related in order to dampen any negative effects they might have on the disadvantaged.

The NHS has been a remarkably popular program over the decades despite, in earlier years, some glaring de facto (and essentially covert) rationing, particularly of kidney dialysis, open heart surgery, and other expensive technologies.[6] Without too much trouble the NHS survived the Thatcher years, when many other public services, such as railroads and airlines, were privatized. In recent years there have been persistent complaints about underfunding, waiting lists, and erratic quality control, regional variations in treatment availability, and lack of incentives to improve care.

As is the case with Canada, there have for many years been voices calling for a greater market role. Their most important breakthrough came in the early 1980s with the introduction of "internal" (sometimes called "quasi" or "social") markets through reforms introduced by the NHS and the Community Care Act of 1990. Conceptualized with the help of Alain Enthoven, their main feature was to introduce a split between the responsibility of purchasing health care and providing it. The aim of the internal markets was, simultaneously, to introduce greater efficiency into the system and to bring in at least a small dose

of competition and various other features to offset the heavy hand of government. Throughout the 1990s, the internal market was the primary means of
allocating health care resources.

By the early 1990s, the first phase of that development had passed and, with
the advent of the Labour government in 1997, various changes were made. One
of them was to abolish GP (general practitioner) fundholding, and another
was the formation of area-based primary care trusts (which have become the
main purchasers of health care services). At the same time, less emphasis was
placed, at least linguistically, on internal markets, to offset anxieties that they
were introducing some fundamental, slippery-slope market features into the
system. The new emphasis would replace the earlier centrality of competition
with that of partnership and collaboration.[7]

The net impact of these market developments on critical indices of quality
and access is hard to discern. The government-dominated nature of the NHS,
and the public and professional support for it, would make it difficult to bring
in strong market measures without a major change of philosophy; and there is
no demand for that. Nonetheless, as Alan Cribb has emphasized, while some
key elements of internal market reforms were dropped by the incoming New
Labour government in 1997, the reelection of that government in 2001 brought
with it a fresh emphasis on internal markets (without using that term), and
there is some renewed anxiety about a gradual slide toward the market and a
slow dismantling of the Beveridge system.

There is also some public discussion of competition, choice, and public-
private partnerships and a recognition of the obvious influence of "managerialism." The latter is introducing into the system new ideas of organization and
decision-making, and carrying with it many familiar market concepts (efficiency, response to consumers, and greater managerial discretion, for instance).
There is also a systematic erosion of the previously well-entrenched boundary
between the public and private sectors. While a strong commitment to public-
sector-managed, and publicly financed, health care remains, Alan Cribb notes
that "at the same time the trend towards elements of internal marketisation as
part of an ideology of managerialism has created significant turbulence in the
cultural and value fields of healthcare."

It is the "bluntness" of those developments, Cribb believes, that has produced significant "cultural effects" in the way the organization and management of health care provision is discussed. Rudolf Klein, a discerning long-
time commentator on British health care, was prescient when he wrote over a
decade ago that "the NHS is . . . likely to remain a self-inventing institution,

responding incrementally both to the evolving and unpredictable pattern of health care delivery and to the ideological biases of whichever party happens to be in power."[8]

Sweden

If the United Kingdom can be considered the fatherland of a state-run health care system, primarily dependent on taxation and direct government management, Sweden might well be characterized as the motherland of the comprehensive welfare state.[9] In the late 1990s, Sweden was spending close to 60 percent of its gross domestic product (GDP) on public expenditures, including of course the health care system. As with other countries over the years, health care expenditures have been heavily dependent on the general state of the economy.

When there has been an economic downturn, the market has been turned to experimentally, and on the supply side since the 1990s (and not too successfully) to help control costs but even more to improve efficiency. There has been, however, no basic change in the funding structure. Like the British NHS, the Swedish system is paid for by taxation, primarily at the local level. It is a highly decentralized, regionally managed system. The central government has the responsibility to make certain the entire system works effectively; county councils at the regional level are directly in charge of most forms of health care; and in 289 municipalities the full range of welfare needs are looked after, including nursing homes and geriatric care.

Swedish health care, in its present form, came into formal existence with the Health Care Act of 1982, but its beginnings can be traced to the creation of county councils in 1862, part of whose responsibility was health care. Just as the health care system is highly sensitive to the general state of the Swedish economy it is no less sensitive to public opinion, because of its dependency on taxation—cost pressures are, therefore, tests of the viability of the values underlying the system. Essentially, Sweden has used three methods of controlling costs: by governmentally imposed caps on spending, by attempted market techniques, such as hospital competition and a greater use of private providers, and by the imposition of copayments.

During the late 1980s and early to mid-1990s, economic pressures led to budget caps, a reduction in hospital beds, and some market experiments. But the market efforts did not go well, at least politically, and during the second half of the 1990s, the term *cooperation* rather than *competition* was tactically used (as in the United Kingdom). The political problem was simply a perception that equity was being threatened as many services deteriorated and, in any case, that the market was not an effective tool for controlling costs.

Over the past decade, Sweden has employed copayments as a peripheral means of controlling costs. One result appears to have been an increase in inequity, with differential self-assessments of health status between manual and other workers, and a concomitant withdrawal of government subsidies for occupational health clinics. Notably, there has been a shift in nursing home costs to patients and the reported impoverishment of some of them. Despite these difficulties, as well as the use by government of more private providers for care delivery, Sweden has been wary of market inroads. During the economically stressed 1980s there seemed to be a swing in public opinion in a market direction, but it gave way in the 1990s to a reemphasis on the public provision of care.

As the European Observatory noted in 2001, "it has been understood that Swedes should not only have equal access to health services, but they should have equal access to high quality health services. Both equity and quality have been important issues in the development of the Swedish model."[10] By and large, moreover, patients have retained considerable choice in meeting their health care needs, and the idea of cooperation rather than competition seems to have struck a responsive chord among Swedish physicians. Underlying all of these developments, however, is a deeply rooted sense of citizen entitlement: it is the obligation of a decent government to ensure citizens' general welfare. That is Sweden's enduring baseline.

Italy

While the United Kingdom and Sweden are often thought of as the model cases of universal health care, other countries have had no less lofty ambitions. Among them is Italy, a country that has gained little international attention for its health care but has worked to attain equitable access to care for its citizens.[11] It is, moreover, one of the southern European countries, which historically have had much weaker welfare policies than in the north. A 1978 reform law established the National Health Insurance (NHI) program. It called for universal access, specifying human dignity, health needs, and solidarity as its key principles. A mixed financing scheme of taxation and statutory contributions was established, ultimately aiming at instituting a wholly tax-based system. A decentralized administrative structure was set up—as in Sweden—at the national, regional, and local levels.

The 1978 reform law soon ran into difficulties, including regional conflicts and deficits (which had to be made up by the central government) and north-south disparities in the quality of, and access to, health care, and resulting from ill-defined legal and administrative responsibilities across the different levels. In 1992–1993 a new set of reforms was put in place, working toward greater competitiveness and increased autonomy for regional authorities in the planning and control of local services and hospitals. Its aim was to decrease federal coverage (that is, funds from the central government), to control costs, to incorporate various incentives to promote efficiency, and to improve the response of patients to competition among providers. A familiar principle of Catholic social ethics, that of subsidiarity—that higher-level institutions should not undertake what lower-level associations can accomplish—was invoked to devolve authority to the most local level possible.

The 1992–1993 reforms were not successful and a new round was introduced in 1998, aiming to find a better balance between economic constraints and equitable access. That reform took the form of even greater decentralization to elected regional and local authorities of health care planning and control. A legislative decree in 2000 made a change in financing, from an arrangement whereby the Italian parliament transferred financial resources to the regions, to one of increased direct regional taxation. The aim was to reduce health care expenditures, but, to avoid inequities, a National Equalization Fund was introduced. Its aim was to guarantee the whole country the realization of "essential levels of health care," much like similar efforts in Canada to equalize care across the provinces (though it has been reported that the wealthier, northern Italian regions rejected this in practice). The net result, together with other reforms, is that the Italian people are entitled to have health care services without incurring further costs or with payment for some services not covered by the NHI.

The market has not been a significant ingredient of recent Italian health care reforms, though efforts have been made to bring some forms of competition into what is a public system. There have been complaints with the Italian system, which sound familiar once one has looked at other taxed-based systems: poor service, waiting lists, queuing for appointments, erratic quality, and regional variations. Private health care services have a large following, with some 35 percent of the population using some of those services, but with a larger percentage, some 50 percent, prepared to choose public services; at the same time, relative levels of satisfaction are not strong. Public opinion surveys indicate also that a large majority would like to have a choice between public and private providers if it would give patients greater choice. But this proclivity does not mean that the public health system should be put into private hands. The public wants more choice but, in the end, a majority is against a market-based system. Nonetheless, a quasi-market was put in place by the 1992–1993 reforms, whereby public and private providers compete on equal terms.

There has been in Italy a steady increase in copayments over the past decade, and they are now among the highest (some 30%) in the European Union. Though a large proportion of the population, about 40 percent or so, is exempt from copayments, they have become an important method of cost containment. We call copayments the "sleeper" variable, not because they are hidden from sight, but because they amount to an important qualification to the concept of universal care, not often fully accounted for when there is talk of universal care and equitable access. An issue widely debated is whether there should be a parallel private system such that those who so choose could exit the public system, pay for their own health care, and be exempt from taxation for the public system. This argument has not had a large following. And when faced with the question of the rising cost of health care, the overwhelming response is not to cut health benefits but to spend less on other things.

The message (familiar to American ears) is, in the words of Pasini and Fasano, that "half the population would like more public resources to be directed to health care but almost none of them is prepared to pay more money for them . . . The general public wants freedom of choice, and at the same time they are loathe to miss out on the security that 'mother' National Health Services has and continues to offer." In the end, Italians "would find it difficult to take on board totally any idea of a health system top-heavy with the influence of the market."

Denmark and France

We conclude this survey with a glance at another market rejector, Denmark, and a borderline case, France. Denmark is a country that has one of the most comprehensive universal, tax-based health care systems in Europe. Rejecting practices otherwise familiar in Europe, it has worked over the years to reduce waiting times, guaranteeing treatment after relatively short stays, and to minimize copayments. Access to physicians and hospitals is free for all Danish citizens and they cannot opt out of the system. Approximately 83 percent of health care financing comes from local taxation. That much said, voluntary supplemental insurance has increased rapidly in recent years, mainly for drug copayments, covering an estimated 28 percent of the population (the for-profit providers of that insurance will not reveal the actual numbers).[12]

The reason for this high figure is assumed to be the many complaints about the government system, particularly what has been widely considered its underfunding. That problem is being addressed by the liberal–conservative coalition government put in place by the 2001 parliamentary election, which has worked to increase funding. In sum, it appears that, while there is private supplemental health insurance, it is not fully welcomed, and is seen as a sad commentary on the public system. Some commentators expect it to diminish in the future, though public-private partnerships are also being explored.

France, in the Bismarckian tradition, presents a different situation and is close to being a market accommodator, except for several reasons: the powerful and continuing role of government in managing the health care system, particularly in imposing price controls on the whole system; the fact that the sick gain increased insurance coverage; and its successful effort in 2001 to insure the remaining 1 percent of the uninsured and to offer supplementary coverage for 80 percent of those below an income ceiling.[13] Yet it also looks like a market accommodator, because the rate of supplemental voluntary health insurance is high, with over 80 percent of the population so covered.

The available private insurance coverage is varied, but mainly used to pay for copayments with the public coverage and for care not paid for by the state system. Copayments are high (with exclusions for the poor and the old): 30 percent for ambulatory care, 35 percent for visits to specialists, and 20 percent for hospital care (for the first thirty-one days or up to a cost ceiling). The French think of their system as one that seeks to synthesize solidarity and some market principles, and is in that sense accommodating to the market. But because of tight government control, its recent efforts to improve universal care, and its efforts to control the market's impact on costs, it can be said to be a market rejector, though a borderline case.

MARKET ACCOMMODATORS
Germany

Germany has the oldest tradition of a welfare state in Western Europe. In recent years, despite high unemployment rates and general economic stress, it has been loath to reduce social benefits, a politically difficult venture with a deeply embedded tradition of generous government programs of all kinds. In that context, arguments about the inefficiency of the German health care system, its excessive bureaucratization, and the threats its costs pose to German economic competitiveness have been vigorous—yet slow in generating reforms.[14] The German health care system, based on private health insurance funds financed by mandatory and shared employer-employee contributions, is among the most costly in Europe (10.6% of GDP). Most of the debates about the role of the market have centered on its potential to control costs by reducing inefficiencies rather than on more transcendent ideological issues. Germany is not a country with a strong entrepreneurial or individualistic tradition. It remained relatively untouched by the market debates unleashed in the 1980s and by the fall of Communism.

That much said, it is also true that the German system has a long-standing commitment to the principles of solidarity and subsidiarity. It is a system that consists of self-administered organizations, but which are heavily regulated by laws imposed by the federal government. Some competition among health insurance funds, and among outpatient and ambulatory doctors, has always been present. The government's role is to regulate the increasingly complicated and bureaucratic legal framework for the relationships among the various organizations. That legal framework also specifies the benefits to be provided by the statutory health insurance, characterized as a legal right. Copayments, save for those below a certain income level, are required and have increased significantly in recent years. The costs of hospital and physician care are worked out by negotiations between providers and insurance funds; patients thus see no bills save for copayments. The majority of doctors outside hospitals are self-employed, and their fee schedule is worked out by negotiations between medical associations and insurers.

Since 1977 various cost-containment schemes have been pursued, but without great success. The Health Structure Act of 1992 worked to bring temporary stability to premium rates by means of obligatory fixed budgets, notably hospital budgets that were forced to compete more vigorously, and by capping fees for ambulatory treatment and pharmaceuticals. But attempts to introduce more thorough reform ran into political opposition and the temporary tactics could not be sustained. A 1997 effort saw a stipulation that, if an insurance fund increases its premium, that would entail an automatic increase in the copayments for services. Further changes in the law since 2000 have aimed to stimulate competition and control costs. The insurance funds were permitted to develop contracts with groups of doctors to provide integrated health care, comparable to American HMOs (health maintenance organizations). The legal changes contributed to reducing costs, for example by bringing about the closing of about 20 percent of hospital beds between 1991 and 2001. Yet even so, by 2003 the premium rate for statutory health insurance had risen to 14.3 percent of wages and salaries, with still more increases expected in the future. Not a welcome development.

While there is, in light of the economic and demographic situation, a general agreement among politicians that radical reform will be needed to manage the cost situation, there is no agreement about its content or direction. Various commissions have made reports, but they differ in direction and scope, with at least one of them—the Herzog Commission—opting for a strengthening of statutory fund competition and allowing insured patients to choose among different options for more or less comprehensive benefits and thus more or less expensive insurance plans. That report would remove dental benefits altogether from coverage, as well as sickness benefits for lost work time (which is where the Bismarck program started in the nineteenth century). Sickness benefits would become the responsibility of employers, taking out special insurance for that purpose.

In 2002, cost containment once again became a serious concern. As with other European countries, economic reform of the health care system is needed. How that is to be done while maintaining the ideal of equal access and high medical standards—and how it is to be done in the context of a general anxiety about market inroads of a more extensive kind—remains uncertain. Though not true of the majority political party (SDP, the Social Democratic Party), there is a readiness to accommodate market ideas and practices, but carefully and not too far.

The Netherlands

The Netherlands has had a long historical tradition of international trade and entrepreneurship, together with a culture far more permissive and choice-oriented than others in Europe (recall its acceptance of euthanasia, prostitution, and the softer recreational drugs). Its embrace of the market, together with a continuing commitment to solidarity, put it in a unique situation.[15] Faced with the same cost pressures as other countries, it seems far less worried about the harms that the market might do than the economic and social benefits it might bring. The title of a health ministry report in 2002, on the need to modernize the national plan for exceptional medical expenses, *Customers Who Choose*, is not easily imaginable in most other European countries. Yet by virtue of firmly wanting to hold on to solidarity and equitable access to care, the Netherlands can hardly be classified as a "market acceptor" country in the same league as, say, the United States or Chile.

The basis of Dutch solidarity can be found in two principles laid down in its constitution: article 1 makes the government responsible for implementing the ideal of equality, while article 22 states the government's responsibility for the population's health. The system itself consists of both public and private health insurance. The public system has two features: a national plan for exceptional medical expenses, and private sickness fund insurance. The government has a central regulatory role, determining health care entitlements and the national health care budget. Private supplementary insurance is available for extra services and is flat rate and risk-related.

Economic troubles began to appear in the early 1970s as health care expenses rose rapidly. In the 1980s, some severe controls were put in place: hospitals were put on a fixed budget (though rarely enforced), hospital beds reduced, and the salaries of health care workers frozen or cut. Waiting lists also began appearing in the 1980s and, together with other system troubles, market proponents had a long list of complaints about the system. There was a gap between supply and demand, lack of patient choice in determining insurance coverage, too few incentives for effective, innovative, and demand-oriented activities, and excessive patient consumption. It was argued that institutional competitiveness, patient responsibility, and greater autonomy all around would create a better, more economical and efficient system.

A 1987 commission then recommended more reliance on market mechanisms, including greater competition, more contractual freedom, and the use of copayments. The political climate of the time favored deregulation and privatization, and sought to reduce government intervention in health care. Then, from the mid-1990s on, a number of market-enhancing moves were made by government: a free choice of sickness funds, the abandonment of obligatory contracting, greater risk-bearing for the sickness funds, and the introduction of a Diagnosis and Treatment Combination system (DBCs, comparable to the American DRG [diagnosis related group] system).

Yet despite this swing to the market in many respects, and a climate favorable to it, there exists a considerable lack of clarity and many contradictory pressures within the government about the concept of the market and of market competition. The term *regulated competition* is used frequently to describe how health care supply and demand should be matched. For health insurers, deregulation and greater competition are sought (though the term *cooperation* is used rather than *competition*). In 2003, a new government of Christian Democrats, Liberals, and Social-Liberals was installed, and announced that a greater call on citizen responsibility will be made. The net effect will be to reduce the size of the health care package, an increased need to obtain private insurance for many services, and an increase of deductibles in the sickness funds. Left unclear is the extent to which these limitations will seriously reduce equitable access and high-quality medicine. What is evident is that the Netherlands is moving, step by slow step, toward a far greater market emphasis—though still within the context of traditional solidarity and social insurance values.

Switzerland

Together with Germany, Switzerland stands at the top of the health expenditure ladder in Europe (11.2% of GDP in 2002). Its health care system is generous in its benefits, strong in its available technology, and provides patients with a wide range of choices.[16] It is a system in the Bismarckian tradition, based on health insurance funds, and stemming from the trade union movement of the late nineteenth century. The funds initially covered salary loss because of illness but moved on over the years to cover medical costs as well. Originally, it was a mandatory program for workers, but that aspect was dropped in 1900 as the result of a public referendum.

Later, by 1918, the sickness fund movement strengthened, though it remained nonmandatory (but with some federal subsidy). Not until 1996 was the principle of mandatory insurance introduced at the federal level (though the cantons were allowed to introduce mandatory insurance and some had done so); coverage by the sickness funds then reached 100 percent and was made compulsory at the canton level. Federal subsidies given to the sickness funds led to a decline of private insurance policies, though private policies remain popular for additional coverage. A mandatory basic coverage is required for all insurance funds and, in theory, insurance companies are not allowed to use risk selection in accepting applicants.

A number of market elements have become part of the Swiss system. Everyone is allowed to change their insurance company once a year and is guaranteed at least the government-imposed mandatory coverage. There is also competition for patients among the funds, but with some evidence of cream-skimming efforts by the funds to attract young and healthy patients, and of foot-dragging in response to applications from sick people. Complaints are frequent about age and health status discrimination in the selection of patients, creating obstacles and harassments for them in gaining entry to funds. Young people are courted, and particularly by being offered HMO coverage, thought to offer less expensive care—and giving at the same time some glamour to the funds by aggressive advertising. Different insurance plans are available, with different levels of out-of-pocket and copayment provisions, and financial incentives of one kind or another are given a strong place in sickness fund options.

A debate on rationing, perceived to be the practice of the sickness funds, was initiated in the mid-1990s, responding to charges of denied or delayed treatment. Waiting times for some hospital services had been increased, but this was not officially acknowledged, though those with commercial private insurance were able to avoid that problem. In the hospital case, it was not the sickness funds that had been at fault but a lack of hospital capacity brought on by budgetary problems at the canton or community level. Individual practitioners' associations, and to a lesser extent HMOs, had by 1999 attracted some 550,000 people, about 7 percent of the population, most of them in good health. For those not part of HMOs, and who are old or sick, the fact of fewer physician visits on their part suggests some access inequities. Some of the abuses of the sickness funds in patient selection have brought them under suspicion, but there is support for the idea that people who keep themselves in good health should be financially rewarded by sickness fund legislation.

In 2003 the parliament rejected a plan to strengthen the sickness funds by giving them (1) greater freedom in contracting, (2) a canton mandate to define the number of caregivers with whom every insurer has to contract, and (3) antitrust legislation to prevent a coalition of too powerful trusts of insurers or caregivers. After three years' debate on the reform in parliament, a vote on these and other measures was delayed until the fall of 2003 out of a fear that, by provoking the opposition of the socialist party and the physicians' and nurses' associations, the public would reject the revised law. The fear was that the sickness funds would be empowered to engage in even more risk selection, and that the financial situation of the lower and lower middle class would not be dealt with adequately. That fear led to the parliamentary failure of the plan. Switzerland has been willing to move well down the market road, farther than Germany, but has hesitated going too far.

Australia and Israel

We want to note, more briefly, two other countries, not European but strongly influenced by its traditions, that can also be called market accommodators. Australia guarantees universal access through a federal government tax-supported financing system but with health care administered and delivered by the states.[17] Australia is interesting in the context of this book because it also encourages everyone to take out private insurance as well. The aim is, among other things, to cover some gaps between government coverage and actual patient costs, to avoid hospital waiting lists, and to encourage people to go to private hospitals. To stimulate the use of private insurance there are also some disincentives (though not severe) for not having such insurance. By 2001 some 45 percent of the population had private insurance, a considerable increase over the 30 percent with such insurance at the end of 1998. A Medical Benefits Schedule determines the kind of care to be subsidized by the government system and the consultation fees for physicians. Physicians are, however, allowed to charge more than the schedule provides, a major reason for the need for private insurance—though various safety-net features are in place such that, if a patient's personal health care expenditures exceed a certain amount, all further costs are paid, up to the 100 percent level.

Although Israel had near-universal health care provided through nonprofit sickness funds, it was not until 1995 that universal care was formally initiated, and then buttressed by a 1996 Patients Rights Law that declared a right to health care.[18] Increasingly after that, financing of the National Health Insurance plan became tax-based and, by 2000, 71 percent of health care financing came from public sources. That money is provided to four nonprofit health funds, each of which allows participants to change funds on an annual basis.

We think of Israel as a market accommodating country for a number of reasons. There is regulated competition among the health funds, and a strong private sector for supplemental insurance, with 29 percent of health care financing coming from that sector in 2000, higher than in most European countries. The private sector covers gaps in NHI coverage and can help with copayments (in the 30% range) and other incidental expenses. Because it is growing, and consists of both for-profit and nonprofit plans, voluntary health insurance provides a way for the government to more easily control NHI budgets, which are capitated.

SECOND-THOUGHT COUNTRIES
Czech Republic

Together with New Zealand, the Czech Republic offers an interesting case study of a country that once headed down the market path, rejecting an earlier tax-financed single-payer system in favor of some market tactics.[19] During the forty years of Communist control there was a tax-based universal health care system, but marked by a low proportion of GDP devoted to health care (4.1% in 1989), covert private payments for better service, and a distinct bias toward superior care for party members.

The Velvet Revolution of 1989 brought an abrupt end not only to the control of Communism but to the existing health care system as well. As happened elsewhere, the country was swept by a market euphoria, for the polity of the society in general and health care in particular.

A government document in the early 1990s, *Proposal for a New Health Care System,* specified that every citizen would have a right to choose his or her physician and health care provider, health policy would be decentralized, health services would be provided in a competitive environment, and mandatory insurance was not to exclude parallel private coinsurance or direct insurance.[20] In addition, during 1991–1992, when the political right had a majority in the parliament, there was a privatization of health care facilities (though not of hospitals) and a fee-for-service policy for physicians, allowing them to open private practices, and a competition among providers (the sickness insurance funds) as well as payers.

Those policies turned out to be a move that raised many unforeseen problems. Formally, the Czech direction was in conflict with a number of international covenants, perceived to be a compromise of the principle of equitable access. Economically, the result was a spate of financial problems. Between 1990 and 1994 enthusiasm for the market peaked. It was followed by a period, from 1995 to 1996, that saw increased debts and insolvency of the public insurance companies (a Bismarckian system had been adopted in the early 1990s) as well as an inability of hospitals to pay for drugs in the face of pharmaceutical industry clout. In 1998, a liberal government came to power and rolled back many of the market practices. There was, as Eva Krizova notes, a nostalgia for the Communist days as well as a resurgence of a traditional Czech egalitarianism. The market was for a time idolized but without an awareness of the actual consequences, the most important of which were an increase in costs and many management difficulties. As it turned out, those consequences brought some longer-standing Czech values back into play.

The present system did not by any means drop all market practices. In principle, patients are allowed a choice of providers and of hospitals, though in practice there are many obstacles standing in the way of making that an efficacious reality. Employers and employees must make mandatory insurance contributions, and only public insurance funds are legally able to receive such contributions. There is no independent private insurance system, but people can buy supplementary benefits from the public funds. To avoid cream-skimming, a public insurance policy is in place to redistribute resources among the funds. While hospitals remain under government control, physicians are permitted to establish private practices and to receive fees based on contracts with the insurance funds. Only 9 percent of hospital beds are private. Health care is free for all patients, and universal health care, based on the principle of solidarity, morally and legally undergirds the system.

Despite the change in direction that came about in the 1990s, there is still considerable ambivalence about the place of the market. There has been great improvement in the system over the years (with 7.1% of GDP now going to health care). A younger generation of affluent people is interested in a more market-oriented system and thus more choice in their health care. There are many complaints about the present system: some continuing inequities, a poor pay scale for physicians and nurses, numerous inefficiencies, and de facto lack of choice. The figure of Vaclav Klaus, an economist and promoter of the market, in and out of power (and now president), is still strong. For the time being, however, the shift back to a government-dominated universal health care system seems secure.

New Zealand

Following the path of some European countries, but especially the United Kingdom, New Zealand put in place in the late 1940s a largely single-payer, tax-based universal health care program.[21] By the 1970s, however, its program was in trouble, with rising costs, system fragmentation, and poor administration. A variety of administrative changes were undertaken. Along the way, in the late 1980s, two reviews of the system recommended expanded market practices, drawing in part on the example of the State-Owned Enterprises Act of 1986, which initiated state activities in the electrical, telecommunications, and postal service sectors. That set of recommendations did not go far at that time, but helped to open the way for a set of radical reforms in 1993. The 1993 reforms have been described as an instance of a "big bang" policy change, where a unicameral political system, such as a parliamentary system, is able to unilaterally put in place massive changes with little place for public debate, compromise, or the need to act incrementally to adjust to political cross currents of a kind found in bicameral governments.

The 1993 reforms, stimulated by a major economic crisis, were put in place in a situation similar to that in the Czech Republic (though with many differences as well). There was a desire, and a perceived need, for radical change, and a fair number of idealistic, even romantic views about the bracing effect of market practices, expected to introduce greater efficiency and more choice. Several standard market mechanisms were put in place, most notably a withdrawal of many government subsidies and increased user charges. Many administrative changes were also made. They included the establishment of regional health authorities (RHAs) to purchase health services for their regions; the establishment of twelve Crown Health Enterprises (CHEs), clustered about existing hospitals, whose aim was to return a profit on their integrated services; the RHAs to contract with a pool of competing providers, including the CHEs; and an independent core services committee to develop a public consensus about which services or users the government should fund.

The big bang did not work, but whether that can be attributed to inherent market weaknesses (surely true in some instances) or a lack of good planning with an eye to outcomes remains unclear. Efficiency declined rather than increased, serious competition was hard to develop, and assorted structural flaws quickly manifested themselves. As one commentator noticed, "while the big bang approach proved effective for getting the market prescription in place, the prescription itself (and perhaps the implementation approach) appeared to be both practically and politically unrealizable."[22] Though many of the market strategies were dropped after 1996, a few remained, and market ideas still have some attractiveness. But these ideas are set in the framework of a single national purchaser (the Health Funding Authority) established in the late 1990s, as well as ongoing efforts to establish health care priorities. There remains a strong desire for greater public sector efficiency and a core of market proponents in government—and steady, unrelenting structural reforms over the years. Waiting times, inadequate funding, cost barriers, and a particularly high level of medical errors remain among the standing public complaints about the system.

THE FUTURE OF SOLIDARITY

The sample we have provided of different responses to market ideas in Western Europe and a few other places makes clear at least one point: whether the concept of solidarity is invoked directly or not, it remains a strong cultural and political reality. Equitable access for all citizens, regardless of their ability to pay, is well entrenched as a value, the benchmark for all reforms. Unlike, say, the situation in the United States, while pressure can be found almost everywhere for an expanded market role, such pressure might be said to be ideologically light in Western Europe and pragmatically heavy. By that characterization we mean that there is a comparatively muted voice from those we have called "the politicals," individuals and groups who equate the fate of democracy and the market, and who are single-mindedly bent on drastically reducing the role of government and strengthening that of the private sector. In Europe, the need to control costs and improve efficiency has been the stronger note.

Cost Pressures

At the end of 2003 the Organization for Economic Cooperation and De- velopment (OECD) issued a survey of cost trends. The OECD is constituted by thirty countries, the majority Western European and North American, with the addition of a few other transitional developing countries. The survey's general conclusion was that "spending on heath care is outpacing economic growth in most OECD countries, forcing government to find new funds or to pass a larger share of the costs onto individuals."[23] The cost increases, averaging 4 percent a year, can be contrasted with the even higher rate of increase in the United States, a 9.3 percent increase in 2002 (and up to 1% of GDP). A *Wall Street Journal* story in late 2003, surveying a number of countries, noted that "conti- nental Europeans . . . face steeper medical bills in the future in their cash- strapped governments." A number of benefit cuts have taken place, though none of them harshly so. Germans will now have to pay for their own dentures and 10 percent of prescription drug costs, and France has reduced reimburse- ments for drugs and various treatments. The same story noted that, despite these economic pressures, private insurers have been slow to respond, uncer- tain just how strong the private insurance market would be in the face of

"recent government changes [that] are mainly nips and tucks to existing benefits within the current system, rather than a profound overhaul."[24]

As we noted, one can find talk in just about any universal health care nation
about a "crisis," or the need for "radical reform." In fact, that kind of reform
rarely happens, and the 4 percent cost increase noted by the OECD, while
posing problems, hardly qualifies as an immediate crisis. But when radical
reform is instituted because of some strong economic anxieties, or some mo-
mentary enthusiasm for change, it may well be reversed (as happened with
New Zealand and the Czech Republic), either because the full implications of
change were not clear or because planning for it was inadequate, or both. If
there is any message that seems to emerge from the European countries, it is
that if cost containment has been the main motivation for the initiation of
market practices (mainly in the name of greater efficiency), there is also a
desire to increase patient choice and to improve the quality of care.

It is worth noting, for more than historical interest, that market activities
increased in a striking way in the 1980s and early 1990s, and at a time when the
health care systems' economic problems were being beset with the woes of
general economic downturns. "Market forces in Health Care," wrote Calum R.
Paton, reporting on a study commissioned by the European Union, "arguably
had their ideological heyday in the late 1980s and early 1990s."[25] But what was
the meaning of that increase in interest and market initiatives? The political
scientist Michael Moran denies that cost containment could explain the interest. One of his points is that such an explanation "flies in the face of evidence
that universalism has been incompatible with cost containment."[26]

That is an ambiguous statement. If by *universalism* one means, typically, a
government-run or financed system, then it is obviously possible for the government to put into effect strong cost-containment policies: reduce hospital
beds, restrict the distribution of expensive technologies, or establish budget
caps. In fact, as the experience of the United States indicates, where there is
no central government management, cost control is almost impossible. And,
as the failed cost-containment experience with managed care suggests, a privately dominated system, subject to political and popular complaints, is in a
poor position to control costs, particularly when that means saying no to professional and patient demands. A unicameral government can often best get
away with that, but so can other political systems with government domination of health care, even if with more difficulty.

More to the point, there was a general expectation in that era that the market
would do better in controlling health care costs than government, just as the

market was good at controlling the costs of many consumer items. There is scant evidence that the market worked in this respect, whether for reasons of imperfect efforts to make it work, ingrained public and professional resistance to market ideas, or deeply entrenched government bureaucracies that could not let their dominance go. At least these are the common reasons given for its failed cost-control aim. In any event, by the early 2000s there was much less optimism about such a market power, even if market practices of one kind or another can be found in every universal health care system—and even if, to cite a paradox noted about the 1980s period, there was a strange fascination with American managed care and managed competition.[27] Managed care techniques have been adopted here and there in Europe on a small scale (Sweden, the Netherlands, and Germany, for instance), but the era of looking to American experiments now seems well over.

The Impact of Market Forces

What did that era amount to? Reporting in 2000 on a study commissioned by the European Union, Reinhard Busse summarizes the evidence from Western Europe behind what he describes as "six pre-formulated hypotheses on the impact of market forces."[28] In each case, it turned out, there was insufficient evidence to verify the hypothesis. That insufficiency suggested, though he did not say so directly, that it is difficult to find decisive evidence in many areas either for or against the benefits of the market, if only because in mixed private-public systems, it turns out, it is hard to disentangle market outcomes and government-induced outcomes. Five of Busse's six hypotheses are of special interest for this book.

Hypothesis 1 was that "market mechanisms increase productivity." Responding to the contention that market mechanisms "increase the productivity and therefore efficiency of the system," the report's conclusion was that, though some increases can be found here and there, there is no "unequivocal evidence" they did so—if for no other reason than the fact that other reforms were usually going on simultaneously, making it impossible to tease out the market variable. *Hypothesis 2* was that "market mechanisms are costly to operate," and the conclusion was that "there is some evidence of increased management costs." *Hypothesis 4* was that "separating purchasing and provision as well as various forms of contracting have led to a greater emphasis on public health." The conclusion: "There is no evidence that, in those countries which have created new forms of purchaser/provider split, equitable health gain has been the primary objective or that, where it has been retrospectively defined as such, equitable health care gain has been achieved." *Hypothesis 5* was that "market reforms have reduced the autonomy of professionals, especially doctors, by creating or 'sharpening' the purchaser/provider split." The conclusion was that, in Bismarckian countries, one result has been "increased use of guidelines and other managerial means of influencing or directing clinical practice"; and that, in Beveridge countries, "overall, it is best interpreted as a means to 'discipline' professionals, especially doctors."[29]

The final hypothesis might be the most important. There have been few, if any, serious claims that an aim of market practices has been to increase equitable access. The European question instead seems to have been: can market practices increase efficiency and control costs without endangering traditional universality of access? *Hypothesis 6* addresses that issue, asking whether "market reforms have restricted access to services in the public sector." The report's answer is that there is no evidence this has happened in any significant way. On the contrary, it would appear that access—also in the name of cost control—has usually been limited by government control of reimbursement rates together with cost-sharing and user fees. "In no system," the report notes, "has rationing or access to public services by income or ability to pay been the key reform."[30]

In these hypotheses and their results, we suggest, three implications can be seen: that market practices are not nearly as effective as government interventions in controlling costs; that if limited in their scope, market practices need not be a threat to universal access; and that in countries with well-entrenched solidarity values, it would take a massive onslaught of market mechanisms to undermine them—an onslaught that has happened with only a few countries and, when it happened, was shortly thereafter reversed. Nothing seems to have happened since the publication of the E.U. report to call either its conclusions, or ours just presented, into question.

Yet the cost problem remains and is gradually getting worse. There is considerable present agreement on the sources of cost escalation: the combination of aging populations, new and more intensively used old technologies, and rising public demand.[31] This is a feature of all affluent, developed countries, with the technological factor taking a leading place. Though European health care costs are not growing nearly as rapidly as in the United States, a function of a greater government willingness to control and cap costs, an inescapable question to ask is: will the cost problem eventually open the market floodgates, perhaps out of desperation, even if the public and government hold their noses

as they bring it about—a tragic choice, so to speak? Cost pressures have certainly been a factor at other times in recent decades, particularly in the 1980s,
and there is no a priori reason to think it could not happen again. Moreover,
if one adds the pressure of globalization and its competitive demands, a younger and more affluent generation in many places with a preference for choice
and consumer discretion, and a more skeptical attitude toward the welfare
state in general, the ingredients may be there for a more wholehearted market
embrace.[32]

While no doubt reflecting an American perspective on the development of
market debates and market advances, it is not hard to imagine a future European scenario. An embrace of the market can come about either because market
ideas become stronger, winning the argument with government, or because
welfare state ideas become weaker, making the entrance of market ideas easier,
or both together. Moreover, market practices can come in by dramatic means, as
happened in a few countries, by great political upheavals, "big bangs," or by
incrementalism, open or hidden. In the latter category would be steadily rising copayments, an increasingly common phenomenon in countries officially
committed to universal care. *Hidden* may not be quite the right word, since
copayments are out there for all to see, but they are not usually openly presented as a market tactic or meant to signal some clear shift to market practices.

Solidarity as a Way of Life

At the heart of European systems and the influence they have had in other
countries is the idea of solidarity, at least at the rhetorical and theoretical level.
There is no clear and fixed definition of the term. "In general," as one study
puts it, "the idea of solidarity is associated with mutual respect, personal support and a commitment to a common cause."[33] We are all in this together,
subject to poor health and the threat of death. We should mutually support
each other against these evils and travails, in part because we are part of the
same national or ethnic community, but in part because we all share the human
condition. "Solidarity," it is noted, "is often juxtaposed against individualistic
and even egoistic behavior . . . associated with the cultural habits, societal
norms and liberal values of the United States."[34] The idea of solidarity has an
important obligatory feature: as citizens we have a duty to financially contribute to its maintenance.

Solidarity is not a notion that has caught on, or been even minimally invoked, in the United States, nor is it part of the rhetoric of market proponents in

any part of the world (and it would contradict the centrality of individual preference in mainline market thought). Solidarity implies a communitarian understanding of the human situation, a need for social interdependence, and a lively awareness of the ways in which disease and illness can overcome our individual economic and social resources. As Richard B. Saltman and Hans F. W. Dubois have put it, "pragmatically, solidarity . . . grows organically out of natural needs and behaviors of communities—it is not an artificial construction that is externally imposed by decree upon an individual or a community."[35] Two comments are in order. The first is that, in the case of Europe, solidarity as a value was a product of nineteenth-century religious and secular thought, not a wholly spontaneous movement. The second is that, as the experience of the United States indicates, market proponents argue in effect that a desire for choice and individual preference satisfaction is a natural need and common human behavior (going back to Adam Smith's observations about human nature).

It is possible, we believe, to think of both the market and solidarity as social constructs, but understanding them not as artificial inventions but instead as the expression of ways of life that took centuries to emerge from different histories and different cultures. Thus while Saltman has observed that European health care systems have become "not simply an insurance arrangement but rather a 'way of life,' "[36] we would want to add that the fragmented market-embracing American health care system is no less a "way of life." For just such a reason both systems are deeply embedded, hard to change, each expressive of different ways of looking at health care and the relationship between the individual and society. That perception lies behind our judgment that the debate about the market and medicine cannot be reduced simply to a struggle between various forms of self-interests and political commitments. In the end, it is a debate about different ways of life.

We advance this line of thought to help account for an inescapable feature of the European scene: the value of solidarity has remained viable and lively even in the face of external and internal threats.[37] By the "external" threats we mean the various cost pressures already noted, and by the "internal" we mean the rise of a younger, more affluent generation, less worried about security than their parents and wanting something more: more choice and an ability to spend more of their own money on health care than their national systems easily make possible. Private insurance becomes more attractive, even parallel private systems, as does faster access to care and the coverage of treatments that

are more of a lifestyle kind than encompassed by traditional health care packages. But these threats have been warded off on the whole, even if there is a
creeping tide of market practices—a slow tide that, so far, does not seem des-
tined to destroy the reefs, jetties, and barriers that have, psychologically and
socially, developed over the years to control the tide. It is the storms that erode
beaches, not the ordinary ebb and flow of the tides, and since the 1980s there
has been no serious economic storm of a kind that sweeps away everything
before it. But some gusty winds are blowing.

They have been gusty enough to lead the Economist Intelligence Unit, oriented to business prospects and opportunities (and part of the *Economist* publication organization), to contend that the time is ripe for a great expansion of
private insurance in Europe.[38] In Europe in 1999, with one exception, private
insurance was a small portion of overall health expenditures. That exception
was the Netherlands, with 33 percent of the population so covered, but with
only 3 percent in France, 10 percent in Germany, 4 percent in Italy, 15 percent
in Spain, and 10 percent in the United Kingdom The conclusion of the Economist Intelligence Unit report was (this was 1999) that "both private medical
insurance and provision should experience explosive growth within the next
decade, despite the fact that public and political support for the welfare state is
as strong as ever." "To date," the report notes, private health care has "been the
preserve of the rich."[39] Though the report presents lots of seemingly persuasive
arguments for why the turmoil in European health care would inexorably lead
to increased private care, as of 2004 it had just not happened. The power of
solidarity seems, in the end, remarkably sensitive to potential threats, again
and again leading European countries to stop short of initiating vigorous market practices and to scale them back when signs of danger were noted.

Another direction may now be emerging, that of "social entrepreneurialism." One of the most distinguished European health care analysts, Richard B.
Saltman of the European Observatory, has noted that European reform efforts
began in the 1980s and, since then, have taken two important directions. One
of them has been to "add micro-economic (institutional) efficiency to already
achieved macro-economic (health system level) efficiency. This has primarily
meant improving management mechanisms in health care institutions. The
other direction has been to find ways of "combining entrepreneurial behavior
with solidarity."[40] By that is meant an effort to develop new organizational
arrangements that "melt" public-private boundaries with the aim of developing social entrepreneurialism rather than individual entrepreneurialism. As

with efforts to develop competition between national health care institutions and planned public markets, especially with hospitals, these are exercises in social markets, with government in the dominant role.

That government domination, committed to solidarity even if some market and entrepreneurial activities are accepted or encouraged, is the most notable and enduring feature of European health care. It is as if the European solidarity systems, whether of the Bismarck or Beveridge type, are saying to market ideas, in effect, "we will sometimes accept you into our house and occasionally even welcome you—just keep in mind that it is *our* house not yours. Do not rearrange the furniture in any drastic way, and be sure to take off your shoes before entering."

We now leave Canada, the United States, and the countries of Europe—all affluent and blessed with a generally healthy citizenry—and move to the developing countries of the world. They are not affluent, and their citizens are burdened with many diseases and disabilities no longer even found in developed countries or—as with AIDS—oppressed by a new and lethal infectious disease with a massive health and social impact. These countries have had, as a result, political histories and health care reform efforts radically different from those in developed countries, and—in the World Bank and International Monetary Fund—major international institutions having an influence in pushing market values with no parallel in affluent countries. No understanding of the role and influence of market thought can be even partially complete without taking account of the emergence, since the 1980s, of a powerful market movement in developing countries.

CHAPTER FOUR

The Market in
Developing Countries

An Ongoing Experiment

Our attention so far has been focused on medicine and the market in affluent, developed countries. Whether market- or government-oriented in their health care systems, however, it can surely be said that money talks. Economic wealth and security together guarantee a decent long life for most of those who have them, however health care is organized. The poor and developing countries of the world have no such benefits. But most developing countries are just that, "developing." With any luck, many of them will move out of their poverty and be more able to deal with the health of their populations; and that has already happened to many countries in recent decades. Given the vastly larger numbers and population growth rates of developing countries, it is fair to say that the future of human health as a worldwide human good lies heavily in their hands. The decisions made about the nature of their health care systems, their priorities and aims, will almost certainly make a greater global difference in human health than what happens in developed countries.

Developing countries are engaged in a great experiment, testing whether and how the market should have a central role and how to balance the market and government. It is a crucial experiment. These countries can look to the experience of the developed countries, where there have been many efforts to find the proper place for market practices, but with mixed success. Now they are trying to find their own way. That way reveals many echoes of the experience and debates that have taken place in affluent countries, but the lack of money, exceedingly daunting health care problems, and often unstable political regimes add considerably to their problems.

APPALLING STATISTICS

For more than a quarter of the world's population, absolute poverty remains the principal determinant of their health status (see tables 4.1 and 4.2). Disease patterns in the developing world are also different from those in the developed world. Noncommunicable diseases, including cardiovascular disease, mental illness, cancers, strokes, and injuries, account for most of the disease burden in developed countries. By contrast, the major causes of morbidity and mortality in the developing world are infectious diseases, with HIV/AIDS, malaria, and tuberculosis, as well as maternal and nutrition-related conditions, high on the list.

Health indicators from developing countries reveal vast global disparities. Women represent 70 percent of the world's poor, and they have less education, longer working hours, and lower life expectancy than men.[1] Maternal mortality is fifteen times the rate of that in industrialized countries. There has been a sharp reemergence of infectious diseases such as tuberculosis, diphtheria, and hepatitis B. Average life expectancy at birth in many developing countries is less than fifty years; the developed world average is more than seventy years.[2] In some developing countries, particularly those worst affected by HIV/AIDS, such as Botswana, Niger, Malawi, and Zambia, life expectancy at birth has fallen to less than forty years. Three diseases—HIV/AIDS, tuberculosis, and malaria—kill around 5.4 million people a year in developing countries,

TABLE 4.1
Gross Domestic Product, 2003

	GDP (U.S. $ billion)	Annual GDP growth rate (%)
Argentina	129.7	8.7
Brazil	492.3	−0.2
Chile	72.4	3.3
China	1400	9.1
Ghana	7.7	5.2
India	599	8.0
Kenya	13.8	1.3
Malawi	1.7	5.9
South Africa	159.9	1.9
Tanzania	9.9	5.6
Zambia	4.3	5.1
Zimbabwe (2002)	8.3	−5.6

Source: Data from World Bank Group, Data and Statistics, www.worldbank.org/data/countrydata/countrydata.html.

TABLE 4.2

Health Expenditures as a Percentage of Gross Domestic Product, 2001

	% of GDP	Per capita (U.S. $)
Argentina	9.5	679
Brazil	7.6	222
Chile	7.0	303
China	5.5	49
Cuba	7.2	185
Ghana	4.7	12
India	5.1	24
Kenya	7.8	29
Malawi	7.8	13
South Africa	8.6	222
Zambia	5.7	19
Zimbabwe	6.2	45

Source: Data from World Health Information, Countries, www.who.int/countries/en/#B.

more than a third of their annual death toll. In 2001, average per capita health expenditures in the developing world as a whole were the equivalent of $98, compared with an average of more than $3,800 in the developed world (see table 4.2).

MARKET EXPERIMENTS

In the face of all these problems, developing countries are struggling with how to deal with health care. Most of the health care reforms in developing countries can be viewed as experiments—different countries testing different market mechanisms and a market-government mix. Some countries have introduced substantial changes to health care systems (because of internal and external pressures), while others have experimented with strategic reforms restricted to only certain sections of the health system. Using selected countries, we will describe how these various health reform experiments, making use of market ideas and practices, have fared under different political and sociocultural systems. We can at this stage disclose one of our main findings: despite the initial optimism brought on by the promise of health care reform, market experiments have not solved—or much helped—the health problems of the developing world. They have, in certain instances, exacerbated the existing health problems because of their emphasis on health care systems (which place a focus on medical care), instead of a focus on health (which would include factors like socioeconomic development, gender rights, and public health strategies).

Where might the story of the market in health care in developing countries begin? One common starting point is the World Bank (the Bank) and the International Monetary Fund (IMF) and their structural adjustment programs and, later, their Poverty Reduction Strategy Papers process. Yet, though important, the World Bank and IMF's role in imposing market mechanisms in developing countries represents only part of the story. Not all developing countries can point to the World Bank as the primary force behind the push for market incentives in health care. Many developing countries had private sectors providing health services well before the Bank and IMF intervened, while some turned to the market because of shifts in political ideology within the countries themselves.

In some African countries, European bilateral funding agencies such the Swedish International Development Agency and the Danish International Development Agency have supported the use of some market mechanisms such as user fees. They have also provided financial, material, and technical support to countries trying market-oriented health care reform.

HISTORICAL BACKGROUND OF MARKET DEVELOPMENTS
Pre-1980s: From Colonization to Independence—
The Era of Government Responsibility for Health Care

Many developing countries have a similar colonial history, characterized by heavy agricultural and mineral trade with colonizers. Economic policies in the colonies aimed to maximize exports with little or no reference to the economic needs of their native inhabitants. Upon attaining independence, the newly emerging nations of Africa and Asia soon became the scene of cold-war skirmishes. The United States and the Soviet Union (and later China) competed for their allegiance, often through economic aid. Even though many countries succeeded in remaining neutral, the political systems of several others became greatly influenced by the ideologies of the countries to which they pledged allegiance. Prior to the 1980s, however, many developing countries had relatively good, and well-distributed, health care.

Zimbabwe, Zambia, Kenya, and Tanzania

We begin our discussion with selected African countries that have been imposed upon or coerced to move toward market-based reform. We pose a basic question: have these countries always been averse to the use of market tools in the provision of health care services, or are their negative reactions more a reflection of their attitudes toward the World Bank and IMF, which brought market-oriented pressures on them, or reactions to the specific pre-scribed mechanisms, or both? Using Zimbabwe, Zambia, Kenya, and Tanzania as case studies, we attempt to answer this question by briefly tracing the his-tory of their health care systems before the era of reform.

Contrary to popular belief, Africans are historically a highly entrepreneurial people. Their entrepreneurship was unique in that they traded as communities rather than individuals; thus the benefits of trade were reaped by everyone who belonged to that particular trading community. For several centuries, many African societies traded freely with Arabs, Asians, and Europeans. From about AD 600 to 1600, for example, Old Ghana derived its financial power from the proceeds of extensive networks of intraregional and export trade in gold, and of import trade in salt, copper, and manufactured goods from Egypt, North Africa, and Europe.[3]

This entrepreneurship was also seen in the provision of health care in Afri-can societies. The traditional African system of health care was interwoven with religion as a way of life.[4] Traditional healers exhibited various market behaviors, often competing with each other. A notable characteristic of the traditional healer's profession was the secrecy of treatment methods. Payment for medical services varied from community to community, but common deter-minants of fee level included severity of the illness, type of disease, time required to treat the patient, and the patient's overall ability to pay for treat-ment. Patients would usually shop around for less expensive services in the area, since there were usually several traditional healers competing for the same demand.

During colonial rule (late nineteenth century to the 1960s), health care ser-vices in most African countries were provided by the colonial governments, to cater to their wounded soldiers; missionaries, to cater to their African converts; industries, to cater to their employees; and private practitioners, to cater to colonial administrators and the settler population.[5] Colonial powers tried to eliminate traditional healers as political and medical authorities.[6]

Following independence, there was much emphasis on what newly formed African governments could do to improve the lives of their citizens who had suffered for decades at the hands of the colonialists. The provision of free or highly subsidized health care services to the entire population was one of the most popular and ambitious policies adopted by these governments. Many of the countries were further inspired by the historic Alma-Ata (World Health

Organization) conference in 1978. It encouraged African countries to focus on community-based approaches to health care. In response, most new states tried to streamline their highly fragmented health systems, making the development of a public health care program an integral part of their long-term national health plans. The majority of countries established centralized, hierarchical health care systems with the government as the main provider of health care services.

Zimbabwe

Zimbabwe was a relatively late starter in the pursuit of a universal health care system for its citizens, attaining independence in 1980 (most African countries became independent in the 1960s). Nevertheless, in the same year, it created a comprehensive national public health care system, complete with provincial medical offices responsible for environmental health, epidemic and endemic disease control, special tuberculosis and leprosy services, health promotion, and school health.[7] In addition, the government doubled the number of rural health centers from about five hundred in 1980 to over a thousand in 1990. These public health initiatives paid off. Immunizations to protect children against diphtheria, measles, polio, tetanus, tuberculosis, and whooping cough increased from less than 25 percent of infants in 1982 to 67 percent in 1988. Life expectancy rose from fifty-five to sixty years, child malnutrition fell from 22 to 12 percent, and infant mortality dropped from 100 to 53 deaths per thousand live births.[8]

Zambia

Similarly, at independence in 1964, the Zambian government expanded medical services throughout the country, with some health progress. Infant mortality was reduced from 123 per thousand live births in 1965 to 85 in 1984. By 1981, the ratio of doctors to population had dropped from 1:11,300 in 1965 to 1:7,110. Most of the doctors (76%) worked in urban areas, where only 54 percent of the population resided.[9] The Zambian government, in its third national development plan (1979–1983), committed itself to primary care as the national health care strategy, with the control and prevention of malaria, respiratory and diarrheal diseases, and measles as its focus. But Zambia was particularly hard hit by the economic crisis that brought down the price of copper (Zambia's main export). By the mid-1990s, Zambia faced a negative growth of its economy, with the government budget for health falling from $29 per capita in 1970 to $2.6 per capita in 1998.[10]

Kenya

Kenya likewise committed itself to providing free health services as part of its development strategy to alleviate poverty and improve the welfare and productivity of the nation.[11] This pledge was honored in 1964 with the discontinuation of the pre-independence user fees in government-run hospitals, and the introduction of free outpatient services and hospitalization for all children in public health facilities. Services in public facilities remained free for all except those workers whose expenses were met by employers. Private health enterprises developed parallel to these government initiatives, with missionary hospitals charging subsidized fees for services offered, and private for-profit facilities moving toward full cost recovery.[12]

In order to meet its "Health for All" promise to its citizens, the Kenyan government constructed new health facilities in rural areas and upgraded existing government health institutions. The government took great efforts to ensure that essential medical supplies and equipment were available throughout the country through the construction of depots in strategically located administrative posts. Rural health training centers were established to provide practical field training in rural health to health officers. The government also expanded and promoted training opportunities and career development for health personnel through public continuing education programs, and assured graduates of employment in the public sector.[13]

These efforts by the government and nongovernmental organizations to increase the population's access to health services translated into marked gains in Kenya's health status. From independence to 1993, the crude death rate dropped from 20 to 9 per thousand, the infant mortality rate declined from 120 to 60 per thousand live births, and life expectancy increased from forty to sixty years.[14]

Tanzania

Tanzania, which gained independence in 1961 under the leadership of Julius Nyerere, committed itself to the path of African socialism in 1967 by announcing the Arusha Declaration. It enunciated long-term goals for Tanzania, including *ujamaa* (familyhood) and self-reliance as well as hard work for the common good.[15] President Nyerere described *ujamaa* socialism as an attitude of mind, the foundation and objective of which was the extended family on the basis of African tradition.[16] Under *ujamaa,* Tanzania placed a great deal of emphasis on the provision of primary care in rural areas and free health services for all.[17] In 1971, the country outlined its National Health Policy, based on the prevailing political ideology. Under this plan, the Ministry of Health expanded services in rural areas through the construction of rural health centers and dispensaries, and the training of health personnel. While the construction of hospitals and the pace of adding hospital beds slowed down, the number of dispensaries, rural health centers, and rural medical aides rose dramatically.[18]

Tanzania's second five-year national plan (1969–1974) was developed on the basis of the 1967 Arusha Declaration, which emphasized the policy of self-reliance and equitable distribution and access to public services.[19] The "village health worker" program was started in the early 1970s to complement the institutionally provided health care services. Tanzania's third five-year development plan (1976–1981) emphasized the need to provide clean water, public health services in rural communities, and training of paramedical staff. At the end of the 1970s, Tanzania developed a twenty-year plan (1981–2000), and its main objectives were to strengthen preventive services, human resources, and community participation.[20] Yet during this time, Tanzania's economic performance was greatly deteriorating, and, despite all efforts under the *ujamaa* policy, Tanzania's economy remained highly inefficient.

Despite marked gains in overall health status in these four countries in the years after independence, the Kenyan, Zimbabwean, Zambian, and Tanzanian health care systems in the pre-reform era became riddled with problems. These problems stemmed from corruption, overemployment of health care personnel in public health institutions, a lack of adequate funding to run these facilities and of qualified health care personnel (many of whom preferred to work in the private sector), poor institutional management, and growing consumer dissatisfaction with the quality of health care services in government-run health care institutions.

There were also chronic shortages of drugs, infrequent equipment maintenance, inadequate logistical support, and a lack of monitoring and evaluation procedures. For households in African countries, this translated into a low confidence in the health care system. For governments, this meant that a large share of public expenditures in health was being wasted, and for private providers that they were often trying to deal with unmet needs with little guidance, assistance, or competition from the public sector.[21]

As if that were not enough, in the same period the fiscal capacity of many African countries to finance health services was further undermined by poor economic performance, the emergence of HIV/AIDS, rapid population growth, and political upheaval.[22] Communicable and infectious diseases remained the major causes of death, and large proportions of their populations did not have access to clean water and basic sanitation facilities. The global economic crisis of the 1990s hurt these countries' economies greatly, and much of the economic and social progress over the previous two decades was reversed. It became clear that widespread reform was needed in various sectors, including the financing and delivery of health care. The question was what direction such reform would take.

Most African countries turned to the World Bank and IMF for financial assistance to help them turn their economies around. The Bank came to their assistance—but only on condition that the countries would engage in Bank-prescribed economic reforms. Between 1980 and 1990, 70 percent of African countries (or thirty-two of forty-five countries) had to implement structural adjustment programs as a lending condition of the IMF and World Bank.[23]

South Africa

South Africa, a middle-income country, presents a somewhat different history than other countries in sub-Saharan Africa. After the formation of the South African state in 1910, health services in the country were characterized by a multiplicity of fragmented authorities and systems responsible for providing health care. The South African health care system was divided according to race, geographic area, the public sector (further divided into local, provincial, and central health authorities), and the private sector.[24] Significant inequalities in the provision of health care emerged between blacks and whites, rural and urban areas, and primary and tertiary health care programs. In 1990 there were approximately twenty-two thousand doctors registered in South Africa, of whom only about a thousand were black. In 1990 the ratio of general practitioners to population was 1:900 in the urban areas as compared with 1:4,100 in the rural areas.[25] Privately financed health facilities, both primary and curative, were accessible to patients (usually white) who had health insurance. In lieu of a national health service plan for all South Africans, the private health sector grew, focusing entirely on patients who could pay for services either out of pocket or through health insurance.

Although there was a sliding scale of payment based on income for medical services at the public hospitals, many people were still unable to pay for health services. The majority of blacks did not have health insurance of any kind. Private purchase of health insurance was far beyond their economic means, and many employers did not offer blacks health coverage as a work-related benefit. Most black South Africans relied on the public health service funded by the government, while whites and Indians obtained their care in the private sector. The segregation of hospital care was one of the most visible manifestations of apartheid practices in health.[26]

In pre-1994 South Africa, therefore, the health care system was characterized by racial discrimination, fragmentation, poor coordination, and duplication of services, with a predominant focus on hospital-based care rather than primary care.[27] From the 1950s to the 1970s, insurance companies providing health coverage increased, and about 40 percent of the doctors in South Africa worked in the private sector.[28] Primary care facilities for poor patients (mostly black), however, did not grow. By the 1980s, the private health sector was very lucrative for health professionals, many of whom left their part-time positions in government-financed health facilities to devote all their time to their private practices or to work in privately owned hospitals.

During this time, tensions became much more apparent between the parallel systems of care: a thriving private health care sector for paying patients, who were mostly white, on the one hand, and a rudimentary, underfunded, and inadequate primary and community health system for indigent South Africans, on the other. By 1990, the infant mortality rate among whites was 7.7 per thousand, while for blacks it was 48.3 per thousand.[29]

The apartheid government, whose rule ended in 1994, was largely indifferent to the plight of the poor blacks in South Africa, resisting several proposals to initiate a national health care system that would guarantee some services to every South African regardless of race. When South Africa established a Government of National Unity in 1994, major reforms of its health care system were geared toward making it more equitable and unified.

China

Before the 1980s, China's powerful Communist government implemented a comprehensive health care system whose principles were "to serve the people, to focus on preventive medicines, and to unite traditional and Western medical services."[30] That policy thus favored prevention over curative care, integrated traditional and Western medicine, and linked health work with mass movements.[31] The government mobilized the population to engage in mass "patriotic health campaigns" aimed at improving environmental sanitation and hygiene.

Health care was provided in both rural and urban areas through three-tiered systems. In *rural areas,* the first tier was made up of "barefoot doctors," peasants who had undergone short training courses in preventive and primary care, and were then sent back to their villages.[32] There was at least one barefoot doctor per five hundred people in rural China. At the next level were the township health centers, which functioned primarily as outpatient clinics for about ten to thirty thousand people each. These centers had ten to thirty beds, and the most qualified members of the staff were assistant doctors. The lower-level tiers made up the "rural collective health system," providing most of the country's medical care. The most seriously ill patients were referred to the third tier, county hospitals, which served two hundred to six hundred thousand people each and were staffed by senior doctors.

In *urban areas,* the first tier of care was provided by street health stations that were staffed mainly by paramedics. If specialized care was necessary, the patient was sent to the second tier, a community health center. The most serious cases were handled by the third tier, consisting of district hospitals. To ensure a higher level of care, a number of state enterprises and government agencies sent their employees directly to district hospitals.

This three-tiered system in both the rural and urban areas was designed to promote efficient allocation of health care resources between primary and tertiary care facilities. For several years, this arrangement provided a structure for efficient patient referral for treatment of health problems, and it brought many health gains. Between 1952 and 1982, China reduced the rate of infant mortality from 250 to 40 deaths per thousand live births, decreased the prevalence of malaria from 5.5 to 0.3 percent of the population, and increased life expectancy from thirty-five to sixty-eight years.[33] Epidemic diseases like cholera, plague, and typhoid were almost eradicated. During this pre-reform period, China's effective health services contributed to development and poverty reduction by diminishing productivity losses from ill health, by increasing the capacity of school children to learn, and by diminishing the frequency and intensity of destructive illnesses that reduced household income and caused increased expenditure.[34]

Despite these gains, there were problems in China's health care system. Poor counties spent far too little on maintenance, equipment, and operating costs, and they hired too many health care workers.[35] Medical training institutes continued to produce many semi-skilled personnel long after the acute shortages had been relieved, and most health facilities employed large numbers of assistant doctors and partially trained health workers with very low work-

loads. Most people had easy access to a health worker, but many of the health
workers had limited skills.[36]

Vietnam

Vietnam's history bears many similarities to China's. Indeed, the northern
part of the country remains heavily influenced by Chinese culture, which dominated it from about 100 BC to AD 900. The south had several strong empires
until the late nineteenth century. At that point, the French conquered the entire
country and divided it into three regions: Cochin in the south, Anman in the
middle, and Tonkin in the north.[37] After World War II, the French withdrew
and the north-south division of the country gave rise to the creation of two
different development strategies along those geographic lines.

The northern Democratic Republic of Vietnam was established as a socialist
state, following Marxist ideology. Like its powerful neighbor China, the northern socialist government implemented radical measures to collectivize land
and industrial property, making the state the chief agent for social and economic development. Social services were organized from the top down, and
the centrally planned services emphasized the construction of facilities, the
training of staff, and the creation of rural services. Health and education were
provided free of charge for everyone. That led to a highly literate population
with improved health status.[38]

Southern Vietnam, by contrast, developed a laissez-faire approach to economic development that eventually led to inequitable distribution of facilities
and resources, and large gaps between the rich and poor.[39] After the Vietnam
war, the country was reunified under the name of the Socialist Republic of
Vietnam. Like China, the new regime established multitiered health care systems that corresponded to the various levels of government; preventive care
was the core element. The unified Vietnam created a national health service
that provided most services (except for the provision of drugs) free of charge.
The government financed preventive programs and government health facilities, while the rural communes financed community health centers and brigade nurses.[40]

Under socialism, Vietnam's provision of public health care services was
considered a state responsibility, implemented by a centralized, hierarchical
multitier health care system. Led by a central ministry, basic health care services were provided free of charge throughout the country's provinces and
districts, and occasionally extending down to the brigade level.[41] Private ac-

tivities in health care were forbidden, and thus legislation and regulations were not necessary. Services were financed entirely from state funds generated at the commune, provincial, and central levels.[42]

Health care in the pre-reform era of the 1980s was thus extensive and mostly equitable, but the system's inefficiency, lack of effectiveness, and poor quality created problems. The high density of facilities ensured geographic access, and free services facilitated economic access, but underpaid health workers in overstaffed, decaying facilities with few drugs, limited supplies, and anti-quated equipment generated neither effectiveness nor quality.[43] More than half of the commune health centers lacked basic equipment such as simple weigh-ing scales and sterilizers.[44] Consumer utilization was low and consumer dis-satisfaction widespread. These factors contributed to some of the reforms that the Vietnamese government pursued in the 1980s.[45]

India

After China, India is the most populous country in the world, with a popula-tion of over one billion people. As in most of their other colonies, the British did not create a formal health care system for India's inhabitants. They estab-lished instead a few medical colleges to produce doctors trained in European medicine to treat the British community in India. Some charitable hospitals and missionary centers were opened, offering Western medical services to the local population. The majority of Indians, however, received their health care from centuries-old indigenous medical systems like Ayurveda.

India gained its independence from the British in 1947 and, despite calls for free health care for all at that time, the drafters of the constitution did not add a right to health care to the list of fundamental rights. They included instead a clause requiring the government to work toward the improvement of public health for all. The first landmark in official health policy of independent India, the 1946 Bhore Committee recommendations, laid the foundations for a com-prehensive rural health service plan with primary health as its core element.[46] That plan called for the development of health centers and hospitals and dis-pensaries in urban and rural areas, where doctors' services could be provided free of charge and drugs dispensed at a minimal cost. Though grossly inade-quate and fragile, a health network was established and, in 1949–1950, the government made a decision to expand services by establishing about twenty-three thousand new health centers in the country.[47]

India's early five-year plans placed a heavy emphasis on public health programs, especially for the eradication of malaria and smallpox. The focus subsequently shifted toward family planning and later toward preventive health care. Primary health centers were developed in rural areas from 1952 on, and public health campaigns, sanitation, and drinking-water programs were also launched.

The private health sector also flourished alongside these developments. India has historically always had a large private health sector, especially for mobile services that included providers of modern medicine as well as traditional practitioners. Before the health care reforms, much of the private sector in health care focused on the provision of health services in nursing homes and medical clinics. In the pre-1980s' reform era, the competitive private sector remained a significant part of the Indian health care delivery system. Part of the reason for this was that the public health system was underfunded, corrupt, and redistributed away from the poor.

Chile, Argentina, and Brazil

After most Latin American countries gained their independence from Spain in the early nineteenth century, the national governments began to assert their nationalism and promote their indigenous cultures. Because of diverse historical processes, each country in Latin America developed its own system of social and welfare protection. They turned social values shared by the population into a complex network of institutions responsible for financing, organizing, and providing social services delivery, and defining entitlement to benefits and services.[48]

Until the 1980s, most countries in Latin America—except the few with an egalitarian tradition of multi-insurance organizations, such as Argentina and Uruguay—had one major government institution managing financial resources and provision for the health sector. Pension systems were often included under the same umbrella. Private health insurance was almost nonexistent.[49] In Chile, Ecuador, Peru, Venezuela, and Colombia, prior to the reforms, each had a national health system that coexisted with a small social security institution. The central authority had three simultaneous missions: maximizing the impact of public financing on the health status of the population, financing and ensuring financial viability of its own providers, and regulating the entire system.[50]

Chile is of special interest since it was the first country to undergo major market-oriented reforms of its social security programs, beginning in 1981.[51]

The first hospitals in Chile were established by Spanish conquerors in the sixteenth century. For the next three hundred years, those institutions that mainly catered to the poor were financed through private donations and run by religious leaders, with little interference from the government. In 1924, a social security system was established in the country, marking the first time the state became involved in providing health to the population. Between 1920 and 1950, state-run health programs were organized around the pension funds. It soon became clear that organizing health delivery systems in that context was not only inefficient but unjust, because health care coverage was limited only to those who received pension funds.

In response to these concerns, the Chilean government launched an ambitious plan, the National Health Service (NHS), in 1952. It aimed at providing free health care to all those who held pension accounts, to blue-collar workers and their families in the social security system, and, for a variable fee, to others. It also provided free health care to the poor—particularly for life-threatening illnesses. It is estimated that 65 percent of the population used the NHS free of charge. A private sector thrived alongside the NHS and adopted a fee-for-service model.

In the 1960s, the government initiated a new program for white-collar employees. The program was paid for by payroll deductions but required users to pay a fee equal to 50 percent of the cost of their care. The program developed its own primary care clinics and laboratories, but it relied heavily on the well-maintained NHS institutions for hospitalizations. Physicians in Chile were mandated by law to work for the NHS for two years after graduation. After that, they had to work for a certain number of hours a week for the NHS, for which they received a modest compensation. Several physicians took advantage of the facilities in the state system to treat their private patients, making private practice lucrative. Health care provision was stratified along blue- and white-collar divisions. Blue-collar workers received direct care from the NHS, while white-collar workers could opt for employer-based government programs or care from approved private providers.[52]

Then everything changed. By the early 1970s, the state-run health programs were in a financial crisis. The political events that occurred between 1970 and 1988 also had a huge impact on Chile's health care policies. Salvador Allende's rule (1970–1973) was influenced by his socialist ideology. Allende nationalized Chile's private copper mines and two hundred major corporations. He introduced sweeping land reforms that expropriated monopoly holdings. Allende proposed as well to create a unified national health care system in

Chile and to outlaw private practice altogether. The latter proposal met with stiff resistance from physicians and led some to organize huge strikes that played a major role in the social turmoil that led to the military coup that overthrew Allende.

When Augusto Pinochet came to power through a military coup in 1973, he quickly dismantled the nationalized structures that had been set up by Allende. At the time, the country was in a state of financial and bureaucratic collapse, and, globally, communist and socialist regimes were on the decline. Led by a group of economists popularly known as the "Chicago boys," Pinochet's government took major steps to reduce state intervention in every possible realm except for the military and police. The new military government also radically cut welfare programs and instituted reforms to strengthen the private sector in order to reduce demands for public services, particularly in health care.

At the beginning of Pinochet's military regime, Chile had small and economically marginal private health care initiatives, composed of solo physician practices that offered primary and secondary care to the upper classes. Tertiary care was often carried out in public hospitals that offered few private wards. Most Chileans sought public services that were poorly financed and erratically administered, indifferent to competition, cost containment, or efficient resource management. That poor track record made it easy for market advocates to make a convincing case that medical care needed to be paid for privately, and that both providers and insurers were and should be in business for profit, each seeking lucrative contractual arrangements. There was nothing wrong with earning money from the sick and the destitute.

At the start of the reforms, Brazil, Argentina, and Colombia (like Chile) also had segmented private-public health care schemes. In those countries, the embracing and accommodation of market mechanisms, and the subsequent growth of the private health sector, served to diminish the role of publicly funded health care services. They were also undergoing the same sort of financing and administrative problems as Chile. Major health care reforms were needed if Brazil, Argentina, and Colombia wanted to attain their articulated goals of efficiency, health equity, and improved quality of health care.

1980s–1990s: THE ERA OF MARKET-ORIENTED REFORM

By the 1980s, the state was the main financier and provider of health care in many countries in Africa, Asia, and Latin America. Under this model, government health facilities received a budget from the state that also paid salaries for health care providers working in them. The state generally funded these services from general taxes. There was, however, room for private sector growth; most of those countries had private providers and clinics alongside state-funded health institutions. Patients seeking care in these private facilities had to pay for the services out of pocket. Middle-income developing countries —Chile, Mexico, Thailand, and South Africa—had health systems that were closer to a Bismarckian system. They gave the state a more limited role in the direct provision of health care. Under that system, employers played a large role in providing health insurance for their employees.[53]

China's system by 1978 was more complex. The government provided only 28 percent of the total health expenditures, excluding the cost of health care for public sector workers.[54] It also funded investments in training, buildings, and equipment, and provided preventive services free of charge. But it charged for consultations, treatment, drugs and dressings, and various consumables. Most people paid these charges out of pocket, but the government and state-owned enterprises paid for their own employees and, in some cases, employees' dependents. Work-related health insurance programs accounted for 30 percent of the total health expenditure in 1978.[55] In the 1960s–1970s, most countries, particularly those in postcolonial Africa, felt that the provision of health care was a governmental responsibility and, as such, could not be turned over to market forces. That was about to change.

The 1980s ushered in an era of major financial reforms that were felt in almost every economic and social sector of many developing countries. For the health care systems, reform encompassed a wide range of actions. They included limitation of government activities, involvement of the private sector, the introduction of market mechanisms, and an emphasis on greater individual responsibility. For most countries these reforms sought to address the scarcity and inefficient use of financial resources for health care as well as poor access to care and goods.[56]

The Role of the World Bank and International Monetary Fund

Although World Bank and IMF policies greatly influenced the move toward the marketization of health care in many developing countries, in some they merely contributed to a process that had already begun. Chile had started developing a market-oriented economy under the Pinochet regime, while India had a long-standing competitive and unregulated private sector providing important health services. In Vietnam, reform of the health care system was greatly influenced by consumer dissatisfaction, and its reform process was not driven by the World Bank at all. That much said, the Bank remains the most important driving force toward health care privatization in many African, Asian, and Latin American nations. Structural adjustment policies, and later processes such as the Poverty Reduction Strategy Papers, have had a profound impact on the social sectors and on social development.

During the Great Depression of the 1930s, most of the world's industrial powers devalued their currencies and erected trade barriers in an effort to buttress income levels in their economies.[57] Those measures contributed to the adverse effects of the Depression, reducing both employment and trade revenues. The economic problems that followed the outbreak of World War II exacerbated those developments. Toward the end of the war in 1944, the major allied governments gathered at the Bretton Woods Monetary and Financial Conference in New Hampshire, intent on reviving international trade in the postwar era. Believing that transnational commerce was the key to both global peace and prosperity, they designed the model for a market-driven postwar economic order. It was predicated on the promotion of multilateral cooperation and interdependence on trade and monetary policy.[58] The World Bank and the International Monetary Fund were established during this conference.

The IMF, a multilateral association of sovereign member countries, was charged with the creation and supervision of an "open and stable monetary system" and the promotion of a more efficient allocation of resources at the global level.[59] The World Bank, a multilateral development institution, was mandated to help finance the rebuilding of Europe's economies. As it turned out, the Bank's initial agenda was entirely overshadowed by the Marshall Plan in Europe. Subsequently, its institutional focus was redirected to economic development in developing countries. The IMF began operations in 1945 and the World Bank in 1946. Today, the Bank's aim is to "reduce poverty and improve the living standards by promoting sustainable growth and investment in people" and to "offer loans, technical assistance, and policy guidance to developing countries."[60] The Bank is the single largest source of external funds for health care in low- and middle-income countries.[61]

Reform Prescriptions

In the late 1970s, under the leadership of Robert McNamara, the World Bank turned its attention to correcting defective public policies in developing countries.[62] Many of them were saddled with large fiscal deficits, an unsustainable balance of payments, and inflation.[63] Under the firm conviction that project-oriented initiatives would be of little use in such unstable macroeconomic environments, the Bank introduced structural adjustment programs (SAPs) as the centerpiece of its lending operations.[64] This form of lending was designed to provide quick financial support to help developing member countries implement less costly adjustments to the prevailing global economic instabilities. In return for financial assistance, the Bank required member countries to undergo a process of structural adjustments. Short-term stabilization measures were not perceived to be sufficient to revive their battered economies.

The IMF and World Bank adjustment policies have two broad components: short- to medium-term macroeconomic stabilization measures designed to deal with budgetary and balance-of-payment problems, and SAPs designed to promote markets so as to allow competition to help improve the allocation of resources. Both programs require market liberalization, the introduction of competition, privatization, and a significant reduction in the role of the state in economic affairs. The World Bank observed that the main factors behind the stagnation and decline in developing countries were poor macroeconomic and sectoral policies that evolved from a flawed development policy that gave the state a prominent role in production and in regulating economic activity.[65]

Interestingly enough, the World Bank had earlier championed "the state," at a time when Keynesian economics was fashionable and the state was perceived to be instrumental in correcting market failures. The perceived failures of this development model, coupled with the attack on big government in industrialized countries in the Reagan and Thatcher years, led to the ascendance of a market-oriented view of the development process and policy.[66] While market advocates did not deny the probability of market failure, they saw government failure as worse.

Increasing the Role of the Market

To enhance their development, poor countries were being asked to increase the role of the market in their public sectors, an experiment that, in particular, mandated reducing the size of the public sector, privatizing public enterprises, and removing government regulations and controls.[67] Although structural adjustment policies operated at the macroeconomic level—seeking to improve overall economic performance—most developing countries seeking financial assistance from the World Bank had to cut back government expenditure and adopt other reform measures to mitigate or compensate for the cutbacks on expenditure. In other words, in some cases, IMF and World Bank lending conditions did not explicitly specify measures to control spending on social services. But in the interest of achieving the bottom-line objectives of curbing deficits and reining in inflation, reductions in spending on public health services were considered inevitable, acceptable, and even necessary consequences of adjustment.[68]

Structural reforms in the social sector involved a radical shift away from the role of the state as one of the providers and guarantor of universally accessible social services to the role of providing essential services in a targeted manner only to those on the margins whom the market would fail to reach. In the health care sector, countries were asked to undertake organizational reforms, contract out services, introduce user fees in health facilities, and promote health insurance programs. Organizational reforms sought to move public hospitals out of the core government bureaucracy into the private sector, aiming to transform them into more independent entities responsible for performance.[69]

Decentralization constitutes one form of organizational reform, seeking to change the organizational and institutional structures of public hospitals. Outside the hospital setting, decentralization seeks to empower lower levels of government to design, finance, and administer health services.[70] Decentralization is not strictly a market reform since it does not incorporate a greater use of market mechanisms. Having said that, there are some organizational reforms that rely on market tools to carry out functions that were traditionally done by central planning authorities.[71] Examples include reforms that increase the decision-making autonomy of public hospitals, and thus expose public hospitals to market pressure, and efficiency-enhancing reforms that require public hospitals to balance their budgets, earn profits, and keep their savings.

Contracting out is another measure that several developing countries are experimenting with. It uses contractual relationships with private providers to deliver health services. The government's role shifts from providing health care to financing it, and also to stimulate competition between providers.[72] Health care services that can be contracted out include clinical services (such as surgical procedures and laboratory tests), nonclinical services (such as pharmaceutical provision, catering, laundry, and equipment maintenance), and administrative functions (such as personnel recruitment and employment, computing, and purchasing). Contracting out can take on various forms, including competitive bidding and internal contracting.

According to the World Bank, contracting out offers four distinct advantages. First, it is a means of benefiting from private sector efficiency while maintaining control over what services are to be provided and to whom. Second, contracting out can confer the benefits of functional specialization. As noted by Ann Mills, "A hospital, for example, is unlikely to have a competitive advantage in all areas required for it to function. A cleaning company may have advantages of size (economies of scales, large pool of skilled managers) and specialization (responsiveness to changing technologies, low overheads). The private sector tends to be better than the state at adjusting to changing factors, prices and technology."[73] Third, contracting out offers greater flexibility to cope with changing demand, particularly with respect to labor, since contract workers can be readily hired and fired. Contracting out also offers a means of distancing the provision of services from the political process.[74]

User fees (copayments) have been arguably the most contentious reform experiment. They are a consequence of the IMF stabilization policies and have been introduced in many developing countries, particularly in Africa, in an attempt to use private funds to supplement or to substitute for governmental budgetary resources for health care. Although user fees were a consequence of SAPs, there were parallel efforts in the international community to increase private contributions for financing of public health services. The WHO's Alma-Ata Declaration of 1978, for instance, required primary health care to involve community participation in financing.[75] The World Bank justified the implementation of user fees in three ways. First, it felt that payment for services would discourage frivolous use of health facilities. Second, the Bank presumed that patients would become more conscious of quality, and demand it, if they were paying for services. Third, it assumed that the greater availability of funds through user fees at the point of service would increase both the availability and quality of services.[76]

Health insurance reforms have also been a part of the World Bank and IMF package of SAPs. The Bank and IMF require countries to encourage the growth of the health insurance industry. They see a potential to raise stable, alternative revenue to fund the cost of health care, and to reduce financial barriers to health care and enhance its redistributive effect. Yet in many developing countries there are no large-scale health insurance plans in either the public or private sectors to adequately test those possibilities. In sub-Saharan Africa, for example, the main beneficiaries are the relatively small middle class, and coverage extends to only about 10 percent of the population.

Some Harsh Criticisms

World Bank and IMF reform prescriptions have received much criticism, some of it harsh. SAPs have been accused of leading countries that have experi-

mented with them to social and political peril. The World Bank and IMF prescriptions have been jointly criticized, not just by outsiders (who see these
institutions as arrogant neocolonial powers), but also by World Bank and IMF
insiders. In a stinging indictment of Bank policies, a Nobel Prize winner for
economics, and former chief economist and senior vice president of the World
Bank, Joseph Stiglitz, wrote:

> Neither [good economics nor good politics] dominated the formulation of policy,
> especially in the International Monetary Fund. Decisions were made on the basis
> of what seemed a curious blend of ideology and bad economics, dogma that some-
> times seemed to be thinly veiling special interests. When crises hit, the IMF
> prescribed outmoded, inappropriate, if "standard" solutions without considering
> the effects they would have on the people in the countries told to follow these
> policies. Rarely did I see forecasts about what the policies would do to poverty.
> Rarely did I see thoughtful discussions and analyses of the consequences of alter-
> native policies. There was a single prescription and countries were expected to
> follow the IMF guidelines without debate.[77]

For most developing countries, there was little public scrutiny or assessment
of borrowing terms during the loan negotiation process, resulting in unten-
able conditions being imposed on countries in an undemocratic and nontrans-
parent manner. Specifically, the World Bank and IMF negotiated conditions
and terms of the loans with small sets of government officials (usually from the
finance ministry, central bank, or planning ministry) in recipient countries
with little participation from other ministries, members of parliament, or the
wider public.[78]

Technically, of course, the World Bank and IMF did not "impose" any conditions—member countries agreed to the terms. Because of the obvious power
imbalance, however, developing countries had no leverage to dispute most of
the terms set by the lending agencies. If countries did not agree to the conditions, they were simply denied access to credit and loans. Faced with overwhelming debt, shrinking national incomes, and no other funding avenues,
most countries agreed to those conditions. Even though the Bank was prescribing macroeconomic reforms that would be felt in almost all the sectors of
recipient countries, they were not given the opportunity to build consensus on
the lending conditions or even to consult with their parliaments and citizens.
Stiglitz described the IMF's relationship with developing countries as one of a
colonial ruler, not interested in hearing the thoughts of its client countries.[79]

The internal dissent within the World Bank and IMF was not just on the market ideology behind SAPs, but also on the process and pace by which countries were being required to make the economic reforms. But few such voices were heard outside the IMF and World Bank (more so the IMF); and they developed a reputation of little tolerance for internal dissent. The firing of Stiglitz in 1999 and the abrupt resignation of Ravi Kanbur, lead director of the Bank's high-profile World Development Report (2001–2002), exposed a growing rift within the Bank.[80] On the one side were those economists who believed that, if poor countries adopted a set of tried and tested policies—conquer inflation, slash government budgets, and open their economies—they would reap the benefits of economic growth. On the other side were economists like Kanbur and Stiglitz who argued that growth was not enough, that quality of growth mattered.[81]

CONSEQUENCES OF MARKET REFORMS
Zimbabwe, Zambia, Kenya, and Tanzania

What has happened under the World Bank and IMF reforms? By the 1980s, many African countries were coerced into entering into loan agreements with the World Bank and IMF to stabilize their economies. With much reluctance (and without extensive public deliberation), our four selected countries began to implement the structural adjustment terms described above. Tanzania, in particular, resisted policy reform until 1986, when it launched its first significant reform aimed at liberalizing the economy.[82] There was widespread concern in Tanzania and other African countries that, once these reforms were implemented, health care would be transformed from a public service to a private commodity—and that the poor would suffer. Because these four countries experienced similar or comparable consequences as a result of implementing structural adjustment policies, we discuss them collectively and include them in the category of coerced marketers (see chapter 3).

Once these African countries started to reform their health care systems, they encountered many problems. For example, although "contracting out" appeared attractive from an efficiency standpoint, the process was demanding institutionally. It involved defining the services to be provided, negotiating contractual terms and conditions, and implementing and monitoring the contract. Those conditions presented major challenges to African hospitals, which had little or no experience with this process. It soon became clear that a number of conditions were necessary for contracting arrangements to succeed, not the least of which was the existence of private sector firms capable of managing public sector contracts.[83] The downsizing of government staff during the privatization process, including health care workers, led to severe personnel shortages. In Zimbabwe, the government discharged eight hundred health care workers and abolished four hundred nursing positions. As a result, patients in government hospitals were forced to wait for up to three days to receive medical attention.[84]

Cost-sharing—primarily user fees—which was supposed to be an important alternative to tax-based financing, seems to have had a socially regressive impact in most African countries, including Zimbabwe, Zambia, Kenya, and Tanzania, partly because they did not have adequate mechanisms to protect vulnerable groups, particularly women, from its negative effects.[85] Several studies found that, even where user fees have been accompanied by some quality improvements, they have had severe effects on the demand for health care by the poor, who get "priced out" of the market. In Zimbabwe, for instance, decreased access to health services and rising morbidity and mortality were documented almost immediately after the advent of user fees.[86]

In Kenya, after the imposition of user fees, attendance in public clinics dropped by about 50 percent. That decline prompted the government to suspend the fees for seven months, during which attendance at government health centers then increased by about 41 percent.[87] Studies of user charges in Zambia also suggest that they have led to adverse effects on utilization of general outpatient care.[88] In Tanzania, it was found that, after the introduction of fees, attendance dropped by 50 percent in three government hospitals in Dar-es-Salaam, hospitals mainly used by lower-income populations.[89] Some studies, however, have suggested that user fees should be seen as only one element in a broader health care financing package, and that there is a greater potential role for fees in hospitals rather than in primary care facilities.[90]

Health insurance programs also met major obstacles. The overuse of health care caused costs to escalate to unacceptable levels. To make matters worse, insurers in many African countries remain reluctant to cover high-risk individuals, and unregulated health insurance has in many cases led to excessive medicalization as health care providers seek to maximize their profits. In any case, less than 10 percent of Africa's labor force is employed in the formal job sector; therefore, the vast majority of people are not eligible for insurance through their employer. In 1997, for instance, insurance coverage ranged from virtually nil in Uganda and Nigeria to between 1 and 6 percent in Zimbabwe, 16 percent in South Africa, and 11.4 percent in Kenya.[91] In Zimbabwe, one half of the cost of premiums is paid by workers and the other half by employers, with both groups receiving tax rebates for part of the payments.[92] In Kenya, the entire premium is paid by employees and the benefits package includes hospitalization costs.[93] Because of urban bias, health insurance coverage in rural areas is inadequate, and few African countries have set up the necessary institutional infrastructure to implement formal national heath insurance schemes that provide national coverage.[94] There is also little information about the coverage and nature of private for-profit health insurance schemes.

All of these health reform measures have affected women disproportionately. In many countries implementing adjustment programs, women and girls had to take on greater responsibility for the health care needs of the extended family, including caring for the sick and elderly to compensate for the lack of access to publicly provided service. At the household level, women have had to cope with the need to compensate for the reduction in the provision of public services.[95] Drastic government cuts in health care spending have also affected the provision of reproductive and maternal health services. Under cost-sharing arrangements, a Uganda study found that women were likely to either forego medical services or resort to home-care treatment.[96]

The Impact of HIV/AIDS

Compounding all these problems is the emergence of HIV/AIDS in Africa. Of an estimated 40 million people worldwide living with HIV/AIDS, approximately 28.5 million of them are in sub-Saharan Africa.[97] HIV/AIDS is almost single-handedly reversing earlier improvements in life expectancy and mortality in most African countries. The disease has been accompanied by an overwhelming increase in tuberculosis cases. The treatment and care of HIV/AIDS patients in African countries has created an unprecedented strain on public health care systems. The costs of AIDS morbidity and mortality alone may already reach 20 percent of the African gross national product. AIDS has put strains on national budgets by reducing economic growth and government revenues, and by increasing the cost of health care and community support. Household budgets in Africa are strained because AIDS reduces working incomes while simultaneously raising out-of-pocket health expenditures. Many African families are thrown into poverty from which they never recover because of the health costs associated with HIV/AIDS.[98]

Because of these limitations, many African countries, including Kenya and

Zambia, are now experimenting with private community-based health insurance plans that are locally developed and district-based, targeting rural, self-employed populations.[99] Yet both orthodox and community-based health insurance schemes in Africa are characterized by low coverage, mainly because of poverty, corruption, poor quality of services, and administrative and financial problems.

In partial response to the negative social impact of SAPs, the World Bank in its 1993 *World Development Report* recommended more sophisticated strategies. The Bank called upon developing countries to pursue sound macroeconomic policies that emphasize the reduction of poverty and the expansion of basic education. It asked governments to reduce spending on less cost-effective interventions and, instead, to double or triple spending on basic public health programs (such as immunization and HIV/AIDS prevention). Despite this emphasis on a government role, the Bank remains insistent on the need for countries to foster competition and diversity in the supply of health services and inputs, particularly drug supplies and equipment. Where feasible, governments (or social insurance) should pay for privately supplied health care services.[100]

Although the Bank has, in response to criticism, stepped back from the active promotion of user fees for basic social services in the developing world, it still argues that well-designed and well-implemented fee structures are potentially useful in mobilizing additional resources for these services in poor countries. User fees, it still contends, have the capacity to improve the quality of health services being provided.[101]

There has been some debate about whether the negative effects on health outcomes should be attributed to structural adjustment, rather than to the effects of the economic crisis, economic mismanagement, sheer bad luck, or other factors causing the crisis. The implementation of spending controls and cost-sharing programs was undertaken in developing countries during periods of economic decline and growing poverty, when social assistance and social services for the poor were in greatest demand. Focusing on adjustment policy as the sole culprit, it has been argued, implies that the alternative would be not to adjust rather than how to adjust.[102]

In response, some analysts have said that it is impossible to distinguish between the effects of adjustment and the effects of the economic crisis. Others have tried to separate the impacts resulting from the economic crisis and those arising from adjustment. The latter approach examines health outcomes before and after adjustment was implemented or compares adjusting to nonadjusting countries.[103] A study in 2000 found that in Senegal, Kenya, Rwanda, and Côte d'Ivoire, child mortality rates had begun to decline before the introduction of SAPs and continued to do so during the reform era. On the other hand, mortality rates started to decline in Uganda, Madagascar, Benin, and Ghana after the introduction of structural adjustment policies.[104]

Response to Criticism

Following the massive criticism of its economic reform programs, and the impact of these policies on social services, the IMF launched a new development process known as the Poverty Reduction Strategy Papers (PRSPs) in 1999. Its aim was to ensure that poverty reduction, not blind economic growth, was at the core of IMF lending policies. The principles underlying this approach are that national poverty reduction strategies should be country-driven, result-oriented, comprehensive and long-term in perspective, and based on domestic and external partnerships.[105] Under this approach, countries seeking bank credit have to prepare a PRSP outlining poverty reduction goals and plans for attaining them. Countries must thereafter demonstrate progress toward these goals before any funds are released. The Bank and IMF encourage countries to seek broad consultation while preparing these papers, particularly from nongovernmental organizations, academic researchers, and analysts and organizations representing poor people in their countries.

The PRSPs do not do away with World Bank and IMF policy requirements altogether. The idea is that the more tightly a government can define its policy targets and timing of actions in the PRSP, the more likely it is these targets will be included in World Bank and IMF terms of lending. IMF conditions are limited to the macroeconomic framework. Although widely seen as a step in the right direction, PRSPs have been criticized: despite giving countries some leeway for priority-setting, the IMF continues to steer them toward free-market macroeconomic policies.[106]

Apart from the PRSPs, the World Bank has also started to support new initiatives, among them health franchising plans. In a franchise, a firm licenses independent businesses to operate under its brand name. Franchisers in the health sector establish protocols, provide training for health workers, certify those who qualify, monitor the performance of franchises, and provide bulk procurement and brand marketing. In Pakistan, for instance, the Greenstar Network franchises private doctors, female paramedics, and pharmacists to provide family planning services and reproductive care in urban areas. Clinics receive subsidized supplies from Greenstar, initial training, and monthly visits from Greenstar doctors.[107] Kenya and the Philippines are also experimenting with this model, but there is a growing concern about its ability to reach the poorest people, as well as about its financial sustainability.

Although the World Bank has increased its funding for health and tried to shift its focus to poverty eradication and social developments, some fundamental problems remain. It is widely believed that new lending for health can achieve little when the debt burden of most African countries is already unsustainable. The conditions attached to the new loans, heavy in their demand, still reflect the same orientation prescribed over the last twenty years.[108]

Most African countries now have a public-private health care system, with the public sector generally accounting for about 54 percent of health expenditures. International or bilateral donor assistance is a major component of health systems support, accounting for more than 15 percent of health spending on average, and more than 50 percent in some countries. Donors typically fund programs for disease prevention and immunization, maternal and child health, family planning, and treatment for malaria, tuberculosis, and HIV/AIDS. Unfortunately, these donor-funded programs are vertical and operate parallel to each other. They often overlap and compete for the limited number of trained health personnel and facilities.[109] Donor funding also depends on political performance; release of funds can thus be unpredictable.

Formal public and private insurance remains limited, and risk-pooling generally takes the form of community-based rural risk-pooling. Several countries focus almost entirely on the financing and delivery of public health services, taking a position of benign neglect toward social insurance, community financing, and other forms of health financing. As a result, these other forms of financing remain insignificant and underdeveloped.[110] In 2001, general government expenditures in health care as a percentage of total expenditure on health were 21.4 percent in Kenya, 45.3 percent in Zimbabwe, 46.7 percent in Tanzania, and 53.1 percent in Zambia. Out-of-pocket spending as a percentage of private expenditure on health was 67.6 percent in Kenya, 52.2 percent in Zimbabwe, 83.1 percent in Tanzania, and 71.8 percent in Zambia.[111] Most poor, rural populations in Africa resort to self-care and self-medication when ill, and they spend a significant portion of their income on indigenous medicines. Public health care facilities remain underfunded, poorly managed, and short on drugs and supplies.[112]

Reestablishing Universal Health Care

Because of the high level of public disapproval among countries implementing market-oriented health reform and the lack of impressive outcomes,
some African countries, including Kenya and Tanzania, are attempting to establish government-managed universal coverage programs for their citizens.
Kenya is currently in the final stages of launching a new national social health
scheme designed to provide a package of health care services for all. Under this
new plan, whose details are still being worked out, a National Social Health
Insurance Fund will be the main mechanism through which all Kenyans, including the unemployed, will be able to obtain coverage. Premiums will be
determined based on income levels. Previously, only people in formal employment were beneficiaries of a state-run compulsory insurance system, which
covered only 25 percent of the population.[113] Tanzania passed a bill in 1999 to
establish a National Health Insurance Scheme for government workers. The
country also introduced a Community Health Fund as a way for communities
to finance primary care. Under this approach, the government aims to improve
the health and well-being of all Tanzanians, focusing on those most at risk
by ensuring that health services respond to the needs of the population.[114]
Whether these countries will be able to adequately fund these reform plans
remains unclear and will surely be influenced by the health of the economy as
a whole.

In the midst of overwhelmingly negative reports about the effects of SAPs in
developing countries, the World Bank and IMF have cited some countries as
economic success stories. Ghana, for instance, received nine adjustment loans
between 1980 and 1994 and, once the stipulated reforms were implemented,
Ghana's economy grew at an average of 1.4 percent per year in the same period.
Mauritius and Thailand are also widely cited as countries where, given the
right conditions, structural adjustment can be a positive measure. One of these
conditions, according to World Bank economists, is political stability. They
argue that the extent of ethnic divisions, and the length of time that a political
leader is in power, can successfully predict the outcome of adjustment loans 74
percent of the time.[115] In response, critics of SAPs concede that the measures
appear to have succeeded in shrinking government budget deficits, eliminating hyperinflation, and maintaining debt-payment schedules in several poor
countries. But while government balance sheets may improve, critics argue,

SAPs have failed to establish a base for sustainable, balanced economic development. The policies have made local industries collapse, increased dependency on food imports, shrunk social services—particularly health care—and fostered a widening gap between the rich and poor.[116]

South Africa

When South Africa became a democracy in 1994, the new African National Congress government inherited a disorganized health system characterized by deep disparity and inequity. Racial segregation of health care had resulted in separate and unequal services for blacks and whites. Health services were fragmented because of the establishment of numerous health services administrations based on ethnicity. Curative care and an extensive hospital-centered health care infrastructure took precedence over preventive health care, and whites dominated the management of health care facilities.

The new government launched an ambitious national health plan with a district approach to primary care as its framework. The plan's main goal is to make primary health accessible to rural populations through decentralized health administrative units based at the district level. As the government tries to streamline its health care systems, the private sector in health remains largely an entrenched culture in South Africa. Health care is, for the most part, dictated by loosely regulated market forces rather than coherent national policy. For better or worse, the private sector has not been affected much by the dramatic changes taking place in the public sector. The market for private patients remains most lucrative and, even though public sector primary care is free in South Africa, about 30 percent of people without medical insurance still choose to pay out of their own pockets for private sector facilities. This is explained partly by the inaccessibility of public services in rural areas and the perceptions of better quality, faster services, and greater privacy in the private sector.[117]

Today, health care coverage is principally financed through employer-sponsored private insurance, and providers and hospitals are privately operated, independent businesses. The public system, which provides basic health services for the poor, consumes about 11 percent of the government's total budget. The large private sector primarily serves the middle- and high-income end, who tend to be members of medical insurance plans (about 18%). The central government remains committed to finding ways to address the inequalities in access and quality, and has plans to develop universal coverage.[118]

One of the biggest challenges the country faces is HIV/AIDS. South Africa has more HIV-positive individuals than any other country in the world: 11 percent of South Africans are HIV-infected; by 2010, adult HIV prevalence could reach 25 percent. Each day approximately sixteen hundred people are infected, and two-thirds of them are aged fifteen to twenty. By 2005 the population size is expected to be 16 percent lower than it would have been in the absence of AIDS. According to UNAIDS, by 2015, population loss to AIDS-related deaths will be 4.4 million.[119] Most of those infected are the poor majority who cannot afford the expensive treatment for the disease. After much pressure from HIV/AIDS activists, the South African government is attempting to develop equitable and sustainable ways to finance the care and treatment of HIV/AIDS for all infected South African—a complex, ethically difficult, and politically charged task.

OTHER FORCES IN THE MOVE TOWARD THE MARKET IN DEVELOPING COUNTRIES

Although the World Bank has been the main driving force in the turn to market mechanisms in health care in developing regions, particularly Africa, there were other factors that led some nations to move toward similar prescriptions for health care reform.

China

In the early 1980s, Deng Xiaoping, China's premier, dismantled the Communist health care reforms and paved the way for China to evolve into a market economy. These changes were not felt in the health care sector alone. There was a marked shift from collective to household agricultural production. Price controls were removed and reforms of state-owned enterprises occurred. A labor market was created, as were new forms of private enterprise ownership; and, in addition, there was a decentralization of the tax authority and public sector financial management.[120]

These economic reforms stimulated unprecedented economic growth. As a result, changes were felt in almost every socioeconomic sector, including health care. In *rural areas,* the government adopted a laissez-faire policy, and rural health care reverted to mainly out-of-pocket financing. The cooperative organizations that formed the basis of rural community insurance programs disintegrated, and many doctors in rural China left to become private practitioners. These programs covered 85 percent of Chinese villages in the late 1970s and financed 20 percent of the total health expenditure. They now cover less than 10 percent of villages and finance 2 percent of total health expenditure.[121] Township health centers and country hospitals are now mainly financed by fee-for-service, out-of-pocket payments. Access to care in rural China is governed by ability to pay, making decent health care virtually unaffordable for most Chinese people living in those areas. The government has since been trying to reintroduce community insurance plans in rural areas, but these initiatives remain severely limited.

In *urban areas,* the Chinese government faces several challenges. Rapid economic growth created greater consumer demand for diversified health services that were not previously affordable—for instance, dental care and cosmetic surgery.[122] Advanced technology, increasing incomes driving demand for better health care, and the lack of effective constraints placed directly on consumers and providers created financial problems for governments and industries providing health insurance to people in urban areas. Policymakers in China realized that they had to address the health care cost escalations. Starting in the 1980s, China began to implement a series of reforms in urban areas.

The first stage of the reform was cost containment. Before 1985, the reforms mostly targeted the demand side—for instance, introducing user fees to make consumers more cost-conscious. From 1985, the focus shifted to control of providers, especially through economic incentives to hospitals. Another supply-side measure was the introduction of limited pharmaceutical lists for which the government would provide reimbursement. These reform measures mitigated China's rapid health care cost escalation, but their full impact has not been felt because the measures lacked important complementary changes in socioeconomic policy, especially in the health sector's price structure. Prices had been set to allow poor Chinese to access basic health care, forcing providers to deliver basic services for prices below actual cost. Providers therefore recovered revenue through charges for drugs and high-technology tests, areas where the allowed fees exceeded marginal costs. This pricing structure led to the rapid increase of high-technology and medical equipment, and an over-reliance on drug prescriptions for provider revenue.[123]

The second stage of reform, starting in 1992, focused on risk-pooling. During this period, China was also reforming its social protection systems. These reforms were implemented in pilot cities across China, using a combination of individual savings accounts and social risk-pooling funds to finance medical expenditures. These reforms have had some measure of success in slowing health care and cost escalation, and in expanding coverage to those who were previously uninsured or underinsured. In 1996, China held its first National Health Conference to develop a major health policy for the next decade. A policy goal that emerged from this meeting was that China would establish a preliminary framework for a comprehensive health system to ensure that every Chinese person will have access to basic health protection.[124] The government resolved to establish constraining mechanisms for controlling health care demand and supply, to actively develop community care, and to develop and improve community-based insurance programs, particularly in rural areas. The lofty goals set in 1996 have not been achieved.

Today China's health system remains administratively hierarchical and bifurcated, with a clear distinction between urban and rural care.[125] There are three formal systems and an informal component:

Government Employee Health Insurance: This program provides coverage for government workers. The government is solely responsible for the financing of this system.

Labor Health Insurance: This program covers employees in state and collective enterprises and their immediate family members.

Rural Cooperation Medical System: Though they were largely dismantled during the period of economic liberalization in the late 1970s, the government has been reviving community insurance programs with assistance from local governments.

Private sector care: In the informal sector, those who are not covered by any of the three programs have to pay out of pocket for their own treatment.

Government coverage of the rural population has decreased from 90 to 10 percent. In 2000, individuals paid for 60 percent of the nation's health care costs (rural residents pay 90% of their medical costs), yet just nine years before, out-of-pocket payments constituted 39 percent of the total costs. On average, the rural health care system provides 1.5 beds and 1.1 physicians per thousand residents. Urban residents, who in 1980 represented 17 percent of the population and today represent approximately one-third, are served by eleven thousand hospitals. On average, the urban system provides 3.5 beds and 2.3 physicians per thousand residents. Since 2000, the government has allowed 15 percent of hospital beds to be cooperatively owned and up to another 15 percent owned privately.[126]

The Chinese urban population has, by and large, accepted these market reforms, particularly because several years of reform of health care in urban areas improved the system, increased the number of doctors per person, and introduced new treatment and diagnostic technologies.[127] In addition, a large proportion of people in China's cities are covered by work-related insurance.[128] In rural China, however, severe problems persist. The vast majority of rural residents do not have insurance and cannot afford to pay for care out of pocket when they fall ill. A 2003 story in the *Wall Street Journal* summarized the concerns of the rural poor in China: "Chinese farmers now fear medical bills almost as much as they do SARS [severe acute respiratory syndrome] . . . through the 1990s, farmers' income roughly tripled, but medical costs soared more than eightfold."[129]

Health reform in China has brought with it a rise in the cost of health services, increased inequality in access to services, particularly rural versus urban, and uneven development of primary care and preventive services.[130] China also has a rapidly aging population that has (or will have) chronic conditions for which there are effective, but expensive, treatments. Because most patients in China are now well-informed about sophisticated treatment options, the government can no longer make prevention its primary policy. It must simultaneously lay equal stress on prevention and clinical care.[131] There have been complaints that the rich are not satisfied with the medical care offered by the government because it is too inefficient, while the poor cannot afford it.

The cost of medical treatment rose by 14 percent each year between 1993 and 2003—a rate faster than the rise in people's income. Widespread dissatisfaction with public providers (mainly high user fees and poor staff attitudes) is driving patients to seek cheaper but lower-quality care from poorly regulated private providers.[132] Market incentives in health care provision have also had an impact among medical graduates. Medical education is still largely funded by the state, but physicians, nurses, and technicians can now decide where to practice, and many opt to go into private practice rather than working within the established systems, where the salaries are quite low.

China is being forced to experiment with more reform measures. In Shanghai, two hospitals are being established with foreign ventures taking a majority shareholding, and two hundred of the city's six hundred hospitals are reported to have entered into cooperative arrangements with foreign hospitals or foreign investment capital.[133] China is also experimenting with pilot rural health insurance programs, under which farmers pay an annual fee of $1.20, which is then matched by local and central governments. Enrollees in this program get reimbursed on a sliding scale, the proportion increasing according to the seriousness of the disease.

Despite these new efforts, serious problems persist in China's health care system, including a lack of public confidence in the system. The unwillingness of people in rural areas to spend even a limited amount of money, without the certainty that they will get something back for it, illustrates this distrust and lack of confidence in the authorities, and in the health system.

India

India turned its economy in a market direction in the 1990s and, in a bid to reduce the budgetary deficit, the government cut social sector spending drastically. The government simultaneously initiated several measures aimed at encouraging private sector involvement in health care. Public health facilities —among them nonclinical services in public hospitals—were privatized or semi-privatized, innovative ways to finance public health facilities through nonbudgetary measures were developed, and the state governments offered tax incentives to encourage private investment in the health sector.

India now relies on the private sector to finance nearly 80 percent of its health care system. Public expenditures for health care are among the lowest in the world, representing about 6 percent of the country's GDP. Private expenditure is at 4.7 percent, with 75 percent of total expenditure being out of pocket. In a population of approximately 1.1 billion, less than 2 million people currently have insurance. The central government plays a limited role in both the financing and delivery of health care, and widespread regional variations in health status and outcomes are linked to the ability of state or municipal governments to provide health services.[134]

One of the most significant trends that has emerged as a result of liberalization in India is the entry of for-profit hospitals and international health corporations into the health care sector, seeking to take advantage of the huge health care demand-supply gap. The Indian economy has seen a significant rise in foreign investment in its health care system. According to the economist Brijesh Purohit,

Health care in India is emerging as a blue-chip industry . . . The earlier image of the private sector in India mainly focused on nursing homes and polyclinics . . . The new market orientation is towards super-specialty care . . . Given the rising costs of health care in the last 5 years, the foreign companies are aiming to capture the potential of the health insurance market for the nearly 135 million people in the upper-middle income segment of the population who can afford health care . . . Besides health insurance, the high-tech, medical, electronic equipment industry has been the other area to attract investment by multinationals following liberalization.[135]

Nationwide, health care utilization rates show that private health services are directed mainly at providing primary health care and are financed from private resources, placing a disproportionate burden on the poor. The central government runs a majority of the rural hospitals and village-level clinics that offer ambulatory, neonatal, and maternal health services. These hospitals and service providers are seen as the system of last resort among the poor.[136]

India's national health care system suffers from a number of problems. It is an overcentralized system with almost no delegation of financial and administrative powers to districts, with a duplication of services, and with a lack of capacity for devising levels of financial management. In addition, India has a complex system of financing, further complicated by the rapidly growing and largely unregulated private sector, and a low quality of services in the public sector. The largest system of mandatory employment-related insurance, the Employees' State Insurance Scheme, covers only a fraction of patients who are potentially eligible. This scheme does not function as an insurer or purchaser, but instead operates directly as a (rather unpopular) health service for lower-income workers.[137]

Vietnam

In 1986, Vietnam did away with three decades of socialism and embraced market ideologies. The Sixth Party Congress proclaimed the *doi moi* (renovation) policy, which set off a powerful set of interactions between economic reform and the health sector in the country.[138] Vietnam did not receive any financial support from the IMF or World Bank, only technical assistance and policy advice during its economic reform process.[139]

Despite the fact that, under socialism, Vietnam's health care coverage was extensive, commune health centers were poorly funded and poorly equipped, and utilization was very low. Consumers became dissatisfied with this system, and they began to lobby for change. Partly in response, the Vietnamese government announced four new health policies under the *doi moi*. First, it legalized private medical practice, which had been hitherto forbidden; second, it privatized the production and sale of drugs; third, the government imposed user charges in public medical facilities; and finally, it created a voluntary health insurance plan.[140] In 1992, the government also mandated, by decree, compulsory payroll-based social health insurance for all government employees, and for workers of state and private enterprises with ten workers or more.[141] This decree also made provision for a system of voluntary insurance for the majority of workers in small businesses and agriculture.

These new polices led to an explosive growth of private medicine and pharmaceutical markets.[142] Vietnam's transition to a market economy has, however, been complicated by the need to integrate the southern part of the country into the economy while managing postwar reconstruction.[143] Vietnam's post-reform health system is complex. On the surface, the country appears to have a two-tier private sector. The first tier consists of a handful of well-established private hospitals located in the big cities, and a second tier is made up of private providers in the urban and rural areas. These private clinics often serve as ambulatory health care providers for middle-income people. There is a third tier that has arisen in Vietnam: mobile practitioners. They are medical officers trained in basic health care, and in some cases retired physicians, who make home visits and offer flexible payment arrangements to patients.[144] These health practitioners are providing an important service in the face of a deteriorating public health sector.

Because compulsory insurance is targeted at the formal sector, virtually all rural inhabitants in Vietnam have no coverage. The government has tried to mitigate this problem by aiming to provide free health insurance to four million people; by 1999 it had been able to insure only two hundred thousand people.[145] Some rural communities are experimenting with private community-based financing programs, with mainly exterior donor support, as a means of increasing access to health services.[146] It is estimated that twenty-eight million Vietnamese people are too poor to pay hospital fees, but not poor enough to have the fees waived. Some 20 to 30 percent of patients from rural areas have to take out loans with high interest rates, sell livestock, or take children out of school in order to pay public hospital bills.[147] The Vietnamese government's expenditure on health as a percentage of total health costs is 28.5 percent.[148] In addition, out-of-pocket expenditure as a percentage of private expenditure on health in Vietnam stands at 87.6 percent.

Now that private practice is allowed, practitioners in Vietnam are moving to cities, resulting in inequalities in availability and quality of services in rural areas. From 1996 to 2000, the number of private facilities more than doubled in forty-four of sixty-one cities and provinces in Vietnam.[149] Preventive services receive a small share of government expenditure.[150] The transition to a market economy in Vietnam has been constrained by a lack of clear rules concerning relationships among enterprises, financial institutions, and government. The introduction of user fees has also created some problems. In a large city hospital in Vietnam, 20 to 80 percent of the running costs are obtained from the users; this money is spent partly on salaries for personnel and partly on other running costs, including materials and equipment. With few facilities to charge for, a simple rural health center in Vietnam does not generate much money. Urban-rural and rich-poor differences have been reinforced and aggravated in the new system.[151]

Latin America

For many Latin American countries, experiments with market ideas in health care came about because of several factors. They included political changes within the countries, consumer pressure for better services, stagnation of economic growth, and reform prescriptions from the World Bank and IMF. As Latin American countries privatized government programs, the public began to participate more in the industrial economy and, with time, became increasingly eager to exert their newly found power as consumers. Public expectations of high quality rose significantly, particularly among the emerging middle class. Daily comparisons with services provided by the private sector left most Latin Americans dissatisfied with the provision of state-run services.[152]

In 1995, Latin American countries, international agencies, and experts from the region, took part in a special meeting to build a regional agenda for health sector reform. Participants in the seminar defined health sector reform as "a process aimed at introducing substantive changes into the relationships and roles performed by the different agencies involved in the health sector. The goal was to increase equity of benefits, efficiency in management, and effectiveness in satisfying the health needs of the population."[153]

Changes proposed for reform of the region's health care system included administrative decentralization of management of funds, deregulation combined with strengthening of the private sector, cost responsibility for large institutions, the introduction of prepaid service plans, and freedom of choice for health care coverage. Some important trends emerged from health sector reform in the region. There was the formal and informal emergence and rapid growth of a competitive profit-making private health sector and health insurance programs. There was also an effort to shift within the public sector from a command-and-control style of resource allocation to one driven by market ideas. This move entailed the transition from a supply-side to a demand-side provider financing mechanism. Finally, there was a change by health care providers from a traditionally professional, self-regulated culture to one that was management-driven and customer-oriented.[154]

Chile

In Chile, health care reforms were introduced by Pinochet's military government as part of a wider economic reform plan whose aim was to dismantle Allende's socialist regime and move toward a more liberal economy. The government-initiated strategic participation of the market in health care services was based on a clearly formulated agenda that included equity in benefits, equitable distribution of resources for health care, increased free choice of providers, and increased efficiency and responsiveness to the needs of the citizenry.[155]

The military government sought to achieve these goals by modifying both the public and private health sectors in the following ways:

- Decentralizing the National Health Care System into regional units that would remain under the administration of the Ministry of Health, but given some financial autonomy to generate and manage their resources.
- Decentralizing primary health care facilities to the municipal level.
- Financing the public health care system with a 7 percent deduction from all salaries and old-age pensions.
- Encouraging the creation of health insurance institutions authorized to compete for the 7 percent mandatory health care deduction. These insurance companies were free to provide health care services directly or to contract out to third-party providers. Many companies established integrated models where the same institution purchases and provides health services.[156]

The emergence of a strong and growing market-oriented health care delivery system introduced important changes. Insurance companies bought and ran their own clinics, they invested in technology, and they became health care providers. Insurance premiums became so costly that people who could not afford to pay for coverage either opted out or drastically reduced their benefits.

As a direct result of these reforms, Chile developed a two-tiered, mixed public-private system, with the wealthy and the healthy in the private system, and the poor and the sick in the public system. These inequalities in health care funding and provision persisted, with public opinion showing dislike for both the expensive private system and the deteriorating public system.[157] The fall of Pinochet, and the return to democracy in 1989, saw renewed efforts to address these inequities by restoring the size and importance of the public health care sector. Between 1990 and 1996, for instance, public health expenditure more than doubled, and public opinion on access to adequate health care is seen to be improving. About 70 percent of Chile's population is currently covered by the public system, with the rest opting for private coverage.[158] The government appears to remain committed to ensuring equitable access for all, regardless of wealth or status, by continuing to increase public health funding and modernizing its public health care services. Although these developments are certainly having a positive impact, equitable health access is yet to be realized in Chile.[159]

Brazil

In the 1990s, Brazil's health care system underwent a massive reform process culminating in the creation of a Unitarian National Health Service covering about 75 to 80 percent of the population (approximately 20% have private insurance). The main thrust of the reform was aimed at decentralizing the national health system by redirecting resources from the federal budget to the state and municipal levels. This new program sought to reduce, to some extent, the inequities between poor and affluent regions in Brazil. The decentralization process has, however, served to fragment national public health programs at a time when one of the biggest problems Brazil faces is the increased incidence of infectious diseases (HIV/AIDS, dengue, and malaria, for example), all of which require strong public health interventions.[160]

Even though the National Health Service oversees basic and preventive health care, the private nonprofit and for-profit health care sectors deliver the bulk of medical services, including government-subsidized inpatient care. This publicly financed, privately provided health system continues to intensify its focus on high-cost curative care. Therapeutic treatment in hospitals takes up much of the health budget, at the expense of health-promotion and disease-prevention programs. Hospital-based assistance, for instance, expanded from 44 percent of municipal health spending in 1985 to 77 percent in 1990, while expenses for primary care decreased from 35 to 3 percent in the same period. Not only have basic and preventive health services for the entire population been reduced, but the public health system also subsidizes expensive, high-technology medical procedures that consume 30 to 40 percent of health resources, and often ends up being used to attend the richer segments of the population.[161]

Argentina

In post-1980s reform, Argentina developed a three-tiered health system designed to provide universal coverage through social security, private prepaid plans, and the public sector. Social security, which represents the largest tier, provides health care financing through multiple Obras Sociales (OS). These are associations linked with trade and professional unions in which membership is mandatory. Public sector agencies operate about 43 percent of the clinics and hospitals, but account for only 23 percent of total health care spending. The public sector provides services primarily to the poor population, and is operated mainly at the provincial and municipal levels through government agencies and programs.[162]

Most spending on health in Argentina is directly transferred from the OS to providers, resulting in overtreatment and excessive diagnostic procedures. In recent times, Argentina's health care system has been facing many challenges because of the government's economic and financial crisis. OS accounts have all but disappeared or have been rescinded by labor groups as a source of funds. This has resulted in a massive influx of consumers into the already troubled national health sector. Under current IMF and World Bank loan conditions, the Argentinean government will not be able to provide substantial subsidies to the OS, resulting in widespread provider withdrawal.[163]

Health reforms in Argentina have reinforced segmentation in health insurance. Mandatory payroll contributions encourage the migration of higher-earning workers to private health insurers. Private insurers attract high-earning, low-health-risk groups, while social insurance and public health care providers cover low-income, high-health-risk groups. In addition to reinforcing inequalities in access to health care, this segmentation limits social insurance's capacity to pool risks. Currently the private sector accounts for a disproportionate and rising share of total health expenditures. In this scenario, improvements in coverage, equity, and cost containment in Argentina are more likely to be achieved by moving in the direction of health systems in which the social insurance principle and that of individual provision can be integrated and complement each other.[164]

Colombia

Colombia's experiment with health reform is widely believed to be one of the market success stories of Latin American health services reform—particularly in terms of providing safety nets for the poor and vulnerable. Colombia enacted comprehensive health sector reform legislation in response to a fiscal crisis in the publicly funded social security system and the fiscal opportunities arising from new petroleum discoveries. Colombia's reform design was to promote "managed competition" among competitive public and private insurance plans. Under this program two regimes were established: a "contributory regime," aimed at people who could afford to pay contributions to the social security system through their employment or independent income, and a "subsidized regime," aimed at people who could not afford to make contributions and therefore have to be subsidized by the government for the total or partial cost of the obligatory insurance. Colombia has achieved much in its reform program. Insurance coverage has expanded dramatically to more than 65 percent of the population. Access to care by the poor has increased, and new insurance and health delivery organizations have been developed. These positive results have, however, been hampered by economic decline, corruption, deficient information systems, opposition from union and professional groups, and political instability in the country.[165]

Cuba

Cuba, finally, provides an example of a country that has repeatedly rejected market mechanisms in its health care system. Cuba finances its health system almost entirely out of the state budget: 86.6 percent of the total health expenditure in Cuba is borne by the state.[166] Benefits include full medical and dental services, as well as prescription drugs. Private out-of-pocket expenditures account for 10.8 percent of health expenditures.[167] Because of the strict embargo, Cuba relies on donations of some medical supplies from Canada, Europe, Latin America, and U.S. nongovernmental organizations. The state also provides financial aid for poorer patients requiring health care.

But there have been problems. The Cuban health care system functioned effectively up through the 1980s. Life expectancy increased, infant mortality declined, and access to medical care expanded. Cuba began to resemble the developed nations in health care figures. In the years that followed, however, the economy contracted some 40 percent, mainly because of the end of Soviet bloc aid and because of unfavorable trade terms. The result was simply less money to spend on the health care system, or on anything else. And because the weakened Cuban economy generated less income from foreign exports, there was less hard currency available to import medicines and medical equipment, all of which contributed to shortages in the Cuban health care system. Although Cuba has invested greatly in human resources, it has not done the same in physical infrastructure. Like many of our selected countries in the pre-reform era, shortages of equipment in hospitals and other health facilities in Cuba continue.[168]

BEYOND MARKET EXPERIMENTS: WHAT NEXT FOR DEVELOPING COUNTRIES?

After tracing the history and organization of health care systems in selected Asian, African, and Latin American countries, as well as their responses to market mechanisms, we find some general trends. Most developing countries in the pre-1980s era, inspired by Western welfare states, and in an attempt to remedy the problems of market failure during the previous fifty years, adopted Beveridge-model health care systems: the state funded health care systems with services produced by a vertically integrated public bureaucracy.[169] In the 1980s and 1990s, the pendulum began to swing back in the opposite direction and, during the Reagan and Thatcher eras, there was a greater willingness to experiment with market approaches in the social sectors, including health, education, and social protection. Some countries, however, particularly those of sub-Saharan Africa, were forced to initiate market reform strategies by World Bank and IMF loan conditions. Today, most countries have a mix of public and private sources of funding for their health care systems.

Have market mechanisms improved health care systems and health outcomes in developing countries? Many critics of market-oriented experiments argue that they have harmed public health, basic services provision, and equity. A 1993 study found that structural adjustment had a negative impact on health indicators such as infant and child mortality in African countries. The study also found that the nutritional status of children declined in adjusting countries and that structural adjustment policies induced a profound change in health policy, resulting in a widening gap between affected communities

TABLE 4.3
Funding Sources of Health Expenditures, 2000

	Out-of-pocket expenditure	Private expenditure as % of total health expenditure	Total government % expenditure on health
Argentina	34.1	45	55
Brazil	38.5	59.2	40.8
Chile	34.3	57.4	42.6
China	60.4	63.4	36.6
Cuba	10.8	10.8	89.2
Ghana	46.5	46.5	53.5
India	82.2	82.2	17.8
Kenya	56.4	77.8	22.2
Malawi	23	52.2	47.8
South Africa	12.6	57.8	42.2
Tanzania	44.1	53	47
Vietnam	68.7	74.2	25.8
Zambia	28.6	37.9	62.1
Zimbabwe	22.2	57.4	42.6

Source: Data from World Health Organization, www.who.int/country/en/.

and policymakers.[170] China's economic reforms, for instance, led to the collapse of rural health systems and a significant increase in inequity of access to care.[171] Chile's health insurance system created a two-tiered system, with private plans spending almost twice as much per capita as public services.[172] Zambia's local districts are receiving less funding than before the reform, and user fees have limited access to health facilities.[173] (Table 4.3 illustrates how developing countries pay for their health care.)

Some take the view that reform experiments have not given enough attention to the political and social realities in the countries, with too strong an emphasis on the content of the reforms and a lack of attention to the actors and processes involved. Professional and business associations in many developing countries have enormous power to control quality, access, and cost decisions in health care systems.[174] These groups also have the ability to stall or change policies, yet they have been, for the most part, sidelined in the health reform process.[175] Externally imposed market experiments, according to some, did not take into account national history, values, and culture.[176] The World Bank and IMF prescriptions were standard in their application, almost never adjusting to the specific local circumstances in individual countries. Implementation of health care reform measures has also been hampered by the lack of institutional capacity in many developing countries. For market ideas to function, health systems must possess a certain level of sophistication in policy analysis, research, information systems, management expertise, and logistics systems. These capacities are simply absent in many developing countries.[177]

Some analysts argue that it is too early to conclude that the experiments with health care reform have been unsuccessful—they have had too little time to be fully implemented, and have not been monitored sufficiently to determine their real impacts.[178] There is generally, however, little evidence of the success of reform experiments in achieving their broad objectives in the developing world. One reason for this might be the lack of information, data, or studies evaluating the impact of market reform in those regions. There are almost no measures of efficiency and quality to determine the real effects of these reforms in developing countries' health systems.

Though a number of proposals to evaluate health reform have been pitched, there remain difficulties in establishing an appropriate yardstick against which to measure change in the various countries.[179] Baseline performance, although used often, may not reveal much, since performance may have changed from that level even without reform.[180] Some scholars have argued that, because of the near collapse of public health systems in developing countries (particularly in Africa), structural adjustment should incorporate successful interventions in health, water, and nutrition. Although health and nutrition programs are generally accepted as necessary and beneficial to the overall well-being and productivity of a population—particularly in developing countries—some international development economists continue to fail to consider health and nutrition essential to development.[181]

In the face of these criticisms, it is important to recall that the welfare state approach also had failed to address many of the health needs that emerged in developing world populations in the pre-reform era, prompting countries to experiment with market-oriented ideas.[182] Today, most low-income countries, particularly those in Africa, do not have functioning public health care systems. Most of these countries give insufficient priority to public health, disease prevention, and maternal and child services, and, consequently, do not allocate sufficient funds to these programs. Developing countries face a dilemma. They have to involve the state in the provision and delivery of health care to provide a safety net for the majority of their population that is poor and vulnerable. Yet such involvement is usually marked by public sector production failure.[183] Similarly, blind faith in the market is no more likely to resolve the complex problems that face the health sector than is a naive belief in government. Developing countries have to find a balance.

How are they trying to do so? Many developing countries are embarking on more reform experiments, including the mobilization of informal resources, and the creation of risk-pool arrangements to cover rural and informal sector workers when the government's capacity to undertake these activities is limited.[184] Some developing countries, particularly those in Latin America, are taking steps to ensure that social insurance and general revenues play a functional role in health financing for the poor.

Several developing countries are engaging in more strategic resource allocation and purchasing arrangements to get the best value for money spent in health care by ensuring that the poor and other excluded population groups get coverage. Governments are also trying to encourage active competition between the public and private sectors on price, quality, and volume when selecting providers. Concrete steps are being taken to ensure that payment mechanisms provide strong performance incentives for the providers selected.[185] Increasing disparities in health care access and utilization can be attributed almost directly to the introduction of market practices in health care systems. Developing countries will, then, have to make political decisions on how much inequality in the health care system can be tolerated by the population for the sake of economic growth. Not an easy call.

We have now looked at the market debates and practices in many parts of the world. Before attempting to assess the evidence of the efficacy of market practices and the various health systems of which they are a greater or lesser part, we turn our attention to the pharmaceutical industry. We have chosen this industry for a closer look because of the growing importance of drugs as a part of health care in all countries and their significant impact on health care costs, and because it is an industry that has fought—sometimes successfully, sometimes not—to uphold market values, to resist government price controls, and to insist on patent protection as a necessary condition of its commercial viability. We might instead have chosen for special attention the medical profession or hospitals, all of which are important everywhere, but in the pharmaceutical industry one can see the most open and striking struggle about the role of market values in tension with other values, social, political, and ethical.

CHAPTER FIVE

The Market Wild Card

Pharmaceuticals

The provision of drugs and other technologies, but particularly drugs, is the market wild card in health care systems. Like the joker in some card games, it can be assigned any value—high or low—depending on how one wants to play it. Some countries want to assign it the highest possible value, notably the United States, resisting price control, upholding the practice of drug companies' charging whatever the market will bear. It justifies its market freedom as a necessity to pursue innovation, to improve health, and to provide a good shareholder return. A monopolistic patent system does not hurt. At the other extreme are countries that are prepared to impose price controls without too much anguish; they believe, it seems, that the health need for drugs trumps standard market principles. In between are countries that assign a somewhat lower medical status to drugs than to physician and hospital care, expect patients to pay a good portion of their costs, and walk a tight rope between population health needs and market freedom. Yet almost everywhere in the world, including the United States but particularly in developing countries, there are now millions of people who cannot afford drugs that will save their lives. The market is given its head. Supply and demand rules (mainly).

What is the proper response of government and the industry to this situation, an enormous human tragedy? Adam Smith proposed, in effect, a compromise position in analogous situations. People were, in his time, starving from an inability to buy corn. He was morally responsive to that problem yet serious about the value of the market as the best way to distribute needed goods. Do not interfere with the market in the sale of corn, he wrote, but provide instead government relief for those unable to pay for it.[1] No such empathy was visible later on, during the Irish famine of 1845–1847, known as the Great Hunger and brought about by a potato blight. The British government initially took a non-interventionist stance, believing it counterproductive to interfere in the food or job market. Protection of a laissez-faire policy was thought more important than the relief of suffering.[2]

In contrast, many countries have established price controls during times of war, as did the United States in World War II (and which led to employer-based health insurance as an untaxed employee benefit: an end run on the price controls). Government price controls are, to be sure, the ultimate repudiation of market values as the highest values, but is it a comparable repudiation if a government uses its monopolistic purchasing power to bargain with the drug industry for lower prices? Is that to be counted as an acceptable market transaction? It seems to us that it is, and in political practice it is regularly done.

We mention this history because the availability and provision of drugs, by now a necessity in good health care, puts the relationship between the market and health care in the starkest, most direct terms. The drug business targets the sick and unashamedly seeks to gain a generous profit from meeting their health needs; it is a business, not a social charity. Unlike the doctor in a traditional fee-for-service relationship, who also sells his or her skills to the sick but has well-established professional moral obligations to them, the drug industry has no countervailing tradition of a duty to put the welfare of the patient above all other values. It is a drug company's stakeholders who have that lofty position, not the patients it treats.

DUTIES OF THE INDUSTRY

That one-sided feature of the relationship between a drug company and its customers does not preclude what might be termed second-order obligations, such as the safety and efficacy of its products, nor does it preclude charitable contributions and philanthropic work. Neither does it preclude the constant claims of the industry that its aims are the improved health of its customers. That may be true enough, but these aims are of logical necessity advanced as voluntarily chosen goals, not built into the very nature of the enterprise the way patient welfare is built into a physician's calling. We want to argue that, by virtue of its crucial role in health care, the drug industry has de facto taken on serious moral responsibilities that can, on occasion, be stronger than its duties to its stakeholders. But that is not the view of the pharmaceutical industry,

even if it can sometimes be pushed, pressured, cajoled, and shamed to temporarily set aside obligations to stakeholders.

The pharmaceutical industry has been, for years, the most lucrative of all
industries, with in the vicinity of a 15 to 20 percent annual profit (figures
disputed by some, we add, though with mixed persuasive success).[3] The industry has claimed for itself all of the rights and privileges that go with a
market-driven for-profit enterprise, notably a right to be free from undue government interference and (save for matters of safety and drug efficacy) from
economic regulation. That claim has been buttressed by reiterated assertions
that, precisely because it is a market-driven enterprise, it is able to be innovative, economically profitable, and an immensely valuable contributor to human health. It defends the high price of its products on the grounds of the
difficulty, economic risk, and expense of developing new drugs.

Many governments, notably in Canada and Western Europe, have been resistant to such claims, but not by flatly denying them. By their regulatory
behavior they have said in effect that the benefits of drugs, their imperative
need in health care, put them in a different market category. It is one that
requires, if not a repudiation of market values—none seem to go that far, particularly in countries where the free play of the market is otherwise acceptable
—then a recognition that its force on occasion must be subordinated to other
goods, in this case that of the equitable provision of health care. That argument
(usually implicit) then joins the ethical and political issue most directly: are
there some societal needs and moral values that transcend those of the market,
however useful it may otherwise be—and is the provision of drugs in that
category? Many nations, it is clear, take exactly that position, and it is no less
clear that, even in the United States, there is considerable uneasiness about a
purely market approach to drug provision, even among those who are ordinarily strong market proponents. Internationally, public pressure, and maybe
some embarrassment, have led the drug industry to make accommodations
with its critics.

DRUGS AND THE INFINITY MODEL

There is another consideration, not so far part of the now-international
debate on the management of drug prices: that of the pharmaceutical industry's
role in feeding the infinity model of medicine, that of a medicine with no
final or finite goals—medicalizing as many of life's problems as possible; selling expensive drugs with marginal benefits, if any, over older, less expensive

drugs; aiming for endless progress wherever it might lead. While there are many doubts about the effectiveness of individual drugs, even granting their great overall benefits, there can be little doubt that, if for profit reasons alone, the pharmaceutical industry will continue to develop new products. Given patent limitations, competition among drug companies, and the development of generics, endless progress is seen as an economic necessity. Together with an explicit premise of market thought—that it is not its task, nor within its power, for the market to determine what count as reasonable human goals, aspirations, or individual preferences—competitive forces and public demand make the drug industry an almost perfect embodiment of the infinity model of medical progress. It is an utterly open-ended enterprise, hospitable to responding not only to traditional medical goals, themselves open to constant modification, but no less to desires for endless human enhancement.

This is partly true of the entire modern medical enterprise, but in the case of the pharmaceutical industry it has behind it a clear and unadulterated profit-seeking aim—not true of most medical practice, which has historically built within it (if erratically applied) an explicitly altruistic aim. Most health care provision does not aim to make the sick want more health care than they need to make them well. Hospitals aim to discharge their patients, and doctors to treat them. Drug companies make the most money from diseases that are chronic, not admitting of cure; and, if one is well in any conventional sense of "well," it is an industry prepared to help us deal with those ordinary stresses and strains of life not traditionally part of the medical model. And why not: if people want something, and it will do them no obvious harm, why not sell it to them? It is not the industry's task, many would argue, to pass moral or social judgment on individual preferences. The line between health-enhancing drugs and lifestyle-enhancing drugs has all but been erased.

The difficulty with a market-driven infinity enterprise is that it admits of no natural or intrinsic limits. It is in principle (though hardly always in practice) resistant to rationing and economic controls. If people want to buy what the drug market can produce, why should they be stopped from doing so? Yet this market momentum, by its own logic—responsive to expressed preferences, good or bad—endlessly forces up costs. Sooner or later they begin to appear unaffordable to health care systems, even if, for some individuals, they can be afforded; and even if some reform schemes are proffered to evade the whole problem by more clever administrative or research strategies.

In short, since there are no *intrinsic* limits to its market drive (as distinguished from external competitive pressures), the pharmaceutical enterprise invites external regulation and control. An impersonal market, responsive only to expressed preferences, many of which it creates with its products, neither can nor will set limits of its own other than those imposed by economic constraints. Moreover, there is likely to be constant pressure to include the expressed preferences within insured or reimbursable programs, by both consumers and the drug companies. They are introduced as a choice to meet an expressed desire; they soon become needs, to be reimbursed. Unlike, say, surgery, drugs have an enormous seductive power, which is why patients want them, even when they are not needed or will do them little if any good. Drugs are little trouble to take, will usually have minimal side effects, and, even if they do no good, are unlikely to do much harm. When they really work to relieve pain or to cure or control a disease, they become irresistible—even when, for economic reasons, they must be resisted.

REGIONAL PHARMACEUTICAL PRACTICES AND POLICIES

In 2003, there was a reported 9 percent constant growth in international drug sales. There are some one million different drug brands on the market, not counting over-the-counter drugs. North America, Europe, and Japan accounted for 88 percent of world drug consumption in 2003. North American sales grew 11 percent, to $229.5 billion; European Union sales by 8 percent, to $115.4 billion; and sales in Asia (save for Japan), Africa, and Australia, by 12 percent, to $37.3 billion.[4]

THE UNITED STATES

The United States has paid special attention to drugs in recent years. The initiative of the Bush administration in pushing for a Medicare pharmaceutical benefit, the first major reform in the Medicare program for the elderly since 1965, was a major political struggle in 2003, barely forced through Congress and leaving in its wake continued debate and recriminations. Conservatives did not like it because of its costs, and liberals attacked it on the grounds that it did not go far enough and was too favorable to market ideas.[5] The fact that the Bush administration had presented the cost of the reform as $400 billion, while later, more accurate, figures showed it would be closer to $534 billion, and then to $720 billion, did not help the administration. As Republican Senator Judd Gregg, who voted against the reform, was quoted as saying: "It's hard to believe you could spend $400 billion and have it be a political loser."[6]

At the same time, the cost of new drugs and the percentage of health care costs devoted to drugs more generally continued at a rapid pace. Those costs in 2002 increased to a rate of 10.5 percent per annum (and are estimated to rise to 14.5% in 2012), continuing a trend of double-digit inflationary increases. Drug expenditures as a proportion of overall health care costs jumped from 7.8 percent in 1998 to 10.5 percent in 2002. Along with growing hospital costs, almost in a neck-and-neck tie, drug costs were a major driver in general health care cost increases. Although, as we note below, there are many calls for a more careful evaluation of pharmaceutical effectiveness, hardly anyone doubts that, overall, drugs have become enormously more important for health than in the past. What might be called the "old medical paradigm," focused on physician and hospital care, has now been expanded to cover drugs as well.[7]

There are some arguments about the reasons for these increases. According to one group of analysts, while new drugs played their role, much of the rise can be traced to intensified use.[8] For another group, it is the impact of new drugs rather than increased prices for old drugs. Whatever the reason (though we lean toward the former, Smith analysis), for all of these cost increases—as a California study in 2001 made clear—some 18 percent of seniors had no drug insurance, while 27 percent of those covered by California's Medigap program were paying $100 a month of their own money to get adequate coverage. Some 18 percent reported either not filling a prescription due to cost or skipping doses to make a drug last longer.[9] The Bush bill will surely make a difference with seniors, but not for younger age groups; and even with seniors, rising drug costs may reduce the value of the benefits.

While hardly anyone doubts the overall health benefits of drugs, new and old (though with much debate—see below—about the specific benefits of specific drugs), the pharmaceutical industry must surely rank near the top in bad publicity and harsh attacks. It is criticized for its high profits, its intense lobbying clout, its manipulation of medical practice and doctors' prescribing practices, its seduction of medical students, its resistance to any and all government price reforms that might weaken its market power, its egregious tax breaks, its dependence on government for basic research (with no compensation to the National Institutes of Health [NIH] for the enormous financial as well as scientific benefit of its basic research), and its harmful effects on university science. Arnold S. Relman and Marcia Angell, both former editors of the New England Journal of Medicine, have been among its most relentless and articulate critics.[10] The wide-ranging critical literature on the industry itself is now almost matched by the literature on conflict of interest that has developed to analyze, and help reform, those conflicts that arise from the actions and publications of academic researchers paid by, or with financial interests in, the drug industry.[11]

Marketing and Lobbying

We will note, in telegraphic fashion, just a few of the mainly familiar arguments that have broken out in recent years about drug industry practices, each one embodying market tactics. A number of medical schools are now trying to resist the incursion of company "detailers," whose job it is to introduce students to drug products, both with sample products and with assorted items ranging from free pens (company name embossed) to free dinners, free speakers, and, for faculty members, trips to lovely destinations to hear lectures (not an excessive number) about the data on new products. One estimate showed that the industry spends about $15.7 billion each year in marketing medications, with $4.8 billion devoted to detailing individual physicians (about $6,000 to $11,000 a doctor per year).[12] One of us has on his desk at this writing no less than five sample products provided by his internist, in each case provided by the doctor along with the words, "see if this does any good." That same author (older by far than his healthy coauthor) has been told by that same internist that he meets at least five detail people a week in his group practice. Of course, the internist could simply say no—but he concedes that he listens because there is simply no time to trace down some definitive analysis in the vast, always growing, pharmaceutical literature.

Washington is a city full of lobbyists, though it may not have reached that magical state where there is one lobbyist for each citizen. The pharmaceutical industry is one of its more active practitioners. The Pharmaceutical Research and Manufacturers of America (PhRMA), the leading professional group for the industry, planned to increase its 2003 budget some 23 percent, to $150 million.[13] Among its stated goals was to spend $15.8 million to combat a union-driven Ohio voter initiative to lower drug prices for those with no insurance to pay for such costs; $2 million to $2.5 million to "generate a higher volume of messages from credible sources" warm to the industry; and $9.4 million for public relations efforts, including many "inside the beltway" efforts. The state government affairs division of PhRMA planned to spend $3.1 million in retaining more than sixty lobbyists in the fifty states.[14]

The direct-to-consumer (DTC) advertising campaign, initiated in a serious way in the 1990s, has, so far as we know, few counterpart in other countries

(New Zealand is one). It might, then, be seen as one of the purest instances of the use of market techniques for commercial gains in the selling of drugs: go after the customers themselves, together with the doctor as middleman, though that doctor was, and still is, the prime sales target. It was a shrewd move, even if it is the doctor who is supposed to pass medical judgment on the drug whose ad the patient has seen. Since apparently well over 80 percent of physicians are likely to acquiesce in the patient's choice—as long as there are no obvious medical harms—it turns out to be a most effective sales technique. Doctors like to please patients, sometimes even when it does the patient no good (and as long as it is doing no obvious harm). The best evidence for that can be seen in the decades-long campaign, not yet wholly successful, to persuade physicians (who already knew better anyway) not to prescribe antibiotics for colds or transitory children's ailments lest they inadvertently build up antibiotic resistance.

Since physicians have for long been wined, dined, solicited, and elucidated on the industry's claim of the efficacy of assorted drugs, one might wonder why further efforts to push the drugs, via patients, were necessary. The simple answer is that they were effective, adding one more sales possibility. A number of studies have tried to assess the benefits to patients of this industry move. The essence of the industry claim is that DTC advertising is a case of beneficial patient information: patients find out about useful drugs they might never have heard about, and (as an implication) perhaps their physician as well. The outcome studies are mixed. One study found that, while 80 percent of advertising was directed at physicians, the ads directed at consumers increased the use of prescription drugs—and that, despite U.S. Food and Drug Administration (FDA) oversight, misleading ads could slip through before that oversight could take effect.[15] Another study could find no harmful effects on drug consumers, comparing those who took advertised drugs and other prescription drugs.[16] An earlier study noted physicians' resistance to the idea of DTC, but mainly offered some ideas about how to safeguard the whole process.[17] The available literature would suggest one conclusion: advertising in general works, well-honed market techniques aimed at consumers work, and efforts to get doctors to go along with patients' requests also work.

Are patients hurt? Probably not. One study found no health differences between patients who took advertised drugs and those who took other prescription drugs.[18] Would it be better if doctors were better informed, if they already knew about what is being advertised to their patients? Yes indeed. Is it wrong for drug companies to advertise directly to patients? Not necessarily. Is the claim on the part of drug companies that DTC advertising is just an innocuous way to educate patients valid? No; of course it is a sales technique that may happen to educate as well. Will the industry keep pushing such DTC advertising? Why would it stop?[19] Will it overcome a widespread impression that there is something slightly unprofessional, even unsavory, about DTC ads? It seems already to have done so. Will the FDA continue to provide oversight of DTC activities? Surely so, but it may not cope well with its lengthy review process, which will be slow to catch misleading sales campaigns.[20] Canada and Europe allow no such advertising.

Responding to Critics

The pharmaceutical industry has hardly been unaware of its many critics. Some of the criticisms are long-standing: that its profits are too high, that it seduces physicians into prescribing ill-examined drugs for their patients, and that it is ingenious in avoiding a government choke-hold on its dubious practices. But the pressure for change has been building up of late, particularly on its prices. A number of U.S. states have entered lawsuits against the efforts of some companies to drag out their patent protection, for excessive profits, or for misrepresenting the "average wholesale price," and a group called the Prescription Access Litigation project has sued a dozen companies because of alleged unfair practices in driving up costs.

In the face of critics of its marketing practices, PhRMA adopted a marketing code in 2002 focused on the relationship of company representatives and health care professionals. Among other things it set rules against entertainment events earlier classified as educational events, and against gifts or offered items worth more than $100, and allows no grants, scholarships, or other forms of financial support offered "in exchange for prescribing products or for a commitment to continue prescribing products."[21] Critics were quick to note that the code is not binding, nor does it prescribe penalties for nonadherence.

Nonetheless, that the code was developed at all was a sign of the industry's growing sensitivity to public and government pressure. It was no less a sign that the industry understood the necessity for some limits on unrestricted market practices. In the end, the pharmaceutical industry, as illustrated by the practices sketched above, has condoned practices that are not in themselves taken to be immoral or illegal in a capitalist society. But it has come to understand that, market freedom or not, it will be judged by moral principles of a higher and more demanding kind than most other market-oriented industries, and that arguments about market freedom will not suffice to justify its marketing and pricing behavior. What seems evident, in fact, is that most of the reforms proposed for the American drug industry will require, to a greater or lesser extent, some compromise of the market freedom it has historically enjoyed.

The Tension over Drug Costs

The real drama of the various proposed reforms of drug provision, whether from liberals or conservatives, lies in the considerable unease with the present situation. It shows a large number of Americans unable to afford prescription drugs or forced to scrimp on their use, and who have become aware of the price of drugs as an important source of rising health care costs. In the Medicare pharmaceutical plan, the Bush administration, with some important bows toward the private sector, was responding to that unease. The private health care industry long ago found ways, with mixed success, of managing those costs: copayments, mandatory generic substitutions, and formularies. The government has found it a harder task in a country that does not like limits, particularly those imposed by government. If efforts to enact government-imposed price controls on drugs have never made any major headway in the U.S. Congress, they are working their way de facto, in various guises, into the American health care system, as are a number of other efforts to better manage the drug problem. We offer a variety of examples, which fall into four categories: cost-effectiveness studies, formularies, parallel purchasing, and government price leverage.

Cost-Effectiveness Studies

There is widespread agreement in the United States and elsewhere that too little is known about the cost effectiveness of pharmaceuticals. Some health economists, such as J. D. Kleinke, like to point to all the savings that drugs have brought about (for instance, formerly hospitalized patients who can now be maintained on drugs).[22] While there is scattered anecdotal evidence to back that viewpoint, the more general consensus is that broad, evidence-based information on cost effectiveness is in short supply.

A study published by the Organization for Economic Cooperation and Development (OECD) in 2003, surveying eleven countries, found a growing number of countries pursuing pharmacoeconomic assessments aiming to "establish the value-for-money of new drugs, to inform decisions on reimbursement and/

or pricing."[23] Those assessments have had mixed success, hindered by a scarcity of experts to carry out the assessments and by inappropriate prescribing. The latter, the study points out, "will require modification of prescriber behavior which is not something intrinsic to pharmacoeconomic assessment . . . If the programme objective is not cost-containment then this may not be a problem . . . [but] it is a problem if the programme objective is value-for-money since, by definition, the value of the product is being reduced through inappropriate use."[24] An American study by Neumann and colleagues concluded, after analysis of 228 databases, that "some drugs reduce net health costs, while others increase them, but the issue depends critically on the context in which the drug is used and the intervention to which it is being compared."[25] To deal with the problem of potentially biased research, noted in the Neumann paper, Uwe Reinhardt and others have proposed federal support of some independent nonprofit information organizations.[26]

Formularies

Formularies are lists of drugs that are approved or recommended by a health plan, hospital, pharmacy benefit manager, or employer. Drugs not on the lists are ordinarily not approved. As the OECD study has pointedly noted, "they become an important tool in controlling drug consumption."[27] Considerations for inclusion in the formulary are a drug's therapeutic benefits and its price. Various mechanisms are used to promote adherence to the formulary: restricting or promoting access to some drugs, preapproval requirements, or classifying drugs in various tiers, aiming to increase copayments for the expensive therapeutic equivalents. An American study of physicians' response to formularies found that half of those surveyed felt they had "a negative effect on the quality and efficiency of medical care," but variables such as participation in capitated managed care plans and having large numbers of patients in health plans with formularies were more favorable.[28] The Academy of Managed Care Pharmacy has developed formulary guidelines, aiming to bring evidence-based standards on quality as well as to evaluate the economic value of drugs relative to alternative therapies.[29]

Parallel Trade

For some years Americans have traveled to Canada to purchase less expensive drugs, a practice characterized in Europe as "parallel trade." More recently, with the advent of the internet, cross-border sales have increased and, most importantly—responding to complaints about high drug prices—the governors of some states (Wisconsin and Minnesota most notably) have advertised prescription medicine prices of Canadian pharmacy web sites on their state web sites. In 2003 Americans spent $695 million buying drugs from Canada, compared with $414 million in 2002. Two-thirds of the 2003 sales came from online transactions, the rest from people traveling to Canada to make drug purchases.[30] Online transactions, one study argued, "are a convenient solution to the issue of limited pharmaceutical access in the United States," but not without safety and other problems—and even worse, it amounts, the author argued, to looking to Canada to solve internal American problems.[31]

Remarkably, President Bush's nominee in 2004 to direct the Centers for Medicare and Medicaid Services, Mark McClellan, announced that he had agreed to facilitate Canadian drug purchases, a position he had firmly rejected when first proposed for the position and during the time he had been commissioner of the FDA. The stated worry then was the safety of imported drugs—though no comparative studies were done to compare the supposed hazards of Canadian drugs against the harm done to people who could not afford to buy drugs at all at American costs or who cut their dosages to save money. In any case, McClellan's shift—almost certainly the result of political pressure—was as good an indication as any of a new politics of drug costs. Despite market considerations of a kind ordinarily attractive to Americans, and formidable industry pressures, the need for less expensive drugs is forcing industry, inch by contested inch, to give way to popular pressure.

Government Price Leverage

Formal legislative efforts to establish price controls at the national level in the United States have traditionally been beaten back in Congress with little effort. But some recent initiatives have shown more concerted efforts at both the state and federal levels to control prices, by using the power of government as a purchaser to bargain effectively and, in some cases, simply to refuse to buy drugs considered too costly. The state of Maine, for instance, following the same path as Kentucky and West Virginia, has a program called Maine Rx. It uses the state's purchasing power to force drug companies to offer bulk discounts on prescription drugs for the elderly, the working poor, and some others. A challenge to the plan by the drug industry, leading to an injunction, was appealed to the U.S. Supreme Court, which overturned the injunction in 2003.[32] The state of Texas in early 2004 excluded Eli Lilly's highly profitable antipsychotic drug Zyprexa from its "preferred drugs" list in its Medicaid program. A committee of doctors and pharmacists said that some less expensive alternatives should be put on the list. This was no trivial matter: national sales of Zyprexa were $4.3 billion in 2003, with state health insurance programs and other public programs accounting for 70 percent of its sales.[33]

In the early spring of 2003, the Bush administration adopted policies to limit what Medicare will pay for prescription drugs, but with some rhetorical wiggling and squirming. As summarized in a *New York Times* story, "the officials said they were not imposing explicit price controls, but stretching dollars to ensure that the government would be a prudent purchaser."[34] But the then-director of the Centers for Medicare and Medicaid Services, Thomas A. Scully, was also quoted in the same story as saying that "it would be much better to have private health plans make these decisions, but I try to be the best price-fixer I can." Around the same time, the Medicare program also expanded coverage of defibrillators, but not to the extent desired by the manufacturer. "Cost," Scully was quoted as saying, "has never really been a factor in these decisions."[35] One might well ask: if not, then why not? And why are price controls pertinent for some drugs but not for some expensive heart disease technologies?

Price Control Creep

As the previous examples suggest, efforts to get around the high price of drugs in the United States have seen what can be called "price control creep," whether of a direct kind, imposed by federal or state health care agencies, or by allowing parallel trade. The drug industry will complain and market enthusiasts will be scandalized, but it is hard to imagine that hard-line opposition to price controls will continue to prevail as effectively as in the past in the face of rising drug costs. Richard Frank, a professor of health economics at Harvard, arguing against price controls, wrote in 2003 that he did not believe "that consumers' preferences should commonly be overridden by cost-effectiveness judgments." His worry was that the latter developments "may be a threat to a major source of technical advance that has improved the well-being of our citizens."[36]

But if cost-effectiveness studies and other ways of controlling costs are to be set aside in the name of "technical advance," then there would be no hope whatever for affordable drugs that are cost effective. And if consumer preference can trump cost effectiveness, then any serious effort to control costs will be badly subverted. But that reality underscores a tension in market theory, that of a clash between efficiency and consumer preference. Not all consumers, one can hardly help noticing, are enamored with efficiency.

The health economist J. D. Kleinke, a well-known advocate for the drug industry, has conceded the necessity for some rationing but has proposed a value-based approach rather than price controls. He would establish a four-tier system: (1) "no copayment for a life-saving drug; (2) a low copayment for a life-prolonging drug; (3) a moderate copayment for a life-prolonging drug; and (4) a high copayment for a life-enhancing drug."[37] Kleinke's conclusion to his article arguing for a value-based approach: "The pharmaceutical industry is a supreme example of the effectiveness of well-financed and highly regulated capitalism, warts and all. Most Americans still have access, 365 days a year, to the astounding miracles that the industry has helped produce. Forty three million uninsured fellow Americans might seem like a small price to pay for the privilege."[38] We suspect that the now forty-five million uninsured may take a different view of the "privilege."

CANADA

For many Americans interested in purchasing less expensive pharmaceuticals, Canada looks like a promised land, one that is nearby but whose drug benefits are denied to them at home. Yet in comparison with many other developed countries Canada is one of the high health care spenders, with only three of the twenty-five OECD countries spending more—the United States, Switzerland, and Germany. Moreover, though there have been calls for reform, drugs are not covered by the Canada Health Act other than for those prescribed in hospitals. While there has been a gradual shift in recent years, 61 percent of drug costs in 2002 were paid either by private insurance or out of pocket, the rest by the provincial governments (the figure was 85% in 1975), but it is still mainly private money.[39] The variation among provinces on government drug support ranges from 22 percent in Prince Edward Island to 48 percent in the Yukon Territories; and there is also variation by education and income level, with those at the bottom end least likely to have insurance coverage. Some provinces, such as Saskatchewan, British Columbia, and Manitoba, provide full public coverage but with a high deductible. While each province has a drug formulary, there is some variation in coverage.

Canada has not been immune from an increase in pharmaceutical costs, spending $15.5 billion (Canadian) in 2002, up 8.6 percent from the previous year. As other countries have done, efforts have been made to trace the reasons for the cost increases. The Patent Medicine Prices Review Board (PMPRB) noted some nine reasons for the trend, ranging through price, demographic, and physician prescribing changes. One reason altogether missing from the list is that of direct-to-consumer advertising, forbidden in Canada. But what are called "indirect ads" are not banned. They are those that identify specific drugs, promote disease awareness, and promote a company rather than its drugs. But ads on American television, available to a large portion of Canada, and on the internet are thought to have some influence.[40]

Canadian drug costs are estimated to be 31 percent less than U.S. costs net of discounts, and 44 percent if discounts are included.[41] How does Canada do it? The answer lies in the ability of the provincial governments to use their buying power, aided by the PMPRB. The provincial governments typically do not negotiate with suppliers, simply accepting or rejecting applications to add new drugs to their formularies. A variety of considerations go into this process, both pharmacological and economic evaluations, with some provincial variation in the standards of judgment (but with a 2002 all-provincial agreement to a Common Drug Review, aiming for some national consistency).[42] Quebec, for instance, will allow suppliers to charge it no more than the best available price in the rest of Canada, while Ontario uses its purchasing power to place flat restrictions on drug prices. The federal PMPRB monitors manufacturers' charges to make sure they are not excessive. It has set a limit price on new drugs as the median price charged in seven comparator countries (all European save for the United States). Nonetheless, a serious problem has been noted in the federal-provincial relationship: "the federal government is almost completely insulated from the impact of its policies because, although it regulates drug prices, it does not buy any drugs. In contrast, provincial governments have no jurisdiction over market competitiveness or pricing, yet end up paying for most of the drug expenditures incurred."[43]

For all of the presently available controls, however, one important estimate is that, because of a failure to take into account discounts by institutional purchasers in the United States, reducing their prices up to 50 percent, "it is likely that *only* those Americans who find themselves without prescription drug coverage are charged prices that exceed Canadian prices."[44] That would, of course, help explain the large number of American elderly taking trips from Maine and many Midwestern states, or placing orders over the internet. The authors of that study add an interesting comment: "Canada's provincial drug benefit programs may also be paying more than a fair price by comparison to institutional purchasers in the U.S. market."

As suggested above, the practice of providing full and inclusive coverage for physician and hospital care might be thought of as the old paradigm. The new paradigm is increasingly coming to include drugs and, at least in Canada, long-term care (a subject that American policymakers have carefully—and no doubt nervously—avoided). As a result, it is hardly a surprise that some important voices have called for the inclusion of pharmaceuticals in terms comparable to those in the old paradigm.

The Romanow report (see chapter 2) concluded that public coverage for drugs is "not the type we have come to expect for Canada Health Act Services."[45] The Kirby report went almost as far: "no Canadian individual or family would ever be obliged to pay out of pocket more than 3% [per annum] of total income for prescription drugs."[46] The much more market-oriented Mazankowski report from Alberta was strikingly silent on the whole problem of drugs. The only reference to it, almost in passing, was that drug needs could be dealt with by "expand[ing] the scope of supplementary insurance." That report, we can recall from chapter 2, urged that patients be called "customers" in the future, and presumably the aim of its supplementary proposal was that it would be easier for those customers to buy drug coverage (though no details were provided).

EUROPE

In November 2001, the German pharmaceutical industry took an unusual step. In order to avoid a 4 percent price cut planned by the Health Ministry, it agreed to contribute $189 million to the German health system.[47] The motivation behind the industry's move was not simply to avoid the cut in prices but also to avoid letting it set a bad European precedent. The fears behind the drug industry's move were not fantasies: everywhere in Europe there is heavy and increasing pressure to hold down drug costs, which have steadily risen over the years. Italy and France were among other countries that have recently imposed price cuts. While still a relatively small proportion of overall costs in most countries (from 10% to 20%), drugs are a highly visible target, and all the more attractive to aim at because a single industry is the source of the prices behind those costs—though the overall cost of drugs to a country will be a function of far more than the manufacturer's prices.

The industry's worries about the future of drug sales and profits in Europe have a double edge. One of them, worrisome to the American industry, is that the virus of price control in Europe will spread to the United States. Who can help noticing that Pfizer's cholesterol-lowering drug Lipitor has a wholesale price for a 10 mg pill of $1.88 in the United States but under $1 in European countries, and that AstraZeneca's wholesale price for Prilosec, for the treatment of ulcers, is $3.69 for a 20 mg pill in the United States but under $1.50 in Europe? Necessity may be, in the case of the United States, the mother of emulation; at least, that is the industry's anxiety.

The other industry worry is the more immediate European market situation. In 1994, the E.U. countries were, as a group, the world's leading pharmaceutical producers, with the United States second. Now the United States is the clear leader, with European producers accounting for only 22 percent of the industry's $400 billion global market. The United States, with fewer people than Europe, accounts for 46 percent of pharmaceutical sales and 60 percent of the profit.[48] A reflection of the European resistance to high prices is that the United States is heavily responsible for the sale of new brand-name drugs (usually a more costly item), some 70 percent, compared with 18 percent in Europe and 4 percent in Japan.[49] An additional worry for European drug manufacturers is that the ten new E.U. member countries—heavily from Eastern Europe and relatively poor compared with Western Europe—will become a new source for parallel market sales. They will be able to resell drugs purchased at government-controlled low costs at a higher price in the richer Western European countries.[50]

"Step-by-step, the profitability of European markets is decreasing, and we're depending on the U.S. more and more," the CEO of a leading French drug manufacturing company has said, ". . . and each year we increase prices a little in the U.S. and each year we have to decrease a little in Europe . . . After a few years down the line, it's a disaster."[51] Yet that "disaster" is the source of some American complaints. As Donna Shalala, Secretary of the Department of Health and Human Services under President Clinton, was quoted as saying in the same news story, the NIH has paid for much of the basic research that lies behind the industry's products, but "in return we get to pay higher prices. It's not fair." "Why," she asked, "should American taxpayers be subsidizing the Norwegians and the French and everybody else?"[52]

We might note that the industry has responded to such unfriendly questions by sometimes arguing that the general profitability of the American drug industry is of great value to the country's economic progress; and that, in any case, its high prices are a main ingredient in the industry's innovations, which benefit the United States but help other countries as well, a win-win situation. It is not as if the United States has stolen drug development from Europe. It is that, because of its market dedication, the United States has nurtured a more favorable research milieu, but one as good for Europeans as for Americans.

The rulings of the various E.U. authorities in recent years, hardly supportive of the industry, raise an issue of more than passing interest: the tension between health policy (health care and public health) and industrial policy (research and development and employment interests). The European countries, for many years the leaders in the pharmaceutical industry—for reasons both of an important historical thread running back to the nineteenth century and the emergence of sophisticated research in German industry, and of supportive academic and government support—have now come into an era that seems to indicate that the earlier balance in its favor has now shifted to an emphasis on the health importance of drugs and the need to keep them affordable. Laments about the decline of the German pharmaceutical industry do not appear to elicit great bursts of sympathy from a German government concerned about rising drug costs and E.U. authorities strongly swayed in the health and solidarity direction.

Yet while nothing might be of greater benefit to the health side of the balance than common pricing in the European Union, that has been an elusive goal. The general aim has been—beginning with the thalidomide disaster of the 1960s—to set a common European standard on matters of manufacturing standards, safety, the licensing of drugs, and the setting of drug prices. With the exception of drug prices, considerable progress has been made. There is, in that respect, a single medicines market. But not for prices. Why the difference? A provocative paper by two distinguished analysts, Gavin Permanand and Elias Mossialos, deals directly with that issue, which the authors describe as "a deadlock." There is, they write, "a dissonance between the principle of subsidiarity (which enables national governments to determine healthcare policy) and the free movement of goods of the single [supranational] market (under which medicines are treated as an industrial good)."[53]

Permanand and Mossialos provide a brief history of what they call the " 'Europeanization' of pharmaceutical policy," moving since 1965 through a variety of stages. The rationale behind each major step of the European community—safety, efficacy, therapeutic benefit—was a common health threat but always requiring a balance with industry policy interests. While there was progress in eliminating tariffs across the E.U. countries, together with the safety issues, that momentum did not carry over to prices. The 1986 Single European Act aimed to establish a single European market for the free movement of all goods, and it singled out the pharmaceutical area as one that was "irretrievably linked to public health."[54]

The fact that, in 1988, the price differential among E.U. countries was up to five times on single products seemed to make the case for common pricing all the more imperative. Nonetheless, the single market idea has not caught on with pricing. Instead, Permanand and Mossialos detect what they believe has been a bias within industry toward the status quo, which, if correct, suggests that the industry believes it is better off with individual country pricing than with E.U. harmonization. But their article was written before the various E.U. court and other decisions that shifted common policy in the health and cost-controlling direction. A Canadian study, focusing on the industry-health tension in the 1990s, brought out how difficult it was to promote "innovative investment and controlling rising health care costs."[55] Ontario—the country's most important center for drug research—as this article and other observers have noted, has offered tax breaks and other supports for the industry and, at the same time, has been considerably less firm on price controls than, say, British Columbia.

CONTROLLING PHARMACEUTICAL COSTS: EUROPEAN STRATEGIES

The most striking difference between the United States and Western Europe is that the latter simultaneously holds on to the deep-seated tradition of universal care—even if with variable proclivities toward market practices—and uses the power of government to ensure its continued existence. Callahan has argued for some years that there is little chance that the United States will ever come to accept universal care unless it is willing also, and simultaneously, to embrace government control of expenditures.[56] Neither part of that argument is attractive to most Americans. But as the European experience shows, you can't have one without the other. Unlike Canada, which has not come close to giving drug coverage parity with physician and hospital care, Europe has for long embraced the "new paradigm" of health care, recognizing the importance of drugs and long-term care for health care. No doubt part of its willingness to do so was that Europe was the heartland for many decades of pharmaceutical manufacturing and sales. There was both an industrial and a health care motive to provide good drug coverage.

What might not have been foreseen was that drug costs would eventually begin outrunning increases in general consumer prices and other health care costs. Well over a decade ago, pharmaceuticals were commanding anywhere from 10 to 18 percent of health expenditures in E.U. countries.[57] In most of the countries, the growth of per capita expenditures from 1990 to 1997 (save for Ireland, Switzerland, the United Kingdom, and Germany) far exceeded the growth in per capita health expenditures.[58] The Netherlands, Australia, Denmark, and Sweden saw an increase of over 8 percent, with 13 percent in Denmark. The United States saw from 1997 to 2002 an average annual increase of prescription drug expenditures from 10.3 to 15.3 percent.[59] In 2002 prescription drug spending accounted for 16 percent of all health spending increases (compared with 32% for hospitals). While there was some correlation between a country's gross domestic product (GDP) and drug expenditures, the OECD study noted that there was enough variation to limit the value of that correlation as a good explanation of the country differences.[60]

Given the European experience with pharmaceutical price increases—and the general willingness in the European health care tradition to use government regulation to deal with difficult cost and managerial problems—it is hardly surprising to find some strong actions to control drug costs. The range of tactics has been wide: patient cost-sharing, positive and negative lists of drugs that will be subsidized, control of the number of products allowed, formularies, profit control (limited to the United Kingdom), price freezes and price cuts, price control, expenditure ceilings, allowing parallel imports, and influencing physicians' prescribing practices.[61]

As the range of means used to control drug prices in Europe indicates, there appear to be few ideological or practical hesitations to using the power of government to keep drug prices affordable. This development has left the European drug industry unhappy, notably the Germans, who have seen their pharmaceutical industry decline in relationship to the United States. The courts and commissions of the European Union have offered them no encouragement. In March 2004, the European Court of Justice approved of a German sickness fund policy that covers patients' cost at pharmacies up to a fixed level. The Court said that drug companies (which brought the case) should not be able to challenge the reimbursement practices under E.U. competition rules. The funds, the judges said, "fulfill an exclusively social function, which is founded on the principle of national solidarity and is entirely non-profit making."[62] The sickness funds, it noted, are not in competition with one another or with private institutions. The scope of this ruling extends beyond Germany. It means that committees of doctors, who set the pharmacy prices and ceilings, can act the same way in other countries with similar institutions.

The European Union Council of Ministers in 2003 voted to uphold a ban on DTC advertising. In 2002 the European Commission had pushed for a relaxation of its standing rule on the subject by permitting those suffering from AIDS, asthma, and diabetes to receive "patient education information" from drug companies (by American standards a mild enough request). The council rejected the request, noting among its reasons that U.S. spending on drugs between 1993 and 1998 had increased by 84 percent, with almost a fourth of that attributable to the ten most advertised drugs.[63]

In April 2004 the Court of Justice ruled against German practices that had blocked the import of cut-rate drugs from southern European countries.[64] The decision supported the discounters, saying that they promote the free movement of goods between European member states and give consumers lower prices. The industry had held that the (parallel) trade is unfair because prices are already set in many cases by national governments; and, as others have claimed, parallel trading already takes $5 billion a year from the industry.

Though the European countries have for years used price controls on drugs, have those control tactics actually worked? Given the steady increase in drug prices in all the European countries—and the use of comparative costs in other countries as an important way of setting drug prices, which can result in all of them rising simultaneously—one might well wonder. In considering reference pricing as a possible means of price control in the United States, Kanavos and Reinhardt have noted that it would face serious political obstacles and, in any case, would be complex to put into practice.[65]

The English health economists Alan Maynard and Karen Bloor have passed a generally negative judgment on the various European means of controlling costs, whether they be that of influencing patients and providers or regulating industry. All are found wanting in one way or another, with the common thread being that of wholly inadequate assessment by an "economics-based medicine." About price control schemes, they note, those that do not "control volume are incomplete"; and it is physician discretion, not price alone, that determines volume. More broadly they conclude about the regulation of the international drug market "that there is little new, and much that is unconsciously replicated, with scant resource to the evidence base. Policy innovations to regulate the market worldwide have rarely been evaluated scientifically."[66]

DEVELOPING COUNTRIES

Drugs offer a simple, cost-effective answer to many health problems in developing countries—provided that they are available, accessible, affordable, and properly used.[67] In 1975, the World Health Organization (WHO) introduced the concept of "essential drugs" as a pragmatic approach to accelerate the positive effects of drugs on health status, particularly for developing countries. An essential drug is defined as one that is clinically proven to be safe and effective; available in a stable, easily managed form; made with only one active ingredient, unless there is a good reason otherwise; designed to meet clearly defined health care needs; less expensive than comparable drugs; and appropriate for a wider range of local conditions.[68]

Under the essential drugs approach, national governments adopt a list of drugs that satisfies the health needs of the majority of the population, and take steps to make them available at all times, in adequate amounts, and in the appropriate dosage forms.[69] The WHO approach also called on governments to centralize drug purchases at the national level, to order only the most essential drugs (mainly generics), and to take advantage of competition on the international market by issuing bids.

The procedure for the inclusion of drugs in essential lists has not been without controversy. The powerful pharmaceutical industry has made attempts to influence entry of its products into essential lists in a variety of ways. These include producing branded generics and justifying higher prices with the claim that brand-name generics guarantee quality.[70] China, generally considered the next great frontier for drug companies because of its sheer market size, also adopted the essential drugs concept in 1994. Since then, foreign pharmaceutical companies, convinced that being on the essential drug roster is a prerequisite for survival in China, have been jostling to have their products listed, and there have been some accusations of drug companies bending the rules by "talking to the right people" in the different Chinese regions and provinces to get their products into lists.[71]

Nearly 160 countries (both developed and developing) have essential drug lists, and usage of these listed drugs grew from 2.1 billion people in 1977 to 3.8 billion in 1997.[72] Despite these gains, an estimated one-third of the world's population still lacks regular access to essential drugs, with this figure rising to over 50 percent in the poorest parts of Africa and Asia.[73] While the total expenditure on health care in many developing countries is not substantial, the proportion spent on pharmaceutical products is great.

After personnel costs, pharmaceuticals are generally the largest item of expenditure in national health budgets in most developing countries. Drug expenditures in developing countries represent between 10 and 40 percent of public health budgets and between 20 and 50 percent of total health care expenditures, compared with an average of 12 percent in developed countries.[74] In 1997, for example, Thailand's pharmaceutical expenditures represented 35 percent of total public and private health expenditures, China's expenditures accounted for 45 percent, while in Mali the percentage was 66 percent and in Indonesia 45 percent.[75]

Drug expenditures involve substantial private, out-of-pocket payments by individual patients, with the poor spending a disproportionate share of household income on the purchase of drugs—sometimes more than twice as much as the richest 10 percent of the population spends.[76] Pharmaceutical products are important not only to consumers but also to health care providers in developing countries. Studies carried out in Nigeria, for example, showed that, when health facilities ran out of commonly used drugs, visits by patients dropped by between 50 and 70 percent.[77] Drug availability thus draws patients to health facilities where they can benefit from other services, including preventive services.[78] Medicines are usually the raison d'être of health centers in many developing countries.[79] As A. Alland wrote in 1970, "The health worker is the adjunct to medicines. You have to see him because it is through him that you will acquire desired medicines. The doctor's value lies in the drugs he gives. After all, the people believe, it is the drugs that make medicine work, not the doctor or nurse."[80]

Developing countries finance and distribute drugs in a variety of ways. Before the post-1980s market reform period described in chapter 4, the World Health Organization's recommended approach—a public centralized system where drugs are financed and procured by government—was the standard practice in most developing countries. Under this system, the total amount spent on drugs, like other health care services, was constrained by government budgets. After market-oriented reforms were adopted in the 1980s, most developing countries, but particularly those in Africa and Latin America, established systems where drugs were supplied by government medical stores or state-owned wholesalers and dispensed by government health facilities, but paid for (in whole or in part) by user fees.

A Thriving Private Drug Sector

Parallel to this system, all developing countries have a thriving private, for-profit pharmaceutical sector, with patients paying the entire costs of drugs by purchasing from privately owned retail pharmacies. Some developing countries also have social health insurance reimbursement systems, where public funding from central budgets and social health insurance premiums are used to reimburse pharmacies or patients themselves for drugs provided through private pharmacies. In some countries, including Kenya, Nepal, and Nigeria, nongovernmental organizations play a vital role in the supply of drugs. In Kenya, for example, two religious organizations established a program with funding from three European countries to supply good-quality essential drugs at a reasonable cost to church-managed health units throughout the country. These units now constitute roughly 36 percent of the country's rural health services.[81]

Most developing countries, therefore, have a combination of public, user fee, and private models of financing of pharmaceutical products. Because of the current pluralistic approach to health care financing in developing countries, different models may be found for different groups in the population. In some countries, for example, fully public financing and supply may be used for the poor and for the treatment of infectious diseases, social health insurance for civil servants and those in formal employment, and a fully private model for populations and categories of drugs not covered by other systems.[82]

In the 1980s, citing the failure of government drug supply systems to provide adequate and efficient services, the World Bank and International Monetary Fund (IMF) instructed several developing countries to include the privatization of sections of the public drug sector as part of the broad health sector reforms (these reforms are discussed in greater length in chapter 4). These international financial institutions saw the problems facing public drug supply as symptomatic of fundamental problems in the national health sector:

1. Lack of incentives for efficient behavior
2. Unclear institutional relationships and responsibilities
3. Political interference
4. Public sector rigidities, particularly bureaucratic staff regulations
5. Absence of competition
6. Inadequate financial resources[83]

In 1994 the World Bank stated that the most important problems facing pharmaceutical markets in Africa were inefficiency and waste. Studies in Nigeria, for example, found that ineffective and even dangerous drugs had frequently been procured by the government, and that brand-name rather than less expensive generic drugs were purchased locally in small quantities rather than in bulk from foreign producers.[84] In response to the World Bank and IMF, several developing countries introduced private sector management methods and elements of competition into the procurement and delivery of pharmaceuticals, including user fees for drugs and revolving drug funds schemes.

Despite the introduction of market mechanisms aimed at improving quality and efficiency, drug procurement and management in developing countries has been plagued with several problems. Surveys from several developing countries show that between 10 and 20 percent of sampled drugs fail quality-control tests.[85] This problem can be attributed partly to insufficient drug-regulatory capacity. Fewer than one in three developing countries are estimated to have fully functioning drug-regulatory authorities, and this has contributed to the growing problem of fake drugs entering the market. A senior pharmaceutical industry executive wrote in the *Lancet:* "Some health officials in Africa have stated that counterfeit medicines are a greater public health threat than AIDS or malaria."[86]

Granted that it is in the pharmaceutical industry's financial interest to check the proliferation of counterfeit drugs, the danger of adulterated medicines in developing countries is a real concern. Approximately 65 percent of 751 instances of counterfeit production reported to the WHO and Interpol over the course of fifteen years occurred in developing countries. According to the WHO, counterfeiting is facilitated where there is weak drug-regulatory control and enforcement; where there is scarcity and/or erratic supply of basic medicine; where there are extended relatively unregulated markets and distribution chains, in both developing and developed countries; where price differentials create an incentive for drug diversion within and between established channels; where there is lack of effective intellectual property protection; and where due regard is not paid to quality assurance.[87]

Continuing Problems

Other problems faced by developing countries include poor storage and distribution facilities. A study in Cameroon found that central medical stores lost 35 percent of their drugs because of poor storage and poor inventory control.[88]

In Cameroon, 30 to 40 percent of all government-procured drugs are thought to be "withdrawn for private use" by staff and, in 1982, an estimated 70 percent of government drug supply in Guinea simply disappeared.[89]

Developing countries also have to confront the problem of an irrational use of drugs. For example, up to 75 percent of antibiotics are prescribed inappropriately even in teaching hospitals, chloroquine resistance has been reported in eighty-one countries, and up to 98 percent of *Neisseria gonorrhoeae* is resistant to penicillin.[90] The costs of antimicrobial resistance are very high—second-line treatment for resistant malaria or meningitis may be fifty to ninety times more expensive than the original treatment. If drug costs are to be affordable and common diseases treatable, it is important for countries to contain such resistance. Prescribing and dispensing patterns in many countries are influenced by sociocultural factors such as patients' demand, the prescriber's attitude to risk, previous prescribing experiences, and drug promotion.[91] Misleading advertisements for pharmaceuticals are commonplace in many developing countries, and also contribute to irrational use and inappropriate prescribing practices.

Because most poor countries do not have adequate regulatory structures, controlling the prices charged for drugs in the private sector is difficult. In Sierra Leone in 1983, the mark-up on private sector sales of chloroquine ranged from 400 to 800 percent.[92] Deregulation of imports and sales of drugs has led to a large black market in several countries in Africa. In addition, many private retail pharmacies are run by unqualified persons who sell expired and adulterated drugs.

The World Bank noted as early as 1994 that informational asymmetries, the separation of financiers from decision makers at the consumption level, and poor management of drug supplies render pharmaceutical markets in most sub-Saharan African countries highly inefficient. There are additional concerns about the desirability of market mechanisms in public drug supplies in developing countries. Because the private sector is so poorly developed, contracting out services may only replace a government service monopoly with a private one—with no real competition taking place. It is also not clear how contractors in developing countries can assure quality; and it can be argued that the profit motive may prompt them to cut corners to reduce costs. If lower costs are attained at the price of lower quality, the result in terms of improved efficiency is unclear.

Competitive contracting can only occur if the government has adequate negotiating and monitoring capacity to ensure the services are carried out according to the negotiated contracts. Many developing countries, particularly those in Africa, do not have such capacity. Another concern is that governments might tend to establish long-term relationships with a private sector company, thereby driving other companies out of the market, resulting in less future competition.[93]

Developing countries are faced with the colossal challenge of trying to keep drug costs down while at the same time ensuring their citizens have the best possible access to quality medicines. Even though all developing countries rely heavily on importation of pharmaceuticals, some countries, like Brazil, China, Egypt, Nepal, Indonesia, Sri Lanka, and India, have sizeable drug manufacturing industries, and their governments are under pressure to develop regulatory instruments to protect and promote local manufacturers in the face of increasing competition from multinational drug companies.[94] In order to strengthen local firms' competitiveness in the regional and global pharmaceutical markets, the governments of Colombia, Ecuador, Nepal, and Venezuela organized and financed training programs in good manufacturing practices for local producers. Some countries also give local suppliers preference in public tendering, as long as the bid price is within 10 to 15 percent of the overseas prices. Because most developing countries limit drug procurement to essential drugs, this means that local manufacturers are encouraged by both volume and a price advantage to concentrate on their production.[95] Some local manufacturing companies in developing countries—particularly those in East and Southeast Asian countries—have entered into joint ventures with multinational companies. For example, India's Ranbaxy Laboratories recently entered into a five-year joint partnership with GlaxoSmithKline to collaborate in research and clinical development covering a wide range of therapeutic areas.[96]

Partly in response to the increasing cost of drugs and the declining availability of public resources for financing pharmaceuticals, a number of African countries are adopting cost recovery and self-financing programs such as those proposed under the Bamako Initiative. Under these insurance programs, communities share in the financing of local health services by buying drugs in bulk at wholesale prices and then using the proceeds to maintain drug supplies and subsidize services. These programs are locally managed and built around facilities, geography, or preexisting groups. At the broader level, these programs are designed to provide protection mechanisms for the poor and other vulnerable groups.[97] The community financing programs are also designed to provide a reliable supply of low-cost essential drugs of good quality, provide good administrative systems for financial management, and ensure strict measures are put in place to discourage overprescribing. Yet these community insurance schemes have encountered several problems, including irrational drug prescribing, financial instability, adverse selection, poor management, and the creation of parallel delivery systems for drug procurement.[98]

Between the Public and the Private

It is increasingly clear that neither purely private nor purely public pharmaceutical systems are likely to be appropriate in developing countries. The solution probably lies somewhere between the two. While competition, flexibility, and the profit motive may make the private sector technically efficient, the concept of essential drugs and a focus on cost-effective treatment may result in greater therapeutic efficiency in the public health sector.[99] It is also well established that, in a free market, access to drugs will be based on people's ability and willingness to pay for the drugs, not on their need for them. Poor people, particularly, are likely be denied access.[100] While there may be some reasons to believe that market mechanisms may improve overall access to and quality of drugs in developing countries, there is little empirical evidence to support this.[101]

Compounding all the domestic problems facing developing countries is the increasing globalization of the international pharmaceutical markets. Today, multinational companies make decisions about pricing of drugs based on factors such as market size, protection of intellectual property, and prices for competing products.[102] When prices for drugs are set at levels aimed at developed-country markets, developing countries have no choice but to either forego purchasing the drugs altogether or buy them at manufacturers' prices, and in so doing place great pressure on their already overstretched health care budgets.

In an attempt to harmonize the way intellectual property is protected around the world, the World Trade Organization passed an agreement in 1995 known as Trade-Related Aspects of Intellectual Property Rights (TRIPS). Countries that join the WTO benefit from a reduction in tariffs when selling their goods and, in return, they must guarantee protection of products and processes by granting patents. The TRIPS agreement set out the minimum standards for the protection of intellectual property. Within this framework, TRIPS contains two "get-out" mechanisms that allow countries to manufacture (through compulsory licensing) or buy (through parallel importing) products covered by patents in exceptional circumstances.[103] Recently, for example, the United States threatened to invoke "eminent domain" to allow for compulsory licensing as a means of reducing the price of Cipro, an anthrax antibiotic used during the anthrax scare in October 2001.[104]

The TRIPS agreement created a sharp division between developed and developing countries, with the latter arguing that, under the agreement, they would be restricted from producing or importing generic drugs as a means of protecting public health in their own countries. The issue is not academic. South Africa was taken to court by the pharmaceutical industry for attempting to pass a law to allow parallel importing and compulsory licensing in the country. Despite the fact that the proposed legislation in South Africa was perfectly compliant with TRIPS, it gave rise to a protracted legal battle between South Africa and the pharmaceutical industry—in the end, delaying implementation of this urgent piece of legislation for more than three years.[105] The fact of the matter is that many developing countries lack the technical know-how to implement the provisions in the TRIPS agreement. Progress has not been helped by the tactics of governments in developed countries aimed at protecting the interests of their large domestic pharmaceutical industries.[106]

TRIPS and the Protection of Public Health

A ministerial meeting in 2001 in Doha, Qatar, provided a breakthrough for developing countries, with the WTO reaffirming that the TRIPS agreement should be interpreted and implemented to protect public health and promote access to health. The deadline for adherence with WTO conditions for the least-developed countries was also extended from 2006 to 2016.[107] The WTO has also recognized the need for differential pricing of essential drugs, whereby prices vary in accordance with national wealth, and with safeguards to prevent parallel importation of these cheaper drugs to high-income markets.[108]

After the Doha Declaration, developing countries still had one issue to resolve: how to provide extra flexibility, so that countries unable to produce pharmaceuticals domestically could obtain generics or copies of patented drugs from other countries. Most developing countries have insufficient or no manufacturing capacities in the pharmaceutical sector, and without a further amendment to the TRIPS agreement, they were certain to face difficulties in making effective use of the compulsory licensing clause. This issue, referred to as "paragraph 6," was resolved in August 2003, when WTO members agreed on legal changes to make it easier for countries to import cheaper generics made under compulsory licensing if they are unable to manufacture the medicine themselves. The decision waives exporting countries' obligations and provides that any member country can export generic pharmaceutical products made under compulsory licenses to meet the needs of importing countries, provided certain conditions are met.[109]

The patent system is profit driven, long defended as a necessary protection of research investments. Pharmaceutical companies rely heavily on patents and go to great lengths to maintain and extend them by introducing new formulations of a patented drug, by applying for second-medical-use patents for drugs nearing the end of their basic patent life, and by filing repeated patent infringement suits that trigger automatic delays in processing the generic product.[110] Patent protection has increased over the last twenty years, but the mean innovation rate has fallen. In the last twenty-five years, almost fourteen hundred new medicines were developed, but only 1 percent were for tropical diseases that kill millions each year.[111]

The much cited "10/90 divide"—with 90 percent of medical research going toward diseases for just 10 percent of the world population—shows the gross neglect of research for diseases afflicting the world's majority poor.[112] The research and development (R & D) pipeline for drugs for diseases like tuberculosis and malaria is virtually empty—even as resistance to drugs for these conditions increases. The bottom line is that the developing world does not represent a profitable market for the international pharmaceutical industry. In effect, the industry is saying that, because of an inability to pay for them, or to properly distribute and monitor them, development of drugs for the diseases of poor countries is a financial loser.

The HIV/AIDS epidemic has served to shift the tide somewhat. While drug companies have a huge stake in maintaining their high prices for HIV/AIDS drugs, they have begun lowering their prices in the face of fierce public criticism from people living with HIV/AIDS, civil society organizations, and international human rights organizations. Offers by generic drug producers such as Cipla and Ranbaxy in India, and by the Brazilian government, to provide African countries with AIDS drugs at much lower prices have served as catalysts to force drug companies to bring their prices down.

With the 2005 passage of an amendment to India's Patent Act to make it compliant with TRIPS, many questions are being raised about India's ability to continue to provide affordable drugs to developing countries. India's former patent law allowed pharmaceutical companies to copy patented drugs as long as they used a different manufacturing process. The 2005 amendment requires India to recognize patents for both processes and products. The amended law provides, however, that all generic drugs already approved for India can still be sold, though sellers must now pay licensing fees. This means that India can still provide generic drugs to poor countries, but it is not clear how prices for these drugs will be affected. As expressed by Leena Menghaney, a health activist in India, "Multinational pharmaceutical firms, which hold patents, could delay issuance of a license to make a new drug by dragging their feet over what should be the royalty amount."[113]

Some of the major pharmaceutical companies that have entered into deals with the WHO to offer substantial discounts for HIV/AIDS drugs in developing countries include Merck & Co., Bristol-Myers Squibb Co., GlaxoSmithKline PLC, Boehringer Ingelheim GmbH, and Roche Holding AG. In 2002, under pressure from activists and generic competitors, Merck offered its new once-a-day 600 mg version of the AIDS drug Stocrin for 95 cents in the poorest countries. The older version of Stocrin, three 200 mg pills a day, costs $1.37 daily in poor countries.[114] However, more than a year after this announcement, Merck has not obtained government approval to sell the drug in African countries, prompting a spokeswoman for Doctors Without Borders to make the following claim: "It appears that this [announcement by Merck] was a calculated attempt to gain media attention for a product launch in wealthy markets."[115]

Perhaps that was too cynical a comment. In any case, in December 2003, GlaxoSmithKline and Boehringer Ingelheim agreed to grant licenses to produce AIDS drugs to four generic companies in India and South Africa. The companies will be allowed to sell the drugs anywhere in sub-Saharan Africa. In return, the two license-granting companies will get royalties of 5 percent of sales. For all the accusations that have been leveled against the pharmaceutical companies for neglecting the plight of millions of people dying of AIDS, they cannot be held solely responsible for the absence of drugs in developing countries, even though we argue that they have a major role to play in trying to provide affordable drugs.

According to the WHO, of the six million people in developing countries who currently need antiretroviral therapy, fewer than 8 percent are receiving it, and without rapid access to properly managed treatment these millions of women, children, and men will die. In Africa, of the 4.4 million people in need of antiretroviral therapy, only 310,000 were receiving the drugs in 2004.

There is some hope on the horizon. In a span of less than two years, new programs such as the Global Fund to Fight AIDS, Tuberculosis and Malaria, the United States Presidential Emergency Plan for AIDS Relief, and the World Health Organization's Three by Five Program, which aims to treat three million people in five years, have been initiated. Global funding for HIV/AIDS in resource-constrained countries has, as a result, increased from just over $300 million in 1999 to an unprecedented $3 billion in 2002 and $4.7 billion in 2003, with additional funding promised by foreign governments and international donor agencies.

Other institutions, such as the William J. Clinton Foundation, the World Bank, and UNICEF, have stepped up to help countries gain access to inexpensive generic AIDS drugs. In January 2004, the Clinton Foundation announced that it had brokered deals for two American diagnostics companies to provide testing machines as well as chemicals and training in a dozen African and Caribbean countries at discounts of up to 80 percent.[116] Hidden in this announcement, however, was the requirement for recipient countries to submit large, irrevocable purchase orders, pay in cash, and show that they will keep the cheap drugs from being diverted and resold in wealthy countries—a tall, and financially questionable, order for most of the countries involved in the proposed deal.

Despite some progress in getting drugs, the sad reality for most in developing countries is that helping patients with HIV/AIDS is not just about buying drugs. As succinctly put by Gordon Perkin of the Bill and Melinda Gates Foundation, "Even if we had free and unlimited supplies of ARVs [antiretrovirals] and other essential HIV/AIDS commodities, they still would not be available to the majority of people who need them because of poor infrastructure."[117] To add to those problems, various controversies have slowed up money promised for treatment. The Bush administration has wavered, in its annual budget requests, in ways that have left some uncertainty about its $15 billion commitment. Difficulties have also emerged over the administration's failure to support generics, delaying their acceptance on grounds of possible safety issues. The international Global Fund to Fight AIDS, Tuberculosis and Malaria and the WHO have had trouble raising the money they need. In the meantime, millions continue to die.

SOCIETY AND THE PHARMACEUTICAL INDUSTRY: WHAT DO THEY OWE EACH OTHER?

The relationship between a for-profit corporation and the society in which it exists can be understood as a social contract. A society owes to those who take the trouble to start and financially maintain an industry the right to conduct its business without unnecessary interference by the state. The well-accepted Western reasons for interference are the health and safety of an industry's employees and those who use its products; health, in this broad context, is usually understood in the sense of "do no harm," rather than that of an obligation to improve health. Since an industry's survival and vitality depend on a favorable market environment to sell its products, it is a sensible course for government to use its police and regulatory powers to foster such an environment (by antitrust laws and fair trade laws, for instance). For its part, the corporation owes society . . .

But, just what does the industry owe society? There is no straight answer, no consensus, on that long-debated question. At one extreme are those who believe that, other than producing safe products, for-profit industries owe nothing special to their society. Their duty is to provide a good investment return to their shareholders, those whose money makes the industry's existence possible. Corporate philanthropy, it has been argued, is nice but hardly obligatory; and, in fact, it can be seen as unfair to its shareholders, depriving them of some profit that is rightfully theirs. At the other extreme would be a view of the corporation as a social citizen: it ought to do what it can to benefit the society that houses it, whose laws protect it, whose government services help sustain it, and whose citizen-employees are human beings who are owed a fair wage and a decent working environment. Some share of corporate profits should also be contributed, by taxation and voluntary contributions, to the welfare of the society.

Should the social contract between the pharmaceutical industry and society be different from that of other industries? We believe it should be. By virtue of its importance to population and individual health, it is second only to medicine in its health importance to society. Unlike most other industries, required only to avoid doing harm, the drug industry's self-proclaimed role is that of fostering good health; and for that it has been long and justly honored. The old paradigm of health care, we noted earlier, focused on physician and hospital care. The new paradigm now encompasses pharmaceuticals. Their considerable capacity to help keep people out of hospitals might, ironically, be seen as one important reason for the industry's admission into the center arena of health care.

The most fundamental law of social morality could be put this way: all organizations, nonprofit or for-profit, have a moral responsibility to the welfare of those who will be directly affected by their actions, whether by commission or omission. The pharmaceutical industry is a collection of such organizations. The question, we believe, is not whether there is a special social obligation to those who can be helped by its products—that seems self-evident—but (1) the extent of that obligation, and (2) how a reasonable and fair balance is to be struck between the need of the industry to flourish and the need of the public for the indispensable benefits of its product. But it must be understood that it should not be a perfect balance, as if industry welfare was the moral equal of public health welfare. The latter, with some basic human goods and needs at stake, is more important. That does not mean industry welfare is unimportant, only less important. It also serves human needs and welfare. But in a show-down, health must triumph. By virtue of its success in improving health, it could be said, the pharmaceutical industry got more social responsibility than it bargained for.

We will try to support these contentions by addressing three issues: the importance of drugs for health and the relationship between their health bene-fits and the prices the industry charges for their purchase; the right of govern-ment to interfere with standard market practices in the name of health; and the place to be given innovation for the sake of future health as a rationale for pricing and marketing policies.

The Importance of Drugs for Health and the Price of Those Drugs

The medical historian William G. Rothstein has written an as nearly indis-putable a paragraph as could be written: "Modern Medicine would be incon-ceivable without the many drugs developed in the last half century. Drugs are the most cost-effective and often the only treatment for most infectious and chronic diseases."[118] If that seems a valid judgment of a medical historian, there is also a cadre of health economists who support that judgment.[119] The fact that a number of countries, such as the United States for its elderly popula-tion, and Canada for its entire population, have of late worked to improve publicly subsidized drug coverage provides a political vote for its importance. After all, no country these days is eager to add new categories of expensive public entitlements unless there are powerful political and medical reasons to do so.

At the same time, every country is experiencing a steady increase in the cost of drug usage, with drugs now accounting for 10 to 20 percent of most nation's health care spending; and the use of drugs and their attendant price becomes all the more important in the poorer countries of the world, even more depen-dent on drugs than the more affluent countries. Because of those prices, the most market-oriented country in the world, with no price controls—the United States—has a large portion of its population with no insurance for drugs, and

even the new Medicare changes will still leave some elderly people in a difficult situation trying to pay for them. The situation of developing countries is
far worse, with tens of millions of people unable to afford drugs that can save
and greatly improve their lives. The medical need for drugs is now endemic,
and the inability of many people to pay for them is no less endemic.

The Right of Government to Interfere with the Market in the Name of Health

There are two ways to give people the drugs they need. One way is, through
taxation, to give people what they need and to increase taxes to whatever point
it takes to make that possible; in short, to use taxation to avoid interfering with
the industry's market freedom. But there is a political limit to how high taxes
can be raised and, we note, it is usually political conservatives who object to
high taxes, usually the same group that defends the drug industry's market
freedom and the prices it charges.

The other way is for national governments to use their state power to control
the price of drugs, most directly by price controls. As we have seen, European governments—however deferential to the market in other sectors—have
shown little hesitation to impose price controls, and thus to keep the provision
of drugs within an affordable range for their universal health care systems
(though almost always requiring patient copayments). The E.U. courts have of
late issued rulings supporting the right of various governments to manage and
control drug costs. In no case, so far as we can make out, has the market been
treated as something sacrosanct, necessary under all circumstances for the
common good. Europe has treated the market as a valuable economic tool, not
as ideological high ground to be defended at whatever the social cost (the view
of those we have called the politicals); and it is the health of the public that is
the final test of how, when, and where to deploy market practices.

Evidence for the utility of the market in developing countries, particularly
those that have little if any regulation of drugs, is hard to come by. While the
pre-reform health care systems in Africa had their own serious limitations,
mainly a lack of money, they represented a concerted effort to make the most of
their limited funds. The market reform era of the 1980s saw decline rather than
progress, with the World Bank pulling back in many ways from its initial
market enthusiasm in health care. As for the United States, the opposition to
price controls at the federal level remains strong, but it is the result of history
and tradition, a deeply ingrained pro-market and antigovernment strain. But

there has been no serious suggestion that price controls would violate the U.S. Constitution and, as noted above, there are many signs of a trend toward price controls at the state level and, here and there, in some federal health controls.

Three forces are at work in that direction: the need for and cost of drugs; the touting, by the industry and its advocates, of the growing importance of drugs for the health of the public; and challenges to the patent system. By claiming enormous health benefits, the industry unwittingly sews the seeds of that very market restraint that it fears. It says, in a loud and proud voice, that everyone needs and benefits from its products, but in a soft and defensive voice it claims that an inability of many to pay for its drugs is not its problem. Yet times are changing. As a historian of the industry has noted, observing its development as a social force, it "has changed from a commercial endeavor to a quasi-public one. Its relationship with society should reflect that fact."[120] The "Accountability of the Pharmaceutical Company," as the title of an article by a staff member of the Norwegian Institute of Pharmacotherapy put it, is increasingly broader and deeper than in the past.[121] And the evidence we have noted of a gradual tearing down of the wall against price controls, even in the Unite States, tells its own story. The patent system is not likely to be overturned in the near future, but some articulate voices can be heard showing that its monopoly pricing creates economic distortions, that its marketing practices lead to misuse of drugs and waste and to a distortion of the research process.[122]

Innovation: The Future versus the Present

At the core of the pharmaceutical industry's public case for high prices and market freedom to sell them has been the cost of innovation—and thus its constant progress in the war against illness, suffering, and death. There is hardly any word used more repeatedly in the literature of PhRMA than "innovation," or any argument more reiterated than the industry's great success in the past in producing it or the need in the present for high profits to keep it going. PhRMA companies, the trade association PhRMA has said, "are leading the way in the search for new cures."[123] Not prominently mentioned, actually not at all, has been the need for innovation as the key to industry return to stockholders and its historical place as one of the most profitable of all major international industries—even if not at the moment.[124]

Never directly confronted by the industry and its market supporters is a moral puzzle: why is the health of those who in the future—whether those already sick or who will be at risk eventually—will gain from the innovations generated by its research given a higher value than the health of those people in the present who cannot afford to buy already available drugs? Why are those whose lives will be saved in coming decades by cancer drugs now in the pipeline more important than the lives now being lost for lack of available AIDS drugs? Leaving aside altogether the long-standing complaint that much of the innovation is for so-called "me too" drugs, with small chemical changes and marginal health benefits, one can at least ask why it is more important to bring them to market than to make available what has already passed through the research pipeline. Even if the industry claim that the marginal benefits of drugs with small variations give physicians more choices in treating patients is accepted, why are marginally inferior drugs, that everyone might be able to afford, worse than marginally beneficial drugs that many will not be able to afford?

To ask such questions is not to deny the necessity of research for the industry, of new products to keep it alive in the face of patent limits and competition, and of the potential health benefits of new drugs. But it is to question, first, the mantra of innovation as if it inherently justifies all efforts to resist price controls, and second, the economic contentions lying behind that mantra, as if nothing else than the present level of profit and industry marketing will ensure its bright future. Nor is it our intention to deny the industry claim that, particularly with the developing countries, it is impossible for it to give everyone everything they need. They will not be able to provide affordable AIDS drugs for all or to spend large amounts of money on drugs for various tropical diseases for people who will not be able to pay for them, or who live in countries that do not have the infrastructure to properly deliver them and monitor their use. But our intention is to question whether the industry is doing *everything* in its power to overcome those obstacles, in its pricing behavior or in its cooperation with national governments and international humanitarian agencies.

Research Costs

There are three important contentions here. The first is that, according to industry sources, it costs approximately $800 million to bring a new drug to market. But other studies estimate a realistic cost of about $100 million for most drugs and up to $400 million for a few.[125] The second is that American research, supported by higher American prices, pays for most of the world's pharmaceutical research. That is wrong. Most of the large European countries have strong research efforts, and there is no evidence that (1) the branches of international drug companies in those countries only break even because of

American research, or that (2) all of the most important research takes place in the United States. At least four other countries devote a larger percentage of their GDP to drug R & D than the United States (and do so with price controls in place), and U.S. research in recent decades is hardly the only source of new drugs.[126]

The third contention is that it is innovation, the creation of new drugs, that is the most expensive kind of research. That is also wrong. For one thing, the majority of "new" drugs are variations on already available drugs, with marginal benefits, if any; and research costs for those drugs are lower than for genuinely new drugs. For another, the National Science Foundation published a report in 2003 showing that only 10 percent of American drug income is devoted to R & D, and only 1.7 percent goes to research for genuinely new, breakthrough drugs.[127] The NIH, moreover, accounts for most of the basic research of importance to the industry, a solid (and free) contribution by taxpayers to industry profit.

Drug Prices

Drug prices and profits are inextricably linked. The industry claim has been that its high prices in the United States are necessary to pay for the high costs of discovering new drugs, mainly carried out in the United States, and they in turn are necessary for the innovation that is the key to future health. We have said enough already to suggest that it is a weak claim. The last step needs to be taken: that of showing that the industry does not require the high American prices, to sustain either the American market or any other market in the developed world.

Consider the following facts (or so we construe them). In the United States itself, institutional buyers of drugs are able to gain major discounts from pharmacy prices (up to 50% off manufacturers' prices) by buying in quantity and bargaining for what they buy. But their success in bargaining not only indicates the power of market bargaining, but also makes clear that the industry has judged it can live with a lower profit margin from those sales. It has no less made clear, by its behavior, that it can live with the lower prices paid for drugs in Europe and Canada. If it could not make a profit in those countries, or with many American institutional buyers, why would it sell to them at all? Because the American prices are so high, subsidizing everyone else? But since the industry will not provide a breakdown of its gains and losses in specific countries, we are asked to simply accept its claims as proof. They are not proof at all, and there is no empirical reason, given the publicly available evidence, to accept them. One study, for that matter, concluded that drug imports from Canada to the United States might actually be a source of industry profit, or at the least a break-even result.[128]

More than that, no case has ever been made why the pharmaceutical industry needs to have the highest profits of any industry in order to return a fair share to its stakeholders. We mean by a "fair share" one that aims to strike a balance between what is owed to stakeholders for their investment and what is owed to those in need of drugs. Other industries have flourished with a much lower profit margin—witness, for instance, the computer industry. A drop from a 20 percent profit margin to, say, 10 percent or less would hardly solve the problem of all those who cannot afford drugs. Yet it would help, and, in any case, would be an important symbolic action to show that the industry was taking health needs with greater seriousness—which its sporadic and charitable activities do only in a token way. A willingness to lower its prices would make its claim of the need for various partnerships, public and private, to pay for drugs all the more plausible—with the industry taking the lead, and making a serious financial sacrifice to do so.

Open Financial Information

The most reasonable aim, we believe, would be to ask industry to open its books to public inspection, company by company. They would then be asked to determine (1) just what would happen to their companies if profit margins were set at different levels (for instance, the effect on their research capabilities, on sources of capital, on their stock offerings, and on stakeholder loyalties); and (2) just what the loss to future health would be if they sacrificed investments in innovations in favor of making financially available the products they already have. But the main message to the industry should be something like this: you have shown us how important your products are for health, but you have never allowed outsiders to judge whether your practices result in all of the health they might, and now, not just in the future. If you want to maintain a reasonable balance between your industry interests and the public's interest in their health, you had better show us—with hard numbers—where that balance might reasonably be struck.

If the industry continues to refuse to open its books for public inspection and debate, then it is almost certain to see an escalation of a pattern of pressure that is already evident, first in Europe and Canada, but now in the United States as well. The industry will be subjected to persuasion to lower its prices. If that does not work, it will be shamed into a change. And if that fails, then the government will step in to control prices with whatever regulatory means it can command.

What ought to happen as well would be a change in the infinity model of progress that now commands the drug industry—a model, it might be said, that meets no public opposition. But it is a model that guarantees that the industry will support a form of progress that turns all desires into needs, that constantly escalates what counts as good health, and that refuses, in the name of the market, to pass any social judgment on what people are prepared to buy. It was Adam Smith who stressed the importance for the market of a foundational culture that aims to use the market to promote a good society. The infinity model of drug progress, where, too often, only private preferences are catered to, is a recipe for the constant development of innovations that will do human life little good at a high price, hard to pay for even in affluent countries, and all but unaffordable in poor countries.

With our country studies and our examination of the pharmaceutical companies behind us, we next turn to an attempt to answer an obvious question: what can one conclude from the market argument about the efficacy and impact of various market practices throughout the world, and about the relative strength and quality of health care systems that have, or have not, given a place to market strategies? No one in his or her right mind, we think, can try to answer that question without some degree of trepidation. There is no end to distinctions that can be made in determining what counts as good evidence in often radically different social and political contexts, in trying to assess the meaning of that evidence, and in cutting one's way through a jungle of empirical, political, and economic arguments that mark almost every step down the road to some kind of clarity. Or maybe the proper analogy is trying to make intellectual progress in an area marked by trench warfare on every front—and with more than enough mud to clog every analyst's footsteps. Whatever the proper analogy, on we go, over the top of the rampart.

The Value of the Market

What Does the Evidence Show?

Arguments about the market and health care seem interminable, lasting many decades now, seemingly resistant to any decisive outcome, much less consensus. Why is that? Is it possible that the evidence on the market's value is ambiguous, open to various divergent interpretations? Or that it is confusingly mixed, with some positive and some negative evidence? Or that the standards of judgment on the evidence differ, whether for technical economic reasons or reflecting ideological proclivities? It is time for us to come to some conclusions. What can one make of the various health care market practices in different countries throughout the world, and which kinds of health care systems seem to have achieved a viable balance between government and the market?

Our aim is to assess the evidence that might allow a reasonable answer to that last question, and along the way to note some of the technical and ideological arguments that help to explain divergent judgments. What will satisfy those who want to give a high place to efficiency *and* equitable access will not likely satisfy those who are looking to affirm some political values, notably choice, a diminished government role, and market dominance. Nor will the latter be satisfied with a solidarity perspective, embodying as it does a communitarian rather than individualistic premise, inclining them in a government direction. All we can say about that possibility is that there are some important international data that shed light on the organizational and ideological arguments.

Our approach will be to look at health care and the market at two levels, one of which might be called tactical and the other strategic. By speaking of a *tactical level* we mean to encompass the most common market practices, singling out six of them: competition, copayments (user fees), private health insurance, for-profit versus nonprofit institutions, medical savings accounts, and physician incentives. What are those practices typically trying to accomplish and what is the evidence for their efficacy? By the *strategic level* we mean the way those practices are melded together in different proportions within health care systems and are meant to serve the underlying social and cultural ends of various societies. Once again, we note, the U.S. data and debate will receive much but not all of the attention, as the heartland of market debate and practice.

MARKET PRACTICES: THE TACTICAL LEVEL

No concept is closer to the heart of market theory than that of competition. Even if one agrees that, in the economic organization of society, competition can be of great value—a point underscored by the demise of Communism and top-down command economies—does it follow that it is equally applicable to all the institutions of society and, most notably, the organization of health care? Kenneth Arrow, as noted in chapter 1, was thought to have shot the fatal arrow into the heart of that assumption. He argued that health care—given the uncertainty of medical outcomes and lack of patient information (among other failings)—could not qualify as a perfect instance of a market; the theoretical conditions necessary for it will never apply. Market failure will be endemic in any effort to organize health care according to the niceties of market theory.

But why use those niceties to decide on the value of market practices in general or competition in particular? Mark Pauly, we recall, suggested that the way to frame the market debate is to compare "imperfect markets and imperfect government."[1] That makes sense in an imperfect world made up of imperfect social theories implemented by imperfect human beings. Anyone can lose an ideological argument that pits high theory against actual practice; and market activities, like much else in life, cannot escape the roar of what William James once called "the blooming, buzzing confusion of experience."[2] But, then, nothing in life can escape that roar, and it may be intellectually puritanical to demand more of the market (or of government) than of the rest of life.

Yet we no less agree with Pauly's frequent economic sparring partner, Thomas Rice, that neither government nor market should be given an a priori preference. "Rather," Rice has written, "all alternative policies being considered would start on an equal basis. Then, empirical evidence would be gathered to determine the likely effect of each alternative."[3] That makes sense also, and if Rice's approach is embraced, then the door is open to some market practices—even if "the market" writ large is on the whole rejected as the best way to manage health care. Moreover, as we tried to make clear in earlier chapters, market practices can be, and are, used within both Bismarckian and Beveridge universal health care systems: the market as useful tool, not as an ideological marriage partner. Market practices, that is, can be used within health care systems without being used to finance those systems. We turn now directly to competition.

COMPETITION
Managed Competition

Competition first appeared in U.S. health care in a serious way with the emergence of prepaid group practice, whose history goes back to the 1930s.[4] Groups of physicians competed for contracts with employers and individuals to provide comprehensive health care for a per capita advance payment. Thus was introduced the forerunner of the HMO (health maintenance organization) movement, the idea of capitated payments for patient care and competition among the group practices. While it is not clear what that early group competition did for the cost of care, if anything, it served effectively to help combat the opposition of American organized medicine to anything other than individual fee-for-service medicine.[5] During that same period, many physicians began actively to market their services and to promote their individual practices. By the mid-1980s, some 40 percent of American physicians were using market techniques to attract new patients, a practice that has never stopped (though it is not overtly price competition, but something close to it—that of gaining a larger share of the available patient market).

Alain Enthoven's 1970s "consumer choice health plan" (later known as managed competition) might be called a child of its time, an effort to develop a plan for universal health care that would also be competitive and consumer-oriented.[6] Put most simply, managed care aims to promote competitive private health care providers, and then use government to manage the competition to keep it viable and effective. It was also, in the late 1970s, part of a trend toward a demand-side policy, with employers required to offer alternative group plans and employees given incentives to buy the best among them—and to bear the extra costs of the most expensive ones.[7]

The key competition in Enthoven's plan would be between fee-for-service medicine and one form or another of prepaid group practice and other innovative arrangements. State-sponsored purchasing cooperatives would be responsible for encouraging and supporting meaningful price competition among providers and a range of choices for people in selecting a provider. But managed competition did not really get off the ground, even though (as Enthoven has noted) some employers worked to give their employees choice about health plans, as did the federal and (some) state governments and universities for their employees.

To what extent, if any, it stimulated meaningful price competition among those institutions taking part is not clear and seems not to have been thoroughly investigated. In any case, President Clinton, though considering the idea of managed competition, finally rejected it in Enthoven's form as the basis of his ultimately ill-fated universal health care plan. A more recent Enthoven paper refers only to "employer policies" (without any suggestion he would abandon it for a universal care system), having employers "increase competition by offering employees a wide choice of carrier and plan designs."[8]

Health Maintenance Organizations

If managed competition as envisioned by Enthoven did not take off as national policy, the 1980s and even more the 1990s did see a rapid growth of HMOs, facilitated by Nixon-initiated legislation in the early 1970s. The principal aim of HMOs was not directly to foster competition *among* them, and by that means to contain costs, but to control costs by efficient management and to provide integrated patient care. But there was, by the mid-1990s, price competition among HMOs and other health plan systems: point-of-service plans, preferred provider organizations (PPOs), and indemnity insurance.[9]

Large employers were shopping among HMOs, and the HMOs were seeking to improve their competitiveness by greater market presence and increased size. There was also nonprice competition: network breadth, access, style of care, and technical quality of care. Price was, however, the predominant mode of competition, with some scattered evidence that capitation rates remained unchanged or declined slightly as a result.[10] Competition based on quality of care in that period remained uncertain in the face of a dearth of reliable indicators and measurements, though it was gaining in importance in the late 1990s and continues into the present.

Where there was, during the early 1990s, a concentration of HMOs in a region, and employers who shopped around, competition probably achieved some cost constraints, though not strikingly. Just what did happen to competition over the past few years, as the HMOs lost their power to control their own costs well, remains unclear, as do the health outcomes of that competition. Reviewing the evidence on HMOs and competition in 1997, Eli Ginzburg concluded that "only an unreformed optimist can believe that the competitive marketplace will be sufficiently powerful to restrain and contain future medical care cost increases."[11] Nothing recent in HMO competition would seem to fault that judgment. The loss of HMO power by the late 1990s did the deadly work, and that was in many ways a shame because, for a time during the mid-1990s, HMOs did have the capacity to provide good, well-integrated health care with manageable costs prior to those complaints.

It remains an open question whether, had the external forces and critics been mollified, the costs could have been kept down as the 1990s ended. These worries were effectively anticipated in a study by Bamezai and colleagues who, in a 1999 publication, found solid national evidence of the effectiveness of HMOs in controlling costs and contributing at the same time to more effective price competition among hospitals.[12]

Most evidently, however, American patients, while appreciating good cost management, quickly rebel when barriers to choice are put in their way, as do physicians when they believe their clinical judgment will be second-guessed. Much the same resistance that greeted earlier universal health care proposals surfaced with HMO practices: a rejection of putatively excessive central control that restricted physician and patient choice.[13] If cost control of an effective kind was rejected, the backlash apparently did little harm to HMO membership, which has remained relatively strong.[14]

Medicare+Choice

The Medicare+Choice program was an effort—expected to increase rapidly after the federal Balanced Budget Act of 1997—to increase the number of Medicare beneficiaries enrolled in capitated HMO programs. The hope was that those programs would control costs much better than the traditional Medicare fee-for-service reimbursement method. At the same time, competition among HMOs for those who chose the Medicare+Choice program was supposed to have a healthy cost-controlling benefit as well. A fine idea, a reasonable premise—and a great failure.

After 1998, the number of those choosing the program declined, not increased. Simultaneously, the participating HMOs began declining as well. What went wrong?[15] For one thing, the 2 percent annual inflation rate granted by the federal government for the program could hardly keep pace with an

average 4 percent annual cost-of-living increase. What HMO with any economic sense would want to remain part of Medicare+Choice? For another, it
turned out to be no guaranteed bargain for those elders who had enrolled in it.
There was wide geographic variation in premiums and benefits, no standard
benefit package, and high out-of-pocket payments (which doubled from $976
in 1999 to $1,964 in 2003). There could be no meaningful competition when
HMOs began disappearing from the program, and no incentive for elders to
remain in it when their personal costs for health care were rapidly escalating.

As Thomas Scully, administrator of the Medicare and Medicaid program at
the time, confessed, "We got creamed."[16] Moreover, as Bryan Dowd and his colleagues noted, for five years efforts were made in Congress to study competitive pricing for Medicare+Choice in order to better judge its results.[17] Those
efforts to stimulate research completely failed. Nonetheless, as part of its
2003 Medicare pharmaceutical bill, the Bush administration plans injected a
large amount of federal subsidy into the program, with generous federal subsidies to insurers, in an effort to revive it; and by 2004 many HMOs were once
again signing on. That effort might be renamed Medicare+Choice+Federal Private Sector Subsidy, a strategy that strong market proponents may find self-
contradictory and that the other side may find a private sector giveaway.

Hospital Competition

California is a state of many people and a diverse range of health care institutions, particularly hospitals and HMOs. It has also been, for three decades
now, the site for a variety of studies of hospital competition. The earliest studies date from the 1970s and 1980s.[18] Their findings were not of a kind to please
market advocates. As James Robinson and Harold Luft noted, surveying the
earlier literature and then using 1982 data, "[hospital] costs were substantially
higher in hospitals operating in more competitive local environments than in
hospitals in less competitive environments."[19] That information was, on the
face of it, astounding. How could more competition lead to higher costs, thus
violating settled economic theory on the impact of competition? But it soon became clear that the competition was nonprice competition. The hospitals were
competing with each other not on price but on amenities, quality, and technological prowess as part of what came to be called the "medical arms race."

The situation changed with a 1982 California law designed to control health
care expenditures. It allowed health insurance plans to selectively contract
with hospitals, a law widely imitated in other states.[20] That change made price

competition feasible and, increasingly, efficacious. A steady stream of studies from then on reported successful stories of price competition among hospitals and, simultaneously, greater price competition among HMOs, many of them serving the now-competitive hospitals. Robinson and Luft's interesting 1988 study, however, found that state regulation of costs in Massachusetts, Maryland, and New York on the whole more effectively controlled costs between 1982 and 1986 than California's market-oriented cost-control policy.[21]

As time went on, mixed reports appeared. A California study covering the years 1986–1994 found prices higher in noncompetitive areas, even for non-profit hospitals.[22] A later study, using data from the state of Washington, found that hospital competition did reduce costs and prices, while a national study found that HMOs and PPOs "significantly restrained cost growth among hospitals located in competitive hospital markets."[23] Their data, however, drawn from 1989–1994, predated the steep escalation in costs that appeared in the late 1990s and the fact that hospital cost increases came to exceed pharmaceutical cost increases in 2003. A study of hospital competition in major U.S. metropolitan areas (using 1991 data) concluded that greater competition is "associated with higher rather than lower costs" and that, in any case, price competition among hospitals is not feasible, given geographic and other variables.[24] Another California study, however, for the period 1983–1987, found that hospitals in areas of greater competition had a lower increase of both costs and revenue during that time.[25]

Some Soft Conclusions

Our reading of the literature and data on competition in health care allows only a soft conclusion: it may work here and there in bringing an increase in efficiency and cost control, but most likely only if coupled with strong government regulation designed to make it work. There is no consistent evidence anywhere that an unregulated competitive market can achieve those goals (such as in India and rural China), much less do so while maintaining reasonably equitable access. Moreover, when looking at the European experience, many countries turned to various competitive strategies to control costs, with mixed success. The most effective means always turn out to be government-imposed supply-side restrictions—with the help of demand-side control imposed by government monopsonistic purchasing clout. To control the availability of expensive technologies, hospital capacity, physician supply, physician fees, or the cost of pharmaceuticals works wonders for cost control.

Even relatively successful competition has nowhere had the comparative force of direct government interventions to contain costs.

We conclude this section on competition with the observations of some seasoned health care analysts. In 1998 Richard Freeman, of the United Kingdom, noted that, after a spate of competitive efforts in Europe, the "transaction costs" of competition (the costs, that is, of promoting and regulating competition) "mean that the efficiency gains of competition are used to sustain the system of competition itself." "Even so," he contended, "competition may have served its purpose. It destabilized the existing institutional structures into which professional interests were locked, making possible some shift of authority from doctors to managers and from hospitals to primary care."[26] Richard Saltman and Josep Figueras have argued that competition seems to work best on the supply side (management of provider behavior) and less well on the demand side (management of patient behavior), where it threatens equity and cost control.[27] Thomas Rice contends that the available literature shows that, without the help of some unfounded assumptions, "there is no reason for supposing that a competitive marketplace will result in superior outcomes in the health area," even though he is prepared also to say that it can have some contributions to make.[28]

Alain Enthoven, unwavering in his support of managed competition, in 2002 surveyed his own earlier efforts "to introduce market forces" in the United States and the United Kingdom: "The details are important and must be got right. Not anything that sounds like 'competition' or 'markets' or 'private sector' will necessarily improve economic performance." We might add that his efforts ironically have been more successful in the United Kingdom than in the United States, surely because, as he notes, "the NHS has been under central control for 50 years," while in the United States "proposed legislative changes are held hostage to a great variety of parochial interests."[29] That is an understatement. The fate and success of President Bush's aim of introducing more competitiveness into the new Medicare pharmaceutical program[30]—a legislative initiative he won—will test whether serious competition can successfully be introduced into a major public program in the United States and whether it will do its hoped-for work. One thing is certain about the enabling legislation: the details are confused, with apparently little effort made to get them fully coherent.

The distinguished economist Burton A. Weisbrod wrote over twenty years ago that "we cannot construct wise public policy on health care by applying elementary economic analysis. Competition does have a role to play. Yet the markets for health care and chocolate chip cookies *are* different."[31] Our own impression is that economic theory and ideology, not empirical data, have driven the commitment to competition in many parts of the world. If it works in general, it must work in health care: we judge that reasoning to be the "market fallacy," even if some good things can be said for it here and there. James C. Robinson has argued that competition in the American health insurance industry is declining because of industry consolidation. It is creating "competition without competitors," and is likely, he thinks, to provoke a negative public and industry reaction.[32]

It is, in any case, hard to reject the conclusion of the philosopher Paul T. Menzel, written in the mid-1980s, that competition cannot be judged good or bad in itself without knowing the context and accompanying conditions in which it will be used. To further complicate the issue of competition, moreover, John K. Iglehart, the founding editor of *Health Affairs,* has noted a point that anyone who has tried to make sense of the role of competition in health care can appreciate. At the end of a provocative commentary on the emerging competition between general hospitals and physician-owned specialty hospitals—and facing strong resistance to the spread of the latter from the mainline American Hospital Association—he noted that "a lasting definition of the right kind of competition has proved elusive.[33]

USER FEES/COPAYMENTS

The terms *user fees* and *copayments* (which have the same meaning) include an extraordinarily wide range of charges and policies. They are probably the most important and pervasive form of cost-sharing, even in most of those countries that pride themselves on their universal health care. Copayments have the common characteristic that they require the user of health care services to pay some portion of otherwise free care.[34] Economists are divided about whether cost-sharing can be an effective tool for improving efficiency and containing costs. There is more general agreement, however, that unless it is accompanied by compensatory measures for those with a low income, cost-sharing will be inequitable for both the financing of and access to care. In countries that do not have functioning comprehensive health care systems, the rationale for cost-sharing may be less one of demand management than of revenue raising for the purpose of sustaining and expanding service provision.[35]

The fundamental rationale for the use of cost-sharing is to dampen demand in the presence of public or private insurance. Some economists contend that demand for care exceeds socially desirable levels when services are fully covered by insurance. Cost-sharing measures are meant to force patients to take costs into account to limit excessive demand.[36] An obvious problem, however, is that patients may not be good judges of their health care needs—when, for instance, they would wish to consult a physician or to take a prescribed drug. Cost-sharing may, in short, deter their seeking needed care. To note that possibility is not incompatible with recognizing that full, first-dollar coverage may lead to needless health care. Getting the right balance is not easy. Some policy analysts have argued that there is an inherent conflict in using a tool that raises revenue as a tool to contain costs. This argument, put forcefully by some Canadian health economists, rejects the use of cost-sharing as a cost-containment measure.[37] If it is assumed that the supplier typically induces demand, and that spending (by insurers and patients) is always equal to revenue (of providers), imposing or increasing cost-sharing will not reduce costs. It will simply cause them to be shifted from those paying premiums (including taxpayers in a tax-based financing system) to those unfortunate enough to fall sick and require medical care.

Cost-sharing raises obvious concerns about equity, in terms of both financing and access to care. It can cause inequity in financing because of the potential for the burden of cost-sharing to fall on households with low incomes. It can cause inequity in the consumption of health services by reducing access for the elderly, the young, and the chronically sick.[38] This differential impact of patient charges reflects the economic reality that price is more of a deterrent to use when it consumes a greater percentage of a household's available funds.[39] Reduction in utilization or delays in seeking treatment can lower health status to the same degree that use of health services would have had beneficial health effects.

In the United States, insurance carriers are moving from provider, or supply-side, means of controlling costs to consumer, or demand-side, means.[40] There is a marked shift of health care costs from employers to employees, with health plans and employers instituting copays for services that never previously required them. About 20 percent of U.S. health care costs are paid by patients out of pocket, usually at the point of health care utilization. During the past twenty years, these costs have risen considerably in absolute terms. Many employers have doubled the cost of prescription drug copayments in recent years: from $5 to $10 for generics and from $15 to $50 for brand-name medications.[41] One study found that Americans spend less money on prescription drugs when their employer-sponsored health insurance plans raise copayments for these medications. Increasing copayments from $5 to $10 per prescription cut spending by employees by 22 percent, from $725 to $563 per year.[42]

While noting that the shift toward cost-sharing may create problems in insurance markets, Robinson also found that it may counteract some of what is wrong with the status quo in these markets—most notably, excessively generous insurance for some leading to an overuse of services.[43] According to Robinson, consumer cost-sharing may contribute to bottom-up health system reform after the exhaustion of government and corporate initiatives. In the short term, increased coinsurance and deductibles may cool the demand for physician visits, routine tests, and brand-name drugs, partially offsetting the surge in medical inflation. In the medium term, service-specific copayments, episode-of-care pricing, three-tier pharmacy and network benefits, and other demand-side innovations may help to address the economic challenges of chronic care. In the long term, thin benefit designs may foster a grassroots constituency for affordability and hence for the use of technology assessment and cost-effectiveness analysis in health care.

Of course, Robinson's scenario is speculation only, made more plausible in part, however, by some small decline in costs beginning in 2004. The Harvard health economist Joseph P. Newhouse, with some fresh reflections on his 1970s study of cost-sharing, has recently contended that a complementary employment of high deductibles (for initiation of care) and the tools of managed care (for costly illness episodes) could be useful.[44] The main health care preference of Americans, it might appear, is cost-unconscious choice with some distant third party footing the bill. When faced with the second-best trade-off between cost-conscious choice and no choice at all, however, Americans may grumble but select the former. Jay Gellert, in response to Robinson's thesis, argues that cost-sharing can be designed to improve the cost effectiveness of the system and that active consumer involvement can lead to better value and coverage for what the consumer actually views as necessary.[45]

Most European countries place a variable emphasis on cost-sharing as a tool for either raising revenue or containing costs of services provided by doctors and hospitals. Cost-sharing for pharmaceuticals is widespread, though not usually for the young or the old. Although the objectives of such policies are rarely stated explicitly, their main purpose appears to be to shift some of the cost of drugs to the users.[46] About half of the Western European countries use some form of cost-sharing for first-contact care, and about half also apply cost-sharing to inpatient and specialty outpatient care. The most common forms of direct cost-sharing are copayments and coinsurance; only in Switzerland is much use made of deductibles.

Yet virtually all countries in Europe use some form of an out-of-pocket maximum to limit the liability of individuals or households for medical care costs, and none employs service or benefit maximums. Hence income protection is a strong feature of these systems.[47] In Belgium, for example, people from low-income households receive complete or partial exemption from cost-sharing.[48] Charges are reduced or, for some services, nonexistent for the low-income inactive population comprising widows, orphans, pensioners, and sometimes children.[49] In Austria, people requiring social services or with incomes below a defined level are exempt from pharmaceutical cost-sharing.[50] In France, exemptions apply to patients with any one of thirty diseases defined as serious, debilitating, or chronic.[51] In Finland and Iceland, many preventive care visits are not subject to cost-sharing.[52]

Some Generalizations about Europe and North America

Evidence suggests that cost-sharing reduces utilization but does not contain costs. Intercountry comparison indicates that the United States has lower rates of contact with physicians and lower bed days per capita of population than many other countries (including Canada, France, Germany, Japan, and the United Kingdom), but spending in the United States is much higher relative to gross domestic product (GDP) than in these other countries.[53] The United States also has the highest overall costs. Other countries have lower cost-sharing and higher utilization rates, but lower costs. This does not mean that cost-sharing causes higher costs, but does suggest that measures other than cost-sharing are more effective mechanisms for cost containment.

In terms of equity, based on data from the 1980s and 1990s, Switzerland and the United States were found to have the most regressive health financing systems of the ten Organization for Economic Cooperation and Development (OECD) countries studied. This finding was attributed to their heavy reliance on both private health insurance and private out-of-pocket payments. The latter were found to be regressive in these two countries because, in most cases, cost-sharing obligations apply irrespective of the patient's income.[54] Evidence consistently shows that direct charges deter poor people from using services more than they deter the better-off. These limitations on access may result in adverse health effects for poorer and sicker groups of the population. The Rand Health Insurance Experiment in the 1970s and 1980s found that cost-sharing decreased the use of all kinds of services with little harm to the average person, but did harm the health of the poor and created financial problems for the chronically ill.[55] It should also be kept in mind that only a small proportion of patients in the United States consume a large proportion of health care. For those patients, their high costs mean that even large copayments or deductibles, soon exceeded in their care, will provide little cost-consciousness incentive.

Some Generalizations about Developing Countries

User fees for health services are not new in many developing countries. Some countries in Anglophone Africa, such as Ethiopia, Namibia, and South Africa, have had national user fee systems for years, and since the 1980s there has been considerable growth in the number of African countries implementing some form of user fees, mostly due to World Bank reform prescriptions. User fees have come to be seen as an alternative to tax-based financing for government health services. Several objectives are cited as justifying the imposition of user fees in developing countries:

- To raise revenue
- To improve quality, especially through improved drug availability
- To extend services coverage
- To promote appropriate or efficient use of health services, including the strengthening of referral systems, reduction in frivolous demand, and limits on the growing demands on health services
- To improve equity[56]

The available evidence on the impact of user fees is both limited and equivocal.[57] The most commonly available information focuses on the effects of fees on utilization levels and patterns, and on the level of revenue generation achieved through fees. Some consensus and lessons are emerging from the available information:

Utilization. If there are no other charges, the introduction of user fees reduces health care utilization, particularly for poorer households.[58] In Zimbabwe, UNICEF reported in 1993 that the quality of health services had fallen by 30 percent since 1990, that twice as many women were dying in childbirth in Harare Hospital as before 1990, and that fewer people were visiting clinics and hospitals because they could not afford hospital fees. Attendance at one clinic in northeast Zimbabwe went from 1,200 in March 1991, to 450 in December 1991, following imposition of user fees. In Kenya, the introduction of fees for patients of Nairobi's Special Treatment Clinic for Sexually Transmitted Diseases resulted in a decrease in attendance of 40 percent for men and 65 percent for women over a nine-month period. Failure to treat STDs can significantly increase the likelihood of transmission of HIV/AIDS. Negative effects on utilization can be reduced if patients are given financing options such as paying in kind or borrowing money.[59] There are, of course, other important determinants of utilization: distance to facility, time availability, education, and cultural factors.[60]

Efficiency. Fees have been shown to encourage inefficient provider behavior when the resulting revenue is retained at the point of collection.[61] Lack of coordination within a fee system may generate inappropriate utilization patterns by encouraging greater use of less cost-effective care when lower levels of the health system charge higher fees than higher levels of the system.

Equity. Fees by themselves tend to dissuade the poor more than the rich from using health services.[62] A few studies show that the nature of the payment mechanism is an important influence over its utilization and equity impact. Pure user fee systems are more likely to enhance inequities in access to health care than those that allow for risk-sharing and/or prepayment.[63] Fees do not appear to generate adequate revenue to enable substantial and sustained improvements in health care for the poor. Fees may nonetheless generate considerable proportions of the total nonsalary recurrent expenditures within lower-level, lower-cost, health facilities.[64]

The implementation of sliding scales that could protect the poor from the full burden of fees is usually ineffective. They do not protect the poor and may benefit more wealthy groups such as civil servants, who are exempted from fee payment.[65] Limited available evidence suggests that sizeable numbers of people who require medical attention and have previously obtained it are staying home and, in some cases, dying because they cannot afford to pay.[66] In sum, although user fees may be seen as a critical step allowing the development of other financial mechanisms, their implementation must be tied to a broader package that includes risk-sharing and exemptions in order to limit the potential equity dangers clearly associated with them.[67]

PRIVATE HEALTH INSURANCE

Private health insurance is a means of funding health care where health insurance premiums are paid by an individual, shared between the employees and the employer, or paid wholly by the employer. Premiums can be (1) individually rated, based on an assessment of the probability of an individual requiring health care; (2) community rated, based on an estimate of the risks across a geographically defined population; or (3) group rated, based on an estimate of the risks across all employees in a single firm. The agents collecting private health insurance premiums can be independent private bodies, such as private for-profit insurance companies, or private not-for-profit insurance companies and funds. Government may subsidize the cost of private health insurance using tax credits or tax relief.[68]

Private insurance is generally considered to be a form of privatization, a set of policies that aim to limit the role of the public sector and to increase the role of the private sector, while (in some cases) aiming to improve the performance of the remaining public sector.[69]

Potential advantages of private insurance include

- Satisfying the demands of relatively affluent people to be self-financed, leaving the government to target public resources to delivering health care for the poor
- Mobilizing additional resources for infrastructure that may benefit poor and rich people alike
- Encouraging innovation and efficiency, which may catalyze the reform of the public sector, because of flexibility and the profit motive
- Increasing choice for consumers, allowing them to use their own resources to purchase the coverage and services they wish to have[70]

Potential disadvantages of private health insurance include the following:

- For competition to operate in the health insurance market, people must be able to compare the benefit packages of different plans. If a standard minimum package is not regulated, the potentially positive role of competition based on consumer choice is greatly diminished. Consumers in most countries are likely to be uncertain about the health care benefits being offered when they purchase private health insurance.
- Because premiums can be risk rated, private health insurance tends

to discriminate in favor of healthy, young adults who use little health care. Because of the potential hazards for spreading financial risk among relatively few people, many private insurers only market their plans to groups. Individual insurance therefore tends to be expensive, and poorer people (with a risk of ill health that is higher than average) have great difficulty purchasing health insurance.

• Private insurance coverage is usually much more expensive for older people, since they need relatively more health care. In countries such as South Africa and Chile, retirees drop out of the private sector because of the cost of insurance.

• Community rating is often used as a tool to ensure equity and solidarity. In the context of the voluntary individual purchase of insurance, however, relatively healthy people (good risks) may consider the community-rated premium too expensive and exit the pool to self-insure. That behavior leaves the poorer risks to drive up the community-rated premium and gradually make that insurance less affordable. Without appropriate regulation, there will be market segmentation, cream-skimming, and the exclusion of vulnerable groups.[71]

Given the wide range of advantages and disadvantages, it is not easy to make valid generalizations about private insurance. Yet this issue is of particular importance in countries with universal health care, where, depending on its scope and deployment, private insurance may help or harm the idea of solidarity and equitable access to care. Thomas Rice has noted the importance of distinguishing two features of private insurance: the role of private insurance compared with what is provided under government-mandated coverage, and whether insurers can compete against each other.[72] Moreover, it is important to distinguish between private insurance as a supplement to government-provided care for what is not provided or to gain added amenities (as in the United Kingdom), and private insurance as alternative, parallel insurance for those who choose, in whole or part, to opt out of the government system (a main topic of debate now in Canada).

Here are our summary conclusions:

On equity. Private health insurance contributes to the regressivity of health care financing in the United States and Switzerland. In Germany and the Netherlands, however, mainly affluent people purchase private insurance, contributing to the progressivity of the financing system.[73] On the delivery side, private health insurance creates access based on a willingness and ability to pay, and typically discriminates against the poor, ill, and elderly. Equitable access has also been undermined as a result of greater sophistication in risk-rating, which enables insurers to select preferred risks.[74] The philosopher Allen Buchanan has noted that the conditions necessary for private insurance to be economically viable for those who sell it contradict the necessary ingredients for equitable access, which requires regulation of competition and the availability of generous public funds to fill in gaps in access.[75]

On efficiency. With private insurance, there are no criteria to determine access to care apart from willingness and ability to pay. In most countries, private insurers compete with or parallel the public system. Private health insurance may cover cost-effective services, which the public sector does not deliver because of mismanagement. Private health insurance may cover more rapid access to services or the costs of amenities, such as private hospital rooms, not covered in public insurance packages. Administrative costs may be systematically higher in a health system with competing private insurers than in a monopsonistic system, because of the costs associated with marketing, promotion, and underwriting. In addition, if private insurers operate on a for-profit basis, further revenue needs to be generated to pay shareholder dividends.

Careful regulation can limit the harm that is a potential result of private insurance, mainly by keeping it at a limited level and working hard to make certain the public system does not require private insurance to guarantee good health for the population. At the systems level, financing health care mainly through private insurance is neither equitable nor efficient, and the United States is a clear example of this. Insurance overheads and a competitive market have made the U.S. system the most costly in the world, yet it still fails to cover the health care needs of millions of its citizens. That much said, a modest degree of private insurance can satisfy some desires for expanded choice, as in the United Kingdom, without harm to the public system.

FOR-PROFIT VERSUS NONPROFIT

Investor-owned, for-profit entities play a growing role in the health industry in the United States. The market share of for-profit health plans rose from 25 percent of HMO enrollment in the mid-1980s to about two-thirds by the late 1990s.[76] Hospice programs are increasingly for-profit, up from 13 percent in 1992 to 27 percent in 1999.[77] While only approximately 10 percent of hospitals in the United States are for-profit,[78] the rate of hospital conversions from nonprofit to for-profit status grew rapidly in the 1990s.[79] The increasing role of for-profits in health care is contentious, particularly because of the belief of some that for-profit health care is inherently inimical to the medical tradition of altruism. But even those who do not posit an intrinsic conflict worry about the effect of the profit motive on the doctor-patient relationship and the provision of appropriate care, and worry as well about the relationship of profit-oriented institutions with their surrounding community.[80]

A basic question is whether for-profit health care poses dangers to equitable access to care. The self-evident answer is yes—not everyone may be able to afford the care. But an important question in that context is whether, and to what extent, for-profit providers have any special obligations to provide equitable access—for instance, care of the poor in the neighborhood of a profit-driven hospital. We believe they do, but under one condition only: that they are the only facility available for necessary medical care, or (even more demandingly) they exist in countries that provide no government safety net. In that case, by virtue of their control of necessary and indispensable health services, they have an obligation to provide care up to whatever point will not threaten their economic survival. Where that point should be set will ineluctably pose difficult moral dilemmas, and there is no obvious answer to where that point should be.

Many nonprofit hospitals in the United States have a similar dilemma: they cannot continue to exist if the care they provide to those who cannot afford to pay creates insupportable financial burdens. We want also to note that a special danger in developing countries is that the for-profit sector, catering to the affluent, often draws off the best physicians and nurses from the public system and, compounding the problem, is also likely to siphon off the interest of the affluent (and politically influential) in keeping the public sector strong.

Do for-profit health care institutions, particularly hospitals, have a harmful effect on health care costs, the quality of care, and relationships with the local communities in which they exist?

Health care costs. The studies and data on this subject are complex and sometimes at odds with each other. A study in the *New England Journal of Medicine* shows that all hospital administration costs increased between 1990 and 1994, but they were particularly high for for-profit hospitals.[81] This study concluded that "contrary to the rhetoric of the market, market forces are apparently 'upsizing' administration and that we should perhaps ask whether our experiment with market medicine has failed."[82] Another study shows that per capita Medicare spending rates in the years 1989, 1992, and 1995 were higher in areas served by for-profits.[83] And data collected on the impact of hospital mergers in 1986, 1989, 1992, and 1994 show that prices at for-profit hospitals averaged 10 percent higher in 1994 than nonprofits.[84] A more recent study shows that, over three decades, Medicare has been more successful than private insurance in controlling the growth rate of spending per enrollee. But when outpatient drug prescriptions are removed from the calculations, the private sector's per enrollee cumulative spending growth fell faster than Medicare's in the 1990s.[85] It remains to be seen how Medicare's new prescription drug coverage will affect its ability to contain costs.

Quality of care. American for-profits apparently spend less on overall patient care, provide less preventive care, have higher disenrollment rates, and reject more beneficiary appeals than nonprofits.[86] Patients who have fair or poor health appear to be overall more satisfied with nonprofit plans. There is a study suggesting that for-profit hospitals have a higher risk of death for patients, as well as another concluding that for-profit dialysis centers have an 8 percent increased risk of death over nonprofit dialysis centers.[87]

Yet the authors of a study to determine whether or not the number of high-cost operative procedures was higher at for-profits were admittedly surprised to discover that their data showed that it was not.[88] An article on patient safety in *Health Affairs* found that the profit status of hospitals did not have any consistent effect on that safety.[89] An argument can, however, be made that it is the volume of procedures a hospital does that determines patient risk. Low-volume hospitals tend to have higher mortality rates for certain procedures, and to have fewer nurses and residents. Low-volume hospitals also tend to be for-profit (but they are also found disproportionately in rural areas or in the South).[90]

Community impact. Some research shows that health plans affect local communities in ways that can impede or enhance residents' well-being. Surveys done by the Kaiser Family Foundation in 1997 and 1998 found that people generally viewed nonprofit and for-profit health plans as similar in their ability to provide quality care, but that nonprofits were seen clearly as being "more helpful to the community."[91] A study published in 2003 compared community benefits derived from nonprofits and for-profits: nonprofits were generally more involved in their local communities, particularly in providing subsidies for medical services in the community and supporting community health centers and mental health centers. They were also more likely to target benefit programs to low-income neighborhoods. Yet for-profits were much better at communicating information and notifying enrollees about potential problems with their medical care.[92] Schlesinger and his colleagues concluded their study by stating that policymakers should be alerted that for-profit status among HMOs "undermines practices that may have substantial community benefits."[93]

The information on this entire subject is limited and inconsistent. Some of the studies compare HMOs with different types of ownership, while others look at hospitals, making it difficult to draw general conclusions. But overall it appears that nonprofits do a better job than their for-profit counterparts. In general in the 1990s, for-profit hospitals had higher administrative costs and higher prices, and spent less per patient than their nonprofit counterparts. The HMO enrollees who use health care the most, those with fair to poor health, seem to be happier with nonprofit HMOs. Nonprofit HMOs have more preventive programs, have lower disenrollments, and reject fewer benefit appeals. Nonprofit health care systems have customarily maintained strong ties to local communities. That practice is part of an important philanthropic tradition of providing charitable health services and supporting community-based health services.

MEDICAL SAVINGS ACCOUNTS/HEALTH SAVINGS ACCOUNTS/ FLEX PLANS

In the United States, medical savings accounts (MSAs), at least in their first incarnation, were a failure. They were authorized by Congress in 1996 to allow people to purchase a high-deductible health insurance plan, open a savings account at a bank or other financial institution, and use money from that account to pay the deductible or other out-of-pocket medical costs. The underlying market aim was to increase choice and personal control over health care spending. Like an IRA (individual retirement account), the investments accrue and the owner can withdraw the money tax-free at retirement. Yet by 2002 only eighty-five thousand participants had enrolled in these plans.[94]

The MSAs were discontinued on January 1, 2004. But the general idea was not dead. With a strong push from the Bush administration, a new plan was made part of the 2003 Medicare reform bill, to be called health savings accounts (HSAs). HSAs aim to remedy some of the problems associated with MSAs and have been touted as possibly "the most important piece of legislation of 2003" by the economist Martin Feldstein.[95] HSAs allow anyone under the age of sixty-five who has a large-deductible insurance policy (a minimum of $2,000 for a family) to make tax-free contributions, up to $5,150 per year, to pay for health-related expenses. Individuals or their employers can make annual contributions.

Both MSAs and HSAs were designed to make people more cost-conscious in their use of health care. HSAs were also created as a possible better alternative to another medical savings plan, called flexible spending accounts (FSAs). FSAs allow employees to set aside a certain amount of pretax money deducted from their pay for medical expenses. Approximately seven million people use these accounts.[96] There are two major differences between HSAs and FSAs. With FSAs, the money deducted must be spent in the same calendar year. It cannot be spent in future years, as can be done with HSAs; and employers have low caps on FSAs.[97] Since these plans are relatively new there does not seem to be any research on their impact, although critics of HSAs predict that they will cause some employers to increase the deductibles on their employees' health plans in order to save money. Regardless, HSAs and FSAs have two major drawbacks: they tend to benefit people with large disposable incomes, and they are directed mainly at controlling the demand side of health care. The early response to HSAs was, by the end of 2004, slower than the Bush administration had expected.

South Africa is another country that has experience with private MSAs. Subsequent to the deregulation of the insurance industry in 1994, 20 percent of the population bought private insurance, with approximately half of that consisting of MSAs. Individuals as well as their employers are given tax incentives to contribute. Usually there are no deductibles for hospital or prescription drugs for chronic conditions, though there are high deductibles for outpatient prescription drugs and outpatient care. With such a small portion of the population subscribing to MSAs, it is difficult to assess their impact, but there is some evidence that both insurers and the insured are pleased with the plans.[98] In 2005, however, the government ended the MSA program.

While the United States and South Africa are examples of the use of MSAs in the private sector, Singapore has led the way with public MSAs. Established in 1984, Singapore's MSA program—called Medisave—is compulsory, universal, and managed by the government. Singapore's health care system is often praised because of its ability to deliver relatively good health care at a very low cost of between 3 and 4 percent of GDP.[99] The system consists of three features: Medisave, MediShield, and Medifund. Medisave is managed by the government for the purpose of covering a patient's share of hospitalization costs and some outpatient services. The contributions are tax free, interest bearing, and part of the contributor's estate. Medisave is a key feature of the government's effort to foster personal responsibility for health. MediShield is an inexpensive catastrophic insurance plan to help pay for hospital expenses resulting from a major or chronic illness. Medifund is a government-established endowment fund. The interest from the fund is used to pay the expenses of indigent people who cannot pay into Medisave.[100]

Following the implementation of Medisave, there was a marked increase in health expenditures in Singapore.[101] In 1993, the government decided to implement some controls to hold costs down. The Ministerial Committee on Health Policies stated: "Market forces alone will not suffice to hold down medical costs to the minimum . . . The government has to intervene directly to structure and regulate health."[102] Several controls to restrict supply were instigated at government hospitals. They consist of restrictions on the use of expensive technology, price caps on medical services, lower subsidy rates for hospitals, restrictions on the number of hospital beds, tighter controls on the number of doctors, and limitations on the number of specialists to no more than 40 percent of the medical profession.[103] Mark Pauly has concluded that, while it is difficult to assess the success of the Medisave program together with the catastrophic care policy (MSA/CHP)—there is no similar city-state for the purpose of comparison—Singapore's health care spending has been significantly lower than it would have been had there been no personal savings accounts.[104]

China has also experimented with public MSAs. Like Singapore, the government has implemented supply-side controls on technology and prescription drugs as well as setting fixed pay rates for doctors and hospitals. To date, there are few data on its success, but there are indications that health care costs fell slightly. Yet catastrophic coverage operated at a deficit, and many employers are opting out of the system because of use restrictions.[105]

There is every expectation that the American MSAs are likely to be attractive to people who are healthier and wealthier than most, but for much of the population they are not a viable method for the funding of health care. Without strict government supply-side controls, MSAs do not appear to contain costs. Still, other countries are looking at MSAs. In 2002, Canada had a heated debate about experimenting with MSAs. David Gratzer, an advocate for trying MSAs in Canada, notes Singapore's low infant mortality rate, long life expectancy, short waiting time for surgery, and large numbers of diagnostic machines (compared with Canada). He argues that "all of these experiments with MSAs should catch the eye—and interest—of Canadian health care experts."[106] At the same time, Canadians who are opposed to MSAs point to a study that calculates that, if Manitoba were to have MSAs, the result would be an increase in spending on the healthiest members of the population.[107]

At best, we conclude, MSAs are not likely to have much impact on most health care systems, and seem more a symbol of market ambition than a useful device for holding down costs, improving efficiency and quality, or enhancing equitable access. As with copayments, moreover, MSAs are meant to force people to make their own choices about which health care they want; their aim is to curb unnecessary or personally unattractive care (and thus to do away with the "moral hazard," an excessive use of medical insurance induced by the breadth of coverage it provides). But MSAs and copayments assume that patients know what medical procedures or treatments are good for them, requiring an expertise in making choices that few of us have. As Malcolm Gladwell has perceptively put it, MSAs are "in their governing assumptions . . . the antithesis of universal health care." Of course, if the value of choice is taken to be an intrinsic good, aiming at individual empowerment not equitably distributed health care, then MSAs will be attractive, especially for those who can afford them.[108]

PHYSICIAN INCENTIVES

There are basically three ways to compensate physicians: fee-for-service, salary, and capitation. Historically, fee-for-service was used almost everywhere as the standard way of paying physicians. But in recent decades, in great part because it was believed to encourage the overuse of health care, other methods have been used; and in Western European countries, where they are still used, physician fees are set by negotiation between the government and physicians' organizations. Salaries are often found in HMOs that employ a staff of full-time physicians. Capitation plans characteristically require a prepayment for the potential use of medical services whether any service is actually rendered. The challenge for capitation plans, and thus their attractiveness for cost-control purposes, is to provide an acceptable quality and level of health care within the boundaries of the capitation fee per patient—and the treatment behavior of physicians in that context is of obvious importance.[109]

In addition to these three compensation categories, many providers make use of bonuses, fee withholds, or subcapitation plans to keep physicians from overusing referrals, diagnostic tests, and other ancillary services. Bonuses are rewards for meeting certain criteria, such as a decrease in patient care costs, increased patient satisfaction, quality improvements, and peer evaluation. Fee withholds are delayed payments that are conditioned on performance. A health care plan may, for example, withhold a percentage of the physician's compensation and place it in a fund pool for ancillary services. If there are unspent funds left in the pool at the end of the year, the residual amount is paid to the physician. With subcapitation, a health provider receives a capitation payment for a group of patients and then subcontracts with other providers on a capitated basis to provide services.

The use of incentives has grown tremendously in the United States. Estimates are that about half of all American physicians are part of some type of capitation or withhold plan.[110] Physician incentives are controversial but perhaps unavoidable: all systems have some kind of financial incentives, either explicit or tacit. Fee-for-service systems can encourage doctors to give more care than patients need if the fee is too high. Salaried physicians may not be as productive as other doctors. But most of the controversy focuses on capitation, bonuses, and withholds. Federal and state regulations have been adopted to try to prevent the most serious abuses.[111]

In order to assess the effects of incentives, three major questions can be asked, bearing on productivity, cost control, and behavioral influence. First, do economic incentives actually stimulate physicians' productivity? One study published in 2002 shows that, indeed, financial incentives based on the physician's own production do increase productivity.[112] This study confirms the results of earlier studies.[113] Whether that productivity improves the quality of care, or avoids overtreatment, is not clear.

Second, do financial incentives actually contain costs? A study published in the *Journal of the American Medical Association* in 1998 found that the method of compensation was not significantly related to the use and cost of health services per person. This was the first study to focus on compensation rather than plan payment. The study found that the principal driving forces for use and cost were the characteristics of individual enrollees and the level of health plan benefit coverage. The use and cost of services increased with age, female gender, and wealth of the plan benefits.[114]

Third, do physicians' personal economic interests influence, or even limit, the care they provide their patients? This question dominates the debate about incentives, and the main worry is whether they create a potential risk to patients. Critics of such practices argue that financial incentives may cause a physician to limit or omit important diagnostic tests, accelerate a patient's discharge from the hospital, or avoid referring a patient to a needed specialist. If such abuse occurs, it is difficult in theory to prove, and has not been proven in the few studies that exist.[115] Even so, it remains a concern.[116] There seems to be some agreement that incentive arrangements should not prove too tempting while, at the same time, having some effect on behavior.[117] One important issue that does not get much attention is the effect of incentives on public perception of, and confidence in, physicians' integrity. Even if incentives never actually affect a patient's care, the perception that they might can itself have a harmful effect on the doctor-patient relationship and the necessary trust that it must embody.[118]

There is not enough information to accurately assess the impact physician incentives have on health care. Two things seem certain: first, if too much of the physician's income is placed at risk, his or her decisions regarding patient care will most likely be adversely affected; and second, incentives are not likely to instill public confidence, though this distrust may be ameliorated by full physician disclosure.[119] But both of those points are hardly more than commonsense judgments. This second issue is evidenced by the existence of lawsuits over incentives, the enactment of state and federal legislation restricting their use, and other ongoing efforts by ethics committees to investigate and regulate them.[120] We note that, in early 2005, the federal Centers for Medicare and Medicaid Services announced an experimental program of physician bonuses for improved quality while also reducing costs.

On an international level, Varun Gauri, who is part of the Development Research Group of the World Bank, has discussed the use of financial incentives in developing countries to entice physicians to serve in rural area. He cites one study that shows that, in Indonesia, it takes a bonus of up to 100 percent of the salary to attract medical school graduates to the outer islands. He also argues that incentives tied to performance are very hard to enforce in developing countries due to monitoring problems. His article also points out how, in many developing countries, it is to the physician's benefit not to refer a patient to a specialist (if one could be found) or to another doctor for a second opinion, because then the physician risks losing the patient, and hence income, to the colleague.[121]

MARKET PRACTICES: THE STRATEGIC LEVEL

In this section we first look at health outcomes, technology, and costs in health care systems, focused primarily on comparative U.S. and European data. We then examine data on health care quality, offering a different cut at the success of health care systems. Together, these comparative data offer a revealing picture of two contrasting "ways of life" in the deployment of market practices (to use Richard Saltman's felicitous phrase on the provision of health care). A further advantage of the comparisons is that good data are readily available (even if one takes into account the numerous cautions that economists and policy analysts note in working with comparative health system data). We will draw heavily on the recent European Observatory study *Social Health Insurance Systems in Western Europe,* and it is all the more useful in encompassing much relevant information about the comparative outcomes of those different (but still universal care) systems.[122] Building on those data and earlier chapters, we will draw some conclusions about the relative advantages of government-oriented versus market-oriented health care systems.

Assessing the Strategic Data I:
Health Outcomes and Available Technologies and Services

Life expectancy at birth and age 65. While the gap is not great, the United States lags a number of European countries in life expectancy at birth, ranking number 13 (table 6.1). If there is remarkably little variance among the European countries in life expectancy at birth, the same is generally true of life expectancy at age sixty-five, but in that category the United States does better; after age eighty, American life expectancy is tied with Canadian life expectancy at that stage of life, with the best outcomes in the world. It is not irrelevant to note that Americans over the age of sixty-five are covered by the federal Medicare program, tax-financed. The SHI study (p. 36) revealed no major distinctions between the social health insurance systems and the tax-based systems on life expectancy.

GDP per capita and health care expenditures as a percentage of GDP. The gross domestic product per capita of the United States is far and away the highest in the world and about 10 percent higher than those of the most prosperous European countries (table 6.2) The United States is no less well known for spending more of its GDP, 15 percent in 2004, on health care than any other country, and more per capita as well ($4,370 in 2001) (table 6.3). The comparable health care spending range in Europe is not inconsiderable, ranging from the United Kingdom at 7.6 percent to Switzerland and Germany, both over 10 percent. One important finding of the SHI study (p. 117) was that the social health insurance systems (government-coordinated but privately run) cost more than the tax-based systems by a ratio of 1.16. There was also a decline in the 1990s of public contributions to SHI funding in comparison with the tax-based systems, and between 1995 and 2000 the cost growth rate for the tax-

TABLE 6.1
Life Expectancy at Birth and at Age 65 and Rank, 2003

	Life expectancy at birth	Rank	Life expectancy at age 65	Disability adjusted life expectancy
Market Acceptors				
United States	76.8	13	17.6	–
Market Rejectors				
Canada (T)	79.3	7	18.6	–
Denmark (T)	76.5	23	16.8	70.1
France (SHI)	79.0	3	19.2	71.3
Italy (T)	79.5	9	18.7	71.0
Sweden (T)	79.6	8	18.4	71.8
United Kingdom (T)	78.2	17	17.7	69.6
Market Accommodators				
Australia (T)	80.3	6	18.7	71.6
Belgium (SHI)	77.4	15	17.5	69.7
Germany (SHI)	78.1	10	17.9	70
Israel (SHI)	78.5	10	17.9	69.4
Netherlands (SHI)	78.3	21	17.6	69.9
Switzerland (SHI)	80.0	4	19.1	72.8
Second Thoughts				
Czech Republic (SHI)	75.5	28	16.0	66.6
New Zealand (T)	78.2	11	18.1	–

Sources: Data from Organization for Economic Cooperation and Development, *Health at a Glance: OECD Indicators 2003* (Paris: Organization for Economic Cooperation and Development, 2003); V. M. Freid, K. Prager, A. P. MacKay, and H. Zia, *Chartbook on Trends in the Health of Americans—Health, United States, 2003* (Hyattsville, MD: National Center for Health Statistics, 2003); World Health Organization, *The Atlas of Health in Europe* (Copenhagen: WHO Regional Office for Europe, 2003).
Note: T = tax-based system; SHI = social health insurance system.

based countries was 3.7 percent per year, compared with 2.5 percent with the SHI systems (p. 120).

Diagnostic technologies, high-technology procedures, and hospital utilization. Exceeded only by Switzerland, with 12.9 MRI (magnetic resonance imaging) units per million, the United States has 8.1 per million (table 6.4). More countries exceed the United States in the number of CT (computed tomography) scanners per million—United States (13.1), over against Italy (20.6), Switzerland (18.5), and Germany (17.1). But, with the exception of Italy, there is a rough correlation between these two technologies and health expenditures as a percentage of GDP. The SHI countries (not all of which are included in our tables) have an average of 19.1 CTs and 6.4 MRIs, versus 11.8 CTs and 7.5 MRIs for northern tax-based systems (SHI study, p. 123).

The gap between the European countries and the United States is far more striking in the case of cardiac bypass and angioplasty procedures (table 6.5), with the United States using either two or three times more procedures per

TABLE 6.2
Gross Domestic Product per Capita

	GDP per capita (U.S. $), 2001	Average annual growth rate per capita (%), 1989–2001
Market Acceptors		
United States	35,182	1.6
Market Rejectors		
Canada (T)	28,811	1.4
Denmark (T)	29,216	1.8
France (SHI)	26,879	1.5
Italy (T)	26,345	1.5
Sweden (T)	26,052	1.4
United Kingdom (T)	26,315	1.9
Market Accommodators		
Australia (T)	27,408	2.0
Belgium (SHI)	27,775	1.8
Germany (SHI)	26,199	1.2
Israel (SHI)	19,790	1.5
Netherlands (SHI)	29,391	2.2
Switzerland (SHI)	29,876	0.4
Second Thoughts		
Czech Republic (SHI)	15,143	0.6
New Zealand (T)	21,077	1.3

Sources: Data from Organization for Economic Cooperation and Development, *Health at a Glance: OECD Indicators 2003* (Paris: Organization for Economic Cooperation and Development, 2003).
  Note: T = tax-based system; SHI = social health insurance system.

hundred thousand population (save for Belgium). Yet the U.S. average hospital stay for acute myocardial infarctions is notably shorter than the European average. The United States has many fewer hospital beds per capita than the European countries and much shorter hospital stays (table 6.6). These data may well reflect the successful cost-containment targeting of hospital beds and length of hospital stays that began in the 1990s, though an increase in hospital costs began to appear in 2002, as well as complaints about a shortage of beds.

The European scene shows that the SHI countries have a much higher average of hospital beds per thousand population (7.6) than the tax-based systems (4.8), as well as substantially longer hospital stays (11.7 vs. 8.0 days). Thus hospital costs are much higher in the SHI countries, though whether that is because the systems are more inefficient is not clear (SHI study, p. 123). Though the United States has far few physicians per hundred thousand population (table 6.7), it exceeds all Western European countries in annual doctor consultations per capita—8.9, over against 6.9 for France, 6.3 for Canada, 6.1 for Italy, 5.9 for the Netherlands, and 4.9 for the United Kingdom.[123]

Having presented these data, however, it is important to note that it is exceedingly difficult to show a direct correlation between available technology

TABLE 6.3
Health Expenditures as Percentage of Gross Domestic Product, to 2001

	% of GDP	Increase in % of GDP, 1970–2001 (OECD)	Expenditure per person (U.S. $), 2001
Market Acceptors			
United States	15.0 (2004)	50.4	4,370
Market Rejectors			
Canada (T)	9.7	27.8	–
Denmark (T)	8.6	7.0	2,420
France (SHI)	9.5	–	2,349
Italy (T)	8.0	–	2,032
Sweden (T)	8.7	23.0	1,748
United Kingdom (T)	7.6	40.8	1,763
Market Accommodators			
Australia (T)	8.9 (2000)	37.1	–
Belgium (SHI)	9.0	55.6	2,269
Germany (SHI)	10.7	42.1	2,748
Israel (SHI)	8.8	–	1,671
Netherlands (SHI)	8.9	22.5	2,246
Switzerland (SHI)	10.9	48.6	3,222
Second Thoughts			
Czech Republic (SHI)	7.4	–	1,031
New Zealand (T)	8.2	37.8	–

Sources: Data from Organization for Economic Cooperation and Development, *Health at a Glance: OECD Indicators 2003* (Paris: Organization for Economic Cooperation and Development, 2003); World Health Organization, *The Atlas of Health in Europe* (Copenhagen: WHO Regional Office for Europe, 2003).

Note: T = tax-based system; SHI = social health insurance system.

TABLE 6.4
Diagnostic Technologies (per million population)

	MRI units, 2000	CT scanners, 2002	Diffusion of MRI units, 1990–2000	Diffusion of CT scanners, 1990–2000
Market Acceptors				
United States	8.1	13.1	3.7–8.1	14.6–13.1
Market Rejectors				
Canada (T)	2.5	9.5	0.7–2.5	7.1–9.5
Denmark (T)	6.6	11.4	2.5–6.6	4.3–11.4
France (SHI)	2.6	9.6	0.8–2.6	6.7–9.6
Italy (T)	7.5	20.6	1.3–7.5	6.0–20.6
Sweden (T)	7.9	14.2	1.5–7.9	10.5–14.2
United Kingdom (T)	4.6	6.2	1.0–4.6	4.3–6.2
Market Accommodators				
Australia (T)	4.7	–	0.9–4.7	–
Belgium (SHI)	3.2	–	2.0–3.2	–
Germany (SHI)	6.2	17.1	1.9–6.2	10.1–17.1
Switzerland (SHI)	12.9	18.5	3.9–12.9	12.5–18.5
Second Thoughts				
Czech Republic (SHI)	1.7	9.6	0.2–1.7	2.1–9.6
New Zealand (T)	2.6	8.8		3.6–8.8

Sources: Data from Organization for Economic Cooperation and Development, *Health at a Glance: OECD Indicators 2003* (Paris: Organization for Economic Cooperation and Development, 2003).

Note: MRI = magnetic resonance imaging; CT = computed tomography; T = tax-based system; SHI = social health insurance system.

TABLE 6.5
Cardiac Bypass Procedures and Cardiac Angioplasty Procedures, 2000

	Bypass procedures (per 100,000 population)	Angioplasty procedures (per 100,000 population)	Average stay for acute myocardial infarction (days)
Market Acceptors			
United States	205	363	5.7
Market Rejectors			
Canada (T)	69	97	8.4
Denmark (T)	66	96	6.7
France (SHI)	40	145	7.5
Italy (T)	48	87	9.4
Sweden (T)	73	94	6.6
United Kingdom (T)	41	39	–
Market Accommodators			
Australia (T)	89	114	6.8
Belgium (SHI)	–	262	9.7
Germany (SHI)	90	–	12.6
Netherlands (SHI)	93	74	–
Second Thoughts			
Czech Republic (SHI)	–	–	8.9
New Zealand (T)	103	74	6.5

Sources: Data from Organization for Economic Cooperation and Development, *Health at a Glance: OECD Indicators 2003* (Paris: Organization for Economic Cooperation and Development, 2003).
Note: T = tax-based system; SHI = social health insurance system.

TABLE 6.6
Hospital Beds and Lengths of Stay, up to 2001

	Hospital beds (per 100,000 population)	Average length of hospital stays (days)
Market Acceptors		
United States	350	6
Market Rejectors		
Canada (T)	400	7.2
Denmark (T)	434	6.6
France (SHI)	820	10.8
Italy (T)	450	7.6
Sweden (T)	522	6.3
United Kingdom (T)	417	9.8
Market Accommodators		
Australia (T)	415	6.9
Belgium (SHI)	699	11.5
Germany (SHI)	912	11.9
Israel (SHI)	616	11.1
Netherlands (SHI)	466	12.5
Switzerland (SHI)	618	13.0
Second Thoughts		
Czech Republic (SHI)	852	11.5
New Zealand (T)	620	6.5

Sources: Data from World Health Organization, *The Atlas of Health in Europe* (Copenhagen: WHO Regional Office for Europe, 2003).
Note: T = tax-based system; SHI = social health insurance system.

TABLE 6.7

Number of Physicians (per 100,000 population), *up to 2001*

	Number of physicians
Market Acceptors	
United States	260
Market Rejectors	
Canada (T)	210
Denmark (T)	284
France (SHI)	330
Italy (T)	567
Sweden (T)	287
United Kingdom (T)	164
Market Accommodators	
Australia (T)	240
Belgium (SHI)	419
Germany (SHI)	363
Israel (SHI)	375
Netherlands (SHI)	328
Switzerland (SHI)	350
Second Thoughts	
Czech Republic (SHI)	342
New Zealand (T)	220

Sources: Data from World Health Organization, *The Atlas of Health in Europe* (Copenhagen: WHO Regional Office for Europe, 2003).

Note: T = tax-based system; SHI = social health insurance system.

and its utilization and good health care outcomes. That problem remains one of the important health care uncertainties. The socioeconomic influences on health status, as well as the quality of welfare systems, can make more difference in health care outcomes than does available medical care.

Ways of Life: Government and the Market

Many health care economists say it is not possible to make a judgment of health care systems, that one is "better" or "worse" than another.[124] Different countries, it is noted accurately enough, have different histories, cultures, politics, health care goals, and quality outcomes; and it is particularly hard to say which balance of government and the market is superior. We have fewer reservations about making such judgments than they do, and we will use their research to do so. It is not quite the same as choosing between vanilla and chocolate ice cream; some defensible generalizations seem possible.

To put one of them in negative terms: no country, or its politicians, seems to think—or at least would be willing to say—that a health care system with great health disparities between rich and poor is a good arrangement, or that signifi-

cant differences in access are beneficial for its citizens, or that gross inefficiency and its attendant poor-quality care and high costs is an acceptable state
of affairs. That does not necessarily mean they are seriously prepared to do
anything about it, but it does mean that there is at least a rough consensus
on the right and the left, between market-biased and government-biased proponents, if not about what is right, then what can be judged wrong—though
with different degrees of concern and indignation. Their differences lie in the
market-government balance and the details of the modus vivendi. Earlier chapters, looking at the history and structure of various systems, suggest some of the
reasons for that, but we want to push on a step further.

Our point of departure was suggested by the conclusions of the European
Observatory report on SHI systems, frequently cited above. Their study, the
authors say, does not allow a firm judgment about whether the European SHI
systems are better in general than the tax-based systems, primarily because a
variety of different performances were assessed, with some countries doing
better on some things and worse on others (e.g., equity, access, efficiency,
patient satisfaction). Noting that there is, in any case, a weak correlation between health status and health system activities, equity outcomes were slightly
worse in SHI countries while patient satisfaction was slightly better; no clear
efficiency trend could be discerned. Ultimately, the study concludes, "The
central question that emerges from the available data is whether the apparent
additional satisfaction is justified by the additional money and resources
spent, despite the fact that not much more health is obtained. This requires,
clearly, a societal judgement, leading back to [an earlier main point about] a
'way of life,' a way of understanding the world, and a social policy based on
that societal perspective" (p. 133). While that statement, and the study on
which it is based, bears on a comparison between European health care systems, it has wider implications. The study itself shows that, in just about every
relevant category, from cost control to health status, the European SHI and tax-
based health care systems do *better* than the United States. But when comparing the SHI and tax-based systems with each other, the tax-based systems do
slightly better on equity and access.

Put another way, the American "way of life" for health care systems, heavily
market oriented, produces worse health and inequity, and does so at a dramatically higher cost than the European countries. Yet three prominent American
market proponents wrote in the *Wall Street Journal* in 2004 that, "after a century of American innovations in medical procedures, technologies and pharmaceuticals, the quality of American medical care is the envy of the world."[125]

We have detected no trace of that envy, either in the literature or in trips to other countries, and most Europeans would agree with the sentence that follows that quote: "Yet [the American] health-care system is in deep trouble."

But we think Europeans would be puzzled, even amused, by the authors' next statement: "without a viable alternative policy, politicians will seek to 'fix' our system by recourse to the heavy hand of government. Free markets are a proven way to discipline costs, encourage innovation and increase quality . . . The governmental system will lead to less choice and a stifling of innovation. The free-market solution will enable America to solve its health-care cost problems and capture the promise of 21st century medicine."[126] To this enthusiasm we respond with an analogy. It is as if a tennis player who has just lost a match walked off the court congratulating himself on his many aces and fine ground strokes, shrugging his shoulders indifferently at the scoreboard and eager to get on to the next match where he will show them once again how good he is.

The data presented at the beginning of this chapter, in the sections on the "tactical level" market practices, offer only the most tepid and modest support here and there for automatic, ideology-driven faith in market practices. When one moves to the "strategic level," the notion that the "heavy hand of government" will destroy choice and innovation is a myth. The one (and only) important category the United States leads the world in, that of the life expectancy of those over the age of eighty, is directly traceable to the superior health care available to them through the federal tax-based Medicare program. That fact is, of course, fully compatible with the verifiable fact of the superiority of the European tax-based systems in providing reasonably equitable and accessible care to every citizen. More broadly, every European system provides its patients with considerable choice, controls its costs far better than the United States in doing so, and has high levels of patient satisfaction.

Since the authors of statements about the "heavy hand of government" must surely have some knowledge of the European health care systems, just as they must know that the federal Medicare program has lower administrative costs and a slower rate of cost increases than the private sector, we are left with a puzzle. How is it that market proponents can have such a low faith in government and such a high faith in market practices? Just what evidence is available from *their side* to support that combination?

To see if there are some elements of the debate we have overlooked, we will now introduce a second set of tables, bearing on the quality of health care, combining both outcome data and factors of interest to people, other than health as such.

Assessing the Strategic Data II: The Quality of Care

The quality of health care has come, in recent years, to have an importance almost comparable to that of health outcomes. It may well be that, for some, the quality of a system is even more important than its health outcomes, particularly if the standard of assessment bears on the way people experience and perceive the care they receive, of which better or worse health per se is only one of many possible standards. We present here some information on quality of care, looking at various dimensions of care. An important study by a Commonwealth Fund working group convened in 1999 made use of an Institute of Medicine definition of quality as "the degree to which health services for individuals and populations increase the likelihood of desired health outcomes and are consistent with current professional knowledge."[127]

This seems to us too narrow a definition, placing the emphasis too much on health outcomes. A worry about paying for care, for instance, can be a source of considerable anxiety even when, at least for some, it may not greatly affect their health status; and annoyance, anxiety, or exasperation at waiting lists—even for care eventually received—can influence people's satisfaction with their health care even if no lasting health harm is done.

Table 6.8 does, however, use health outcomes as a standard of quality measurement. Using twenty-one quality indicators, the Commonwealth Fund working group's data show considerable variation. The group concluded that "none of the five countries scores the best or the worst score on all of the indicators . . . no country scores the best or worst overall, and each country has at least one area of care where it could learn from international experience."[128] Table 6.9 presents data from the same five countries on some important general features of their health systems, with respondents passing judgment on the need for major reform and on access in a variety of situations. Table 6.10 takes a somewhat different approach to the need for reform, while table 6.11 goes at the problem of access in a somewhat different way also. Table 6.12 provides a citizens' assessment of their satisfaction with their health care system for some seventeen countries, while table 6.13 presents data on health system satisfaction among the poor and the elderly.

If one combines the information from the first seven tables and from tables 6.8 to 6.13, it is hard to see how, by any but ideological standards, U.S. health care is a good system in comparison with many others. Many health care economists, perhaps restrained by some professional norms, are reluctant to say

TABLE 6.8

Standardized Performance on Twenty-one Quality Indicators in Five Countries

Outcome or process indicator	Standardized scores					Value of indicator for country with score of 100
	AUS	CAN	Engl	NZ	US	
Survival rates (outcome)						
Breast cancer	107	104	100	106	114	75 (H)
Cervical cancer	111	106	100	105	108	70 (H)
Colorectal cancer	116	113	100	123	108	53 (H)
Childhood leukemia, ages 0–15	100	118	109[a]	102	110	67 (H)
Non-Hodgkin's lymphoma	116	107	100	115	109	58 (H)
Kidney transplant	106	113	104	104	100	83 (H)
Liver transplant	110[b]	123	100	–[b]	102	71 (L)
AMI, ages 20–84	134	100	NA	121	NA	11 (L)
Ischemic stroke, ages 20–84	120	124	NA	100	NA	12 (L)
Avoidable events (outcome)						
Suicide, all ages	112	114	155	100	120	13 (L)
Suicide, ages 15–19	162	151	187	100	165	25 (L)
Suicide, ages 20–29	140	149	171	100	154	29 (L)
Asthma mortality, ages 5–39[c]	144	NA	122	100	130	0.7 (L)
Pertussis	100	135	196	NA	191	31 (L)
Measles	187	198	100	160	199	5 (L)
Hepatitis B	167	133	168	167	100	6 (L)
Smoking rate	111	115	100	106	115	27 (L)
Process indicators						
Breast cancer screening rate	117	116	106	100	111	63 (H)
Cervical cancer screening rate	119	115	100	116	140	67 (H)
Influenza vaccination rate, age 65+	125	114	115	100	112	59 (H)
Polio vaccination rate, age 2	113	106	116	100	110	82 (H)

Sources: Commonwealth Fund International Working Group on Quality Indicators; P. S. Hussey et al., "How Does Quality of Care Compare in Five Countries?" *Health Affairs* 23, no. 3 (2004): 89–99. Used with permission.

Notes: Specifications, years, and technical notes for each indicator are in endnotes accompanying the descriptive text. 100 is the worst result; higher numbers indicate better results (in all but "Value of indicator" column). Whether higher (H) or lower (L) rates are considered more desirable, the standardized scores displayed across countries always show how much "better" one country is (in percentage terms) than the index case (that is, the "worst" country, which is automatically assigned a score of 100).

Aus, Australia; CAN, Canada; Engl, England; NZ, New Zealand; US, United States; AMI, acute myocardial infarction; NA, not available.

[a]For this population, the observed survival rate should almost perfectly equal the relative survival rate.
[b]Australia figure includes Australia and New Zealand.
[c]Data are for 1990–99.

which health care systems are better or worse. No doubt if one is comparing various European countries with each other (Sweden vs. France, for instance), such a judgment would be difficult. But, in light of all the money the United States spends on health care, its low ranking in general health outcomes, and its weak level of public approbation, the fact that on a few indicators it does better than other countries hardly suffices to render it judgment-proof, much less to praise it. The authors of this book are provided with a good health care plan by our employer (provided by Oxford): we can gain quick access to good

TABLE 6.9

Citizens' Views on Their Health Care Systems and General Access Problems, by Income Group, Five Countries, 2001

	There is so much wrong with the system that it should be completely rebuilt	Access is worse than 2 years ago	Very or extremely difficult to see a specialist	Very or somewhat difficult to get care in evening or on weekends	Often or sometimes unable to get care because it is not available where you live
Australia					
Below-average income (n = 483)	22%[a]	22%[a,b]	14%[a]	33%[a]	19%[a]
Above-average income (n = 587)	18	17	11	35	14
Canada					
Below-average income (n = 465)	23[a,b]	28	20[a,b]	46[b]	23[b]
Above-average income (n = 558)	13	24	14	36	17
New Zealand					
Below-average income (n = 374)	25[a,b]	20[b]	21[a,b]	22[a]	24[b]
Above-average income (n = 693)	18	12	6	22	16
United Kingdom					
Below-average income (n = 526)	19[a]	20[a]	16[a,b]	31[a]	14[a]
Above-average income (n = 500)	17	17	9	36	11
United States					
Below-average income (n = 545)	35[b]	26[b]	30[b]	49[b]	28[b]
Above-average income (n = 609)	22	18	8	40	15

Sources: Commonwealth Fund/Harvard/Harris Interactive 2001 International Health Policy Survey; R. J. Blendon et al., "Inequities in Health Care: A Five Country Survey," Health Affairs 21, no. 3 (2002). Used with permission.
[a]Significantly different from U.S. below-average income at $p \leq .05$.
[b]Significantly different from above-average income at $p \leq .05$.

doctors, emergency care, specialists, and superb care at nearby university hospitals. But only 62 percent of Americans have that kind of employer-provided care, and it declines every year; and of course, millions have no insurance at all.

Does the market offer some distinct advantages over government control? Not much beyond marginal advantages here and there in some contexts, as far as we can see. We can only guess how market advocates reason their way to conclusions about the superiority of market practices. They could say, but rarely do, that government-run or -supervised health care in Europe works well enough *there* but would not work *here,* because of the American culture and particularly its hostility to government. But to cite that hostility as a reason for

TABLE 6.10
Citizens' Overall Views about Their Health Care System, Five Countries,
Selected Years 1988–2001

	Australia	Canada	New Zealand	United Kingdom	United States
Only minor changes needed					
1988/90	34%[a]	56%[a]	—[b]	27[a]	10[a]
1998	19[a]	20	9[a]	25[a]	17
2001	25	21	18	21	18
Fundamental changes needed					
1988/90	43[a]	38[a]	—[b]	52[a]	60[a]
1998	49	56	57	58	46[a]
2001	53	59	60	60	51
Rebuild completely					
1988/90	17	5[a]	—[b]	17	29
1998	30[a]	23	32[a]	14[a]	33[a]
2001	19	18	20	18	28

Sources: Canada, U.K., and U.S. data collected in 1988, Australia collected in 1990; Harvard/Harris/Baxter Foundation. For 1998, Commonwealth Fund/Harvard/Harris 1998 International Health Policy Survey. For 2001, Commonwealth Fund/Harvard/Harris 2001 International Health Policy Survey. R. J. Blendon et al., "Inequities in Health Care: A Five Country Survey," *Health Affairs* 21, no. 3 (2002). Used with permission.
[a]Significantly different from U.S. in 2001 at $p \leq .05$.
[b]Not available.

its purported likely failure in the United States would beg the question: why, given the European evidence, is there such hostility? Or it may be that a strong government role in human affairs is judged to be intrinsically wrong—an offense against human freedom and dignity. Thus it is characterized invidiously as a "heavy hand"—the fact that it may work well enough in many countries does not undo its inherent wrongness. Or perhaps it is because the market and suspicion of government are so much a part of the American way of life that any other course seems unimaginable. It may also have to do with what we earlier called the "market fallacy," which moves from the undoubted general superiority of market economies over command economies to the conclusion that a market-based health care system would be no less superior—even if we have yet to see it in practice anywhere.

That is just speculation, but what does seem clear enough is that much market advocacy is a mixture of government-bashing and hypothetical promissory notes, the one vying with the other for attention. Commonly missing is an empirical foundation for the vaunted promise of the market for health care. We offer as our evidence for those characterizations three items. The first is the article from the *Wall Street Journal* cited above.

While calling government bad and the market good, the authors of that article propose a number of reforms to get the country on a stronger market

TABLE 6.11
Citizens' Views of Access to and Quality of Care, Five Countries, 2001

Access	AUS	CAN	NZ	UK	US
Very or extremely difficult to see a specialist	12%[a]	16%	11%[a]	13%	17%
Somewhat difficult to see a specialist	23	28[a]	23	22	22
Not too or not at all difficult to see a specialist	60	51[a]	61	53	59
Access worse than two years ago	19	26[a]	15[a]	17	20
Access about the same as two years ago	69[a]	65	71[a]	69[a]	62
Access better than two years ago	8[a]	6[a]	10[a]	11[a]	17
Somewhat or very difficult to get care on nights or weekends	34[a]	41	23[a]	33[a]	41
Often or sometimes unable to get care because it is not available where you live	17	21	18	13[a]	20
Did not fill a prescription due to cost	19[a]	13[a]	15[a]	7[a]	26
Did not get medical care due to cost	11[a]	5[a]	20[a]	3[a]	24
Did not get test, treatment, or follow-up care due to cost	15[a]	6[a]	14[a]	2[a]	22
Did not get dental care due to cost	33	26	37	19[a]	35
Problems paying medical bills	11[a]	7[a]	12[a]	3[a]	21

Quality ratings					
Rated overall medical care as					
Excellent	26%	20%	27%[a]	21%	22%
Very good	37	34	40[a]	32	35
Good	26	32[a]	23[a]	30	28
Fair	8	9	6	13	10
Poor	2	3	2	2	3
Rating of physician responsiveness as excellent or very good					
Treating you with dignity and respect	80[a]	79[a]	84[a]	73	72
Listening carefully to your health concerns	73[a]	74[a]	75[a]	67	65
Providing all the information you want	72[a]	67	73[a]	58[a]	63
Spending enough time	69[a]	62[a]	71[a]	54	58
Knowing you and your family situation	63[a]	59	67[a]	51	57
Being accessible by phone or in person	59[a]	55[a]	64[a]	48	52

Sources: Commonwealth Fund/Harvard/Harris Interactive 2001 International Health Policy Survey; R. J. Blendon et al., "Inequities in Health Care: A Five Country Survey," *Health Affairs* 21, no. 3 (2002). Used with permission.

Notes: Some columns may not add up to 100 percent because each respondent was given the option to say that they were not sure or could decline to answer altogether. For Australia, N = 1,412; Canada, N = 1,400; New Zealand, N = 1,400; United Kingdom, N = 1,400; United States, N = 1,401.

[a]Significantly different from U.S. at $p \leq .05$.

track: elimination of the tax exemption for employer-provided health care; a tax deduction for individually purchased private insurance and out-of-pocket expenses; much higher copayments with that private insurance; reduction of barriers to entry that limit the supply of health professionals; provision of affordable insurance for the chronically ill; and, finally, just "allow market forces to work."[129] Yet for none of these proposals individually, much less collectively, is there any good evidence they would deliver a more cost-effective, cost-controlling, efficient or equitable health care system.

TABLE 6.12

Citizens' Satisfaction with Their Own Health Care System, Compared with Rankings by Public Health Experts, in Seventeen Countries, 1998 and 2000, and 1997 per Capita Health Spending

	Percent satisfied with system[a]	Ranking by WHO overall system performance	Ranking by WHO overall system attainment	Ranking by WHO responsiveness of system	Ranking by per capita health expenditure	Total health expenditure per capita (WHO)
Denmark	91%	16	13	3	7	$1,940
Finland	81	15	14	11	12	1,539
Austria	73	4	7	8	5	1,960
Netherlands	70	8	5	6	8	1,911
Luxembourg	67	7	2	2	4	1,985
France	65	1	3	9	3	2,125
Belgium	63	11	9	9	11	1,738
Ireland	58	10	16	13	14	1,200
Germany	58	13	10	4	2	2,365
Sweden	58	12	1	7	6	1,943
United Kingdom	57	9	6	14	15	1,193
Canada	46	14	4	5	9	1,836
Spain	43	3	12	15	13	1,211
United States	40	17	11	1	1	3,724
Italy	20	2	8	12	10	1,824
Portugal	16	5	17	17	16	1,060
Greece	16	6	15	16	17	964
Rank-order correlation (Spearman's rho)		−0.235[b]	0.233[c]	0.457[d]		

Sources: Eurobarometer 49 (1998); U.S. and Canada data are from Harvard School of Public Health (2000); and total per capita health spending, in 1997 U.S. dollars, is from *World Health Report 2000* (Geneva: WHO, 2000). R. J. Blendon, M. Kim, and J. M. Benson, "The Public versus the World Health Organization on Health System Performance," Health Affairs 20, no. 3 (2001): 10–20.

Note: Countries are arranged in order of citizens' satisfaction: Denmark scored highest; Greece, lowest.
[a] Percentage saying "fairly or very satisfied" with their own health care system.
[b] Correlation between ranking by the World Health Organization (WHO) overall system performance and ranking by satisfaction.
[c] Correlation between ranking by the WHO overall system attainment and ranking by satisfaction.
[d] Correlation between ranking by the WHO responsiveness of the system and ranking by satisfaction.

It is all speculation. That way of thinking is a common feature of market advocates: if we only did x, y, or z, we could control costs, give people real choice, and get government off our back. It is not that, on paper, these are necessarily bad ideas. It is the confidence with which they are advanced that is incredible: a batch of putatively great ideas with no obvious, tested evidence to support them. It is only fair to mention in this context that pro-government liberals have their own set of speculative reforms, some of them untested for their long-term value. Karen Davis, proposing ten supply-side controls to control costs, is an example of this phenomenon.[130] Her list includes reduction in hospitalization of patients with high-cost conditions, negotiation of drug prices, and evidence-based medical guidelines. They are all sensible enough in

TABLE 6.13

Satisfaction with Their Own Health System among the Poor and the Elderly, Compared with Rankings by Public Health Experts, in Seventeen Countries, 1998 and 2000

	Poor		Elderly		Ranking by WHO overall system performance	Ranking by WHO overall system attainment	Ranking by WHO responsiveness of system
	Percent satisfied with system[a]	Ranking by satisfaction	Percent satisfied with system[a]	Ranking by satisfaction			
Denmark	90%	1	93%	1	16	13	3
Finland	78	2	83	2	15	14	11
Austria	73	3	74	4	4	7	8
France	69	4	68	7	1	3	9
Luxembourg	69	5	75	3	7	2	2
Netherlands	68	6	70	5	8	5	6
United Kingdom	67	7	69	6	9	6	14
Ireland	65	8	62	9	10	16	13
Sweden	56	9	66	8	12	1	7
Belgium	54	10	57	11	11	9	9
Germany	52	11	57	12	13	10	4
Spain	47	12	57	13	3	12	15
United States	45	13	61	10	17	11	1
Canada	40	14	48	14	14	4	5
Italy	22	15	30	15	2	8	12
Portugal	20	16	19	17	5	17	17
Greece	18	17	22	16	6	15	16

Rank-order correlation (Spearman's rho)
Poor					-0.154^b	0.25^c	0.361^d
Elderly					-0.279^e	0.299^f	0.471^g

Sources: Eurobarometer 49 (1998); U.S. and Canadian data are from Harvard School of Public Health (2000). R. J. Blendon, M. Kim, and J. M. Benson, "The Public versus the World Health Organization on Health System Performance," *Health Affairs* 20, no. 3 (2001): 10–20. Used with permission.

Note: Responsiveness refers to how responsive a health system is to the nonhealth needs of its citizens. The United States ranks number 1 on this measure, but number 14 in citizen satisfaction.

[a]Percentage saying "fairly or very satisfied" with their own health system.

[b]Correlation between ranking by World Health Organization (WHO) overall system performance and ranking by satisfaction among the poor.

[c]Correlation between ranking by WHO overall system attainment and ranking by satisfaction among the poor.

[d]Correlation between ranking by WHO responsiveness of the system and ranking by satisfaction among the poor.

[e]Correlation between ranking by WHO overall system performance and ranking by satisfaction among the elderly.

[f]Correlation between ranking by WHO overall system attainment and ranking by satisfaction among the elderly.

[g]Correlation between ranking by WHO responsiveness of the system and ranking by satisfaction among the elderly.

theory, even commonsensical, but some are fueled more by hope than evidence. Yet if some of her proposals are relatively untested in American health care, they are overshadowed by the larger and long-running experiment of European health care, whose various features show a clear superiority in almost all categories of health care. Her proposals amount to incremental improvements on the present system, some requiring government management, others a change in patient and physician behavior. The European systems, in contrast, offer a picture of various ensembles of government and market activities, and it is those ensembles that seem to us the final test of the strengths or weaknesses of health care systems.

In *Lives at Risk: Single-Payer National Insurance around the World,* John C. Goodman and his colleagues try to show that single-payer systems fail in terms of access, quality, and cost, but also, and even worse, pose a threat to the lives of their patients.[131] As it turns out, however, they focus on only three countries: Canada, New Zealand, and Great Britain. Other systems that do much better, such as France, Switzerland, and Germany, are not even mentioned. Yet even the countries they choose to examine do better on most indicators than the United States. Waiting lists are a particular target—as is common among most pro-market advocates—and they surely are a weak point in some single-payer systems. Do some people on waiting lists die as a direct result of the delay in receiving needed care? Apparently so, if anecdotal evidence is to be believed, but no hard data seem to exist anywhere on waiting list mortality rates. Nor does every single-payer country have a waiting list problem. An OECD study published in 2003 found that twelve countries identified elective surgery as a high priority for improvement, but seven countries perceived no waiting list problem.[132] In any event, Canada and the United Kingdom have worked in recent years to deal with the problem.[133]

Another item we note is a pro-market collection of essays edited by a prominent health care economist, Roger D. Feldman, with a foreword by Mark V. Pauly *American Health Care: Government, Market Processes, and the Public Interest.*[134] Notable in Pauly's foreword is a note of caution and a repeating of his point, noted in chapter 1 of this book, about the difficulty of trying to compare "real and imperfect markets with real and imperfect governments," and that "the assurance of adequate care is the one that most requires government" (p. x). Feldman, however, is less modulated. The Clinton health care failed because people don't trust government to manage their medical care. From this viewpoint, the primary failure of the academic literature is its failure to offer a cogent analysis of why government health care does not work. Do the European solidarity systems, with their strong government regulation, universal coverage, and good quality indicators, show that government control "does not work"? Even in the United States it is hard to know what to make of an assertion of that kind in the face of the success of the Medicare program and the experience of the Veterans Administration health care system, and of course that of numerous European countries. In response, we say: just take a look at the evidence we cited earlier and at the tables we have presented.

Pauly characterizes the discussion in the Feldman book as "hopeful, but much of it is avowedly tentative" (p. ix). He is right, save for the most untentative government bashing that surfaces repeatedly in the book. But beyond that, with the aim of reforming government health care regulation, there are proposals for improved medical savings accounts, greater freedom for health care contracting, better price competition, much looser health care provider licensing requirements, reform of Food and Drug Administration advertising restrictions, private industry certification of the safety and efficacy of medical devices, and a restatement of arguments against price control.

There is surely something to be said for some of these proposals, which we do not mean to dismiss out of hand—though some of them sound far-fetched. But it is hard to find a balancing role for government in any of them. Moreover, exactly the same critical commentary we offered in the preceding proposal applies here as well—they are essentially schemes with little or no evidence to demonstrate their systemwide efficacy. When not displaying outright hostility to government regulation, silence seems the usual response in these essays to any positive role that government might play. Yet in a confession that seems implicitly to reject the notion that Americans hate government, the conservative legal scholar Richard A. Epstein wrote in his contribution that, "in the end, one despairs of doing anything sensible through the political process. Of all the alternatives, market solutions seem socially most desirable, and politically least feasible."[135] For our part, we offer a parallel observation: of all the alternatives, government-run programs seem socially most desirable, and politically less feasible.

Alain Enthoven, our third example of market advocacy, is far less pessimistic than Epstein. With more empirical support for his proposals than most market advocates, he cites a number of changes he believes are feasible. Citing the experience of Harvard, Stanford, and the University of California, the Wells Fargo Bank and Hewlett-Packard, the Federal Employees Health Benefits Program and the California Public Employees' Retirement System, as members of his "honor roll" of organizations that "follow a reasonably good approximation to the managed competition model," he believes that some feasible changes would "create a health care economy in which market forces are strong enough to deliver efficient health care systems."[136] They include requiring employers to offer their employees multiple, wide, informed individual choices; management of competition; and fresh efforts to apply antitrust laws to health care.

If some of those changes are feasible, the fact still remains that nowhere in the United States has Enthoven's model, in its full scope, been tested. It seems to us one of the *theoretically* more plausible plans. But it can hardly be used to demonstrate, other than hypothetically, that the end result would be superior to any one of the European systems, which are up and running with already visible results, or that it would be superior to the "Medicare for all" idea—which he believes, more or less fatalistically, will eventually triumph—but which he says would be inefficient.

In sum, it is hard not to conclude that the animus against government, and the untested faith in the market as the remedy for health system problems, reveals a profound bias rarely well defended. No doubt its deep roots in American culture make it hard to dislodge; and counterevidence seems to have little impact, particularly among the politicals. Yet we have presented bits of evidence earlier, here and there, that market enthusiasm may be slightly waning and that pressure in a government direction is increasing—but we do emphasize "bits" only. The point is not that the European systems should be—much less could be—brought wholesale to the United States. More simply it is that those systems demonstrate that government-dominated systems of different kinds can be effective, providing high-quality care at a lower cost and with a higher quality than in the United States, and in countries with a wide variety of governments, histories, and cultures (think only of the differences between Italy and Sweden, Norway and France).

As we will suggest further in our final chapter, there are some useful market practices to be learned and adopted without aiming for a full system transplant. For the developing countries, most of which are in no financial condition to emulate the European systems in their full scope, there are many more individual practices and policies to borrow from than are available from the example of the United States. But the market, we conclude, has a potential only at the margins of government-run systems. It might in some circumstances make those systems work more efficiently, but it shows little promise of serving as the bedrock of any health care system *as a whole.* Instead of arguing from a baseline of market enthusiasm, for the most part untested, to American reform, it would be wiser to use European systems as the baseline, making use of what works there and rejecting what does not. As our chapter on European health care makes clear, there are many ways of organizing universal care systems. If European countries can innovate in adopting such systems, so can the United States.

If this chapter has presented our findings and analysis, there is still one more step, that of laying out our reading of the implications of the evidence we have set forth and making some suggestions about the future. Newt Gingrich, the American conservative politician and an advocate of a greater market dominance in health care, has reputedly said that foreign policy is a far less complex area than health policy. If we agree with him on little else, he is right on target with that insight.

CHAPTER SEVEN

The Future of the Market in Health Care

Undercurrents from the Past, Riptides from the Future

Most people want decent health care to be readily available at an affordable price. When they hurt, they want a doctor to look at them, a nurse to care for them, drugs they can afford, and a hospital to take them in if they need medically necessary surgery or complex care. Increasingly in developed countries, they also want their personal preferences, variable though they may be, respected. When all is lost, the battle all but over, they want long-term or nursing home care, and without beggaring them or their family. As the diversity of the world's health care systems shows, there are many ways of attempting to satisfy these desires, and many ways as well of judging just what counts toward their achievement.

The terms *decent health care, readily available, affordable price,* and *medically necessary* are all contestable. At least one reason why health care can never be a technically perfect market is that of its murkiness to most people: complex, usually in flux, short of meaningful information, full of medical uncertainty, and suffused with political and social arguments. What is clear for most people is often that their health system is not clear. That is one reason why health care reform is so difficult, full of too many variables to be put together in some perspicuously coherent way, able to go in many possible directions, few of them fully predictable in their outcomes.

It is not for nothing that wide-scale health care reform has been so difficult in the United States, with its tripartite constitutional government, its longstanding debates about the relationship between the market and government, its plethora of interest and advocacy groups, and its deeply ingrained individualism. Canada and the European countries have had an easier time of it, by virtue of their welfare state traditions and with the force of parliamentary governments that can act decisively to bring about social change. But the possibility of noticing these national traits—sometimes easier from the outside than from the inside—makes another point clear: the force of history and tradition in the shaping of health care systems.

The European health care systems, with their strong solidarity commitments, are traceable back to the nineteenth century and have been reconfirmed over the decades despite periodic financial stress. The failure, by contrast, of the United States to achieve universal care despite many attempts to do so, the intensity of its market proponents, and (perhaps perversely) the fact that Americans seem more to take pride in the quality of their high-technology medicine than to feel shame at the forty-five million uninsured, all bespeak a tradition as deep and enduring as that witnessed in Europe.

If it is comparatively easy to characterize the American and European systems with some broad strokes, that is less easy to do with the developing countries of the world. Too often their health care systems have not grown out of deep cultural roots but were superimposed either by colonial powers or, in their aftermath, by authoritarian and often repressive governments, or by well-meaning, but not necessarily helpful, international agencies such as the World Bank.

MAKING JUDGMENTS: GOOD AND BAD HEALTH CARE SYSTEMS

For our part, attempting to look into that uncertain gray zone that is the future, two conclusions seem supportable: on the best and worst kind of health care systems, and on the threatened future of the best.

The Best and Worst Kinds of Health Care Systems

We do not hesitate to say that the best health care systems are found in Canada, Western Europe, and a few other countries in the same tradition. They are systems run along Bismarckian or Beveridge lines. Their strength lies in their universality, with coverage for all; in their quality for the money spent, producing high levels of health for significantly less per capita than the United States; and in health outcomes that are the best in the world. All of them have their faults—waiting lines in some places (notably Canada and the United Kingdom), some technological scarcity here and there, a mixed record on some quality items, and sometimes less than adequate drug and long-term care coverage.

But most of them are looked upon favorably by their users, only a small proportion of whom believe their system needs radical overhaul. As long as the systems adhere to their solidarity and universal care commitments, little harm seems done in their effort to find some market practices to make them more efficient. If those practices have done no notable good, neither have they done any notable harm. The key is to hold on to the principles of solidarity and universality, allowing market practices only to the extent that they do not undermine those principles. In that context, the market may bring benefits within a context that limits its possible harms.

The worst kinds of systems are those where the market has triumphed in its harshest form, as in rural China, India, and many African countries. That result has for the most part come about not because of the outcome of a theoretical or political debate about the idea of the market, but as a way for governments in poor countries to get the burden of health care off their back. The result too often is a disorderly and unregulated market, a laissez-faire situation, one likely to induce financial fear when illness strikes and certain to promote inequitable access to care. When the market is the dominant reality in developing countries, there is almost always the lack of a decent government safety net. The available private care favors the affluent, draws the better physicians out of the public and into the private system, and achieves none of the potential benefits of the market (at least in theory), those of meaningful competition on choice, quality, and price. More than developed countries, the developing countries are heavily dependent on drugs in their health care, but suffer great deprivations in getting them. They are at the mercy of an international pharmaceutical industry that gives up high profits only when shamed into it by public opinion, or forced into it by government power; and that does not happen enough in developing countries.

As for its health care system, the United States is not the best or anywhere near the worst. It is not near the top in health outcomes, but it is at the top of per capita health care expenditures. Yet if one is fortunate enough to have good private insurance from an employer and live in a large metropolitan region, the available medical care can be superb, equal to the best in the world. In light of that uneven record, it is impossible to say with a straight face that its heavy dependence on private care, and its willingness to use market practices, have led to an overall system that is better than those found in Canada and Western

Europe. The market has been tried in the United States, but it is hard to find notable triumphs that the rest of the world is eager to emulate.

The Threatened Future of the Best Health Care Systems

Market ideology within health care systems has never had the sway in Europe that it has had in the United States. For the former, the attraction has been that of better managing cost pressures, beginning sharply in the 1980s, fluctuating during the 1990s, and strong again in the new millennium. For the latter, with a heavier measure of ideological influence, but with even more worrisome cost increases, the market continues to beckon, spurred by the George W. Bush administration.

Those cost increases, beyond ordinary cost-of-living increases, are common in developed countries. There is considerable agreement among many health care economists on their most immediate causes: the adoption of new technologies and the intensified use of old ones, and rising public demand. In the United States, the estimate is that from 40 to 50 percent of the cost increase can be traced to the impact of technology, with comparable, if not quite so intense, developments in Europe and Canada.[1] A number of studies have suggested that the aging of a population does not, in and of itself, exert as much pressure on costs as popularly thought.[2] But when that demographic shift is combined with a more intense use of technology for elderly patients (common everywhere), the impact can be considerable and is bound to increase in the future.

Less well explored has been public demand, but there is good reason to believe that one result of medical progress and technological innovation is to constantly raise the standard of what counts as decent health care. As with some ancient mathematical problems that have lacked solutions for many centuries, no society has managed to come up with a consensus on the meaning of "medical necessity" as a baseline for minimally acceptable health care. The reason for that is in part that progress stimulates a constant change of perspective and cultural expectations. Coronary by-pass surgery for those over eighty-five would have been unthinkable even thirty years ago; now it has become routine, just as kidney dialysis has become routine for those over seventy. Both are now considered medically necessary if there are no obvious medical counterindications—and age per se is less and less one of them.

Taken together, these cost-enhancing ingredients, now well mixed, presage likely trouble in the future for health care in developed countries. There is always the possibility of increased efficiency from better management techniques and evidence-based medicine, but it is unlikely that they can for much longer significantly stem the tide of rising costs. That means that universal health care systems (not to mention the United States, with its own problems) will have a problem on their hands, which even the strongest underpinning of solidarity will have trouble managing. The only consistently effective method of cost control is on the supply side, with government using its strong hand to deny needed and desired medical care or a greater adoption of market practices to relieve the pressure on government—or, most likely, some of both.

While competition can be stimulated, and will probably work here and there, the most attractive, least politically troublesome approach is likely to be an increase in copayments, something already noticeable in many countries. This tactic might be understood not as a rejection of universal care but as a hollowing out of its contents. Politically, governments can boast that they are holding on to the old solidarity values, but in practice they will be thinning out its benefits. Exceptions can be made for some segments of the population—the aged and the poor, most notably—but even those exceptions can be hollowed out by setting more stringent rules on qualification for them.

The (Possibly) More Promising Future of the Developing Countries

As matters now stand, most developing countries have poor health care systems, and made all the worse by misguided efforts to give the market a stronger role. The failure of that effort is now being acknowledged, if only tacitly. The next step is to begin reintroducing strong public health systems, aiming to deal effectively with the most basic health need for good sanitation, nutritious food, and at least a rudimentary primary care system. In many countries, that kind of system did exist prior to the 1980s "reform," and it is possible (one can say no more) that it could be brought to life again. It is also possible that, with sufficient public and political pressure, and some change of heart, the pharmaceutical companies could be cajoled or coerced into changing their research and marketing practices to be more helpful to the developing countries with their heavy dependence on drugs.

If the important international monetary agencies, together with private foundation contributions and with help from the governments of developed countries, would throw their weight behind the creation of even minimal forms of universal health care in developing countries, that would be a major and hopeful movement. Most important in the long run will be a continuing improvement in the overall economic and social welfare of those who live in poor countries. There are many signs of health improvement, most of which have little to do with health care: declining mortality rates for all age groups (save for sub-Saharan Africa, because of AIDS), the emergence of a chronic illness problem associated with aging (an ironic sign of progress in mortality reduction in the elderly), a great improvement in education and literacy rates, an improved social status for women, and a gradual movement toward more open, democratic societies.

Those trends represent slow, glacial shifts, but of a kind that even now serve as an antidote to the unregulated market habits and practices now rampant in so many developing countries. To move health care back to government, and to begin regulating the worst market practices, would be much more than simply icing on the cake of socioeconomic progress. It is a necessary ingredient in solidifying that progress and helping to avoid a reversal of the trend. Since, at the moment, developing countries have no choice but to accept a finite model of health care, not the high-technology infinity model of the developed countries, hanging on to that model will be critical to efforts to develop good health care systems.

TWO WAYS OF THINKING ABOUT HEALTH CARE REFORM

There are, we want to argue, two distinct ways of thinking about health care reform, even though they can and should overlap. One way of thinking, most conspicuous in debates about health care reform, can be termed management-oriented and the other value-oriented. By a *management orientation* we refer simply to efforts to change the workings and details of health care systems, attempting to make them better achieve the political ends set for them. Systems can be tinkered with, moderately changed, or overturned altogether in favor of some other arrangement. Most, if not all, proposals for health care reform around the world fall into the first two of those categories. Their aim is not to change underlying values of the deepest kind, but instead to change the way those values are implemented in delivery systems. The main thrust of the market debate has been to deal with the question of whether market practices produce better, more efficient systems than government control. Thus it has remained mainly in the management arena, whether the various combatants want to embrace a market or government approach or some combination of both. The five proposals for reform of American health care, outlined in chapter 2, mostly embody a management approach, however different their details and underlying ideology.

That management debate has paid little attention to such matters as the meaning of health, illness, and death—our finitude—and how they are best understood as part of the human condition; those issues are ordinarily well outside its ordinary scope of market arguments. By a *value orientation* we mean a focus on just those issues, not on how to organize and manage health care systems, but on their moral and value premises. Those premises are usually unspoken or at least not examined with the kind of nuance and attention to detail given to organizational and management tactics.

We have already, from time to time, looked at one of the value premises of contemporary medicine, that of its infinite aspirations, its unrelenting war against illness and death, its reluctance to set any boundaries to medical hopes and dreams. That premise, we believe, is well overdue for critical examination, and particularly in light of the power of market ideas to foster and promote that premise. An alternative set of values can be described as finite medicine, which understands that health is not necessarily the highest human value— save for society-destructive epidemics such as AIDS, high childhood and maternal mortality, and various tropical diseases—and that sickness and death are a permanent part of the human condition.

There is still another value premise, also promoted by market ideas—though more implicitly than explicitly: that the key to ever-improving health lies in organized health care systems, in the way we deploy knowledge and technology within the domain of scientific medicine and institutional arrangements. But that view, promoting the notion that the secret to better health lies in medical progress heavily deployed through technologically oriented health care, is no longer plausible. Throwing increasingly expensive medicine at illness and death will, sooner or later, become an economic dead end. An alternative view centers on prevention and a reduction in behavior-related causes of illness and death, and on the far greater role played by socioeconomic conditions in advancing health than by organized health care systems.

THE PLACE OF THE MARKET IN THE FUTURE OF HEALTH CARE
The Managerial Perspective

We turn first to the managerial perspective, which we have most heavily analyzed in this book. In that context, we have distinguished two strands of market thinking, the instrumental and the political. The instrumentalists are primarily health care economists, and many are European solidarity-committed administrators, oriented toward helping health care systems work in the most efficient and efficacious way; and equity is a concern of many if not all of them. The politicals, by contrast, see the market as a necessary partner of a democratic society; each needs the other; while equity is not ignored, choice and freedom as values are the dominant note, and even at the cost of some equity.

The instrumentalist approach is by far the most valid. It has a variety of virtues. It wants to bring its economic skills to the well-functioning of health care systems, recognizing their complexity and using various monetary and regulatory techniques to help bring out their highest potential. It is an approach that does not have a built-in political agenda, and that makes it suitable to work with diverse political regimes. Most important, it wants its theories and approaches to be supported with solid empirical evidence: what works and does not work to advance the goals of health care? And then, because of its lack (for the most part) of a professional political agenda, and the high place it gives to evidence, it can promote change and nuance, cutting through special interests and resisting political pressure that aims to have health care systems serve ends other than health. There are many market proponents in this camp, but they agree with and abide by the rules of good analysis and sensible proposals: be prepared to experiment before jumping in, insist on good evidence to test present and proposed policy—and grant the need for an important government role, at the least to provide a safety net and to regulate market practices.

Does the instrumentalist approach have some shortcomings? It can be insensitive to cultural currents and considerations, cutting through them just a bit too smoothly. Too much efficiency may not, for instance, well serve the doctor-patient relationship, dependent on trust and intimacy, and may not easily be amenable to tight regulation or even oversight. It can no less be indifferent to the nature of medicine and the appropriate goals of medicine, its instrumentalism serving health care systems rather than well-grounded notions of the relationship between health and human welfare. Its professional ambivalence toward equity, considered more in the realm of ethics and politics than economics, may not always make it suitable to work closely with health care systems where that is the highest and most indispensable value, even if inefficient. Equity can be messy and not necessarily the least expensive way for government to go.

But these drawbacks are far less than those that burden the approach of the politicals to the market. Its most striking drawback is precisely the heated conviction, a kind of single-minded and dogmatic faith, with which it is hawked. Its distrust of government means that market failure is not seen as an important kind of failure, never enough to legitimate government as the superior custodian of health care. Better to tinker with the market, swallow some failure, rather than move dangerously toward that great—and allegedly discredited—leviathan, a centralized health care system managed by "big government."

Hardly anyone among the politicals explicitly says that a government-run single-payer system is the Hayekian road to serfdom, though President George W. Bush in his campaign speeches came close to doing just that. They are more likely to claim it is clumsy, inefficient, bureaucratic, and insensitive to individual preferences. The European health care systems provide the best possible evidence that this need not happen. But that ideological stance remains the flavor of, say, editorials in the *Wall Street Journal* or articles in the *Weekly Standard* touting medical savings accounts, defending high drug prices, and poking holes in any reform proposals that do not embody market deference. The way of government is doom, so say the politicals, and the way of the market is liberation.

The instrumentalist approach, a bit cool and analytical in principle, sees the need to find evidence to support health care strategies, to look carefully at the details of health systems, and to accept the reality of complexity and uncertainty in reform proposals. No such hesitations burden the politicals. It is choice, competition, and a minimal government role they want. That no one can find anywhere in the world a good example of a market-dominated health care system that is superior to the government-controlled universal health care systems of Canada and Europe seems beside the point.

Of course, there is a response to such skepticism. The market has never really been tried has it? Or allowed to succeed when it might have done so? And in any event, it is the right way to go for people who would be free and have choice about their health care. It is hard to argue with that kind of faith, but we believe it to be not the god that failed, though it has for the most part, but the god that has not been examined with a cool and skeptical eye—and perhaps never will be by the ideologically driven.

Making Second Best Work

Let us make our argument clear at this point. Our ideal health care system would be government managed and regulated, financed either directly by taxation or indirectly by mandated employer/employee contributions—that is, either a Bismarckian or Beveridge plan. It would give pharmaceutical coverage, and long-term and mental health care, parity with physician and hospital care. It would leave considerable administrative and priority-setting obligations in the hands of local or regional authorities, and it would require a central place for citizen consultation. The role of the federal, or central, government would be overall monitoring of health care results and health status, public health programs, evidence-based medicine research, and the determination of an appropriate level of federal support. Its principal obligation would be to make certain every citizen had good health care coverage, and it would work to equalize health care financing among the various regions of the country.

Our idea of an ideal system, it should be evident, is nothing other than a composite portrait drawing upon already successful universal health care systems. In the American context, the "Medicare for all" proposal comes the closest to our ideal—even though its scant provision for market practices probably renders it politically implausible. Our second-best choice would be Alain Enthoven's managed competition plan—though its complexity and a government management of the competition probably render it politically implausible also.

We will not attempt here to add more details to this composite portrait, but with one important exception: that of finding an appropriate place and level for market ideas and practices. We move in this direction for two reasons. One of them is that we do not believe it likely, given its history, culture (that deadly hyperpluralism), present federal debt burden, and current level of health care costs, that the United States will embrace government-managed universal health care in the foreseeable future. Thus the only meaningful issue is where and how to use market practices to make the present imperfect system a little less imperfect—while simultaneously working incrementally for expanded government coverage to deal with the uninsured and with market failure. The other reason is that we expect Canada and the European countries to find that the steadily rising costs, with no end in sight or even imaginable, will push them further in a market direction. How should that prospect be handled? As for the developing countries, their need is for health care systems that begin approaching universal care ideals. They should be exceedingly reluctant to pursue market practices at this historical moment, most of which would increase inequity in their situation. These practices can be tried when the countries are well down the road to universal care, even of an inadequate kind because of a lack of money.

In other words (and leaving out the developing countries), if universal health care will be difficult to maintain as an ideal, at least in its present form, what is a good *second-best* strategy? We realize that, in the eyes of many of those devoted to maintaining and advancing universal health care, it is considered unhelpful and politically damaging to express pessimism about the future and to even consider extending the scope of the market further; that is, don't give up the good fight and don't make any concessions, much less those that will grease a slippery slope down the market abyss. But it seems to us a form of blindness to deny the likely course of events in the future and to refuse to begin thinking about them. We say "likely," not inevitable. History surely teaches us, too often in a confounding way, that the future cannot be known, failing to follow even our most well-grounded projections and predictions. But we say "likely" because no one has presented a plausible picture of the future that shows promising ways of dealing with the triple economic threat of aging societies, a steady stream of new and expensive technologies, and ever-rising public demand.

We now want to suggest some criteria that should be used in judging the deployment of market practices, and we follow that with some specific proposals in light of our findings in the previous chapter on some key market practices.

Criteria for Deployment of Market Practices

Population Health. Market practices should not be introduced unless they show a serious promise of improving population health. By that we mean that they are a plausible means of reducing national mortality and morbidity rates. A highly seductive and politically attractive argument of "choice" advocates is to point to the likely benefits for individuals of high drug prices, or new heart technologies, or innovative cancer treatments. But even if market practices could be limited to particular groups of patients, population benefit should always take precedence over individual benefit when everyone will bear, directly or indirectly, the cost and other burdens of those benefits. So, the important question is: what will the market practices do for all of us together, not just for you or me?

Equity. The principal, and well-recognized, danger of market practices is that they will increase health inequities, giving those with economic resources an advantage over those without. Perfect equity is probably nowhere possible (the wealthy can always fly to another country to get the care they want), and the affluent and well-connected will no doubt always extract more from their health system than others. Nonetheless, market practices should never be used without their differential impact being transparent to the public and without strenuous efforts to minimize any inequities by government subsidies for those who cannot take advantage of market choices. The fact of expanded choice because of market strategies should not be allowed to overshadow the hazard of inequity, the main effect of which is to eliminate choice of any kind for those unable to pay for it.

Regulation. Market practices should not be introduced into health care systems in the absence of an effective regulatory system to monitor and control their activities. The abuses of market practices in health care are well known—monopolies, cream-skimming, hidden discounts for favored customers, and so on—and they must be controlled, not the least in order that markets function in an optimal way as markets. Beyond that, markets need regulation to minimize inequities (as noted above). It is not simply a shame that laissez-faire market practices are dominant in some developing countries, not allowing government health care systems to get off the ground or shrinking those already in existence. The utter lack of regulation of those markets invites the worst kind of abuse, as even the most avid market proponents are likely to concede.

The Use of Market Evidence. When market mechanisms are proposed for implementation, it is imperative that the public, health administrators, and legislators know the historical track record of those practices. That record should include when and how they were used, the extent of their use, and the results of their use. As noted in the previous chapter, many proposed market mechanisms often have little or no hard evidence behind them, or have evidence of such a limited scale as to raise questions about their more general applicability; they are thus essentially speculative schemes, which may or may not work in practice. Particularly important is whether the proposed mechanisms have been employed on a national scale, as distinguished from a regional or local scale. If market-oriented and government-oriented policies are to be compared and evaluated, market advocates should recognize that, in Canadian and European health care, there are decades of evidence available on the efficacy of government-oriented policies. If market proponents cannot offer comparable practice, in scope and depth, that should be made clear.

Market Experiments. If proposed market mechanisms do not have a solid, empirically grounded track record to be called upon in their favor, then they should always be designed and introduced as experiments. They should, moreover, be designed in a way that lends itself to national extrapolation; that is, if the experiment shows a certain market practice to be useful at a regional or state level, any extension of it to a larger, or national, level should have behind it evidence that such an extension would be workable on a larger scale.

In light of the possibility that market practices may be helpful to the development of equitable and economically sustainable health care systems, they should be encouraged. It seems to us inappropriate, however, for the government to subsidize market practices or experiments, as has been done as part of the Bush administration's Medicare pharmaceutical program. Such a subsidy would undermine its validity as a market practice or experiment. Market advocates have long claimed that their ideas have been given too little opportunity to be tested, and that seems to us a valid claim. Hence, such testing should go forward, but only in ways that will make possible as decisive an evaluation as can be devised.

Supply-Side Controls

The management and regulation of consumer and patient demands, what economists call the demand side, has nowhere proved a wholly satisfactory way of controlling costs—the problem that bedevils most health care systems. Waiting lists, on the one hand, and copayments, on the other, can make some difference, but the former can have some undesirable health effects and surely engender patient dissatisfaction almost everywhere (and particularly in Canada), while the latter can discourage the poor from seeking the care they need. Moreover, since much patient demand is heavily physician driven, attempts to influence that behavior have some extrinsic limits.

Thomas Rice has usefully examined the main assumptions lying behind a market advocacy of controlling health care demand rather than health care supply.[3] Each of us is not necessarily the best judge of our own health welfare, much less of whether our judgment will be conducive to the welfare of others. Even a minimal degree of reflection on our own experience should bring that point home to us. Few of us, in any case, will have the necessary medical information in many instances to make good health choices. Nor can most of us know in advance the results of our choices, many of which pose counterfactual questions: would the problem have gone away if left untreated? Would the result have been different if I had gone to a different physician or to a specialist rather than a primary care physician? In much the same vein, Rice raises questions about our supposed rationality, about the notion that our actions reveal our true preferences, and about the belief that social welfare is maximized when individuals maximize their own good.

Nothing Rice says is meant to deny individual freedom and preference satisfaction a place in health care. It is only to argue that a health policy that aims to manage a system by controls on patient demand not only does not work well but is dependent on dubious assumptions. And they are all the more dubious when used to show the supposedly inevitable and necessary failure of government-dominated policies in bringing better health or greater efficiencies. Regulating the behavior of individual health consumers and patients has proved in the end to be, at best, only modestly effective and usually accompanied by some untoward health outcomes.

The same cannot be said of supply-side regulations, aiming to control the production and distribution of health care products rather than their consumption: "What we see in health policy throughout the world . . . is the reliance instead on supply side policies . . . capitation, DRGs [diagnosis related groups], utilization review, practice guidelines, technology controls, and global budgets . . . None of these policies arise from the competitive model, nor would any be shown by economic theory to result in superior outcomes. Nevertheless, most countries rely on them, and many analysts would argue that [they] have resulted in superior outcomes in the health services marketplace."[4]

We earlier noted the success of the European countries in regulating drug prices as well as the growing pressure in the United States to move in a similar direction, either directly (through price controls) or indirectly (by the use in the United States of government buying power or allowing purchases from Canada). Generally speaking, however, government efforts to control the supply of hospital beds and expensive technologies in the United States have failed to work well or have been rejected out of hand. The resistance of various political and economic interest groups usually proved to be the undoing of such efforts. Nonetheless, when they are in place in a strong way and free of interference, they do work to restrain costs and improve quality, as the evidence from the European countries shows.

Is it even conceivable that the United States can cope with fast-rising costs without using similar restraints? Unlikely. Are there any alternative *demonstrated market practices on a national scale* that have shown a similar capacity? None that we have been able to discover. Whether the American way of life in health care can transcend its government phobia and its indifference to Canadian and European experience with supply-side controls remains, unfortunately, an open question.

The Value Perspective

We have argued that, within the management perspective, there may well be some room for useful market practices so long as certain conditions are met. The most important condition is that they be either within universal care systems, designed to make them operate more efficiently, or in those systems that are incrementally moving in a universal care direction. Yet the pursuit of health encompasses much more than the organization and management of health care systems, whose main function is usually that of taking care of those already sick.

There are at least four important value dimensions that receive little attention in most market debates: the appropriate goals of medicine, health care, and the doctor-patient relationship; the place of prevention in the promotion of health; the relative importance of organized health care systems in improving population health status; and the way medical progress is understood (and, in particular, how the infinity model of progress should be evaluated). In each case, we believe, a market perspective has little to contribute and, in some instances, is positively harmful.

Appropriate Goals of Medicine, Health Care, and
the Doctor-Patient Relationship

By its emphasis on choice, its eschewing of visions of the common good (much less social solidarity), and its focus on individual preference as the (almost) final arbiter of political acceptability, the market cannot be considered to advance many important features of good medicine and good health care. It is not that it rejects such considerations; they simply don't play a significant part in the calculus of market theory at all, whether instrumentalist or political. Three such considerations are important: what ought to be the goals of medicine, as a research and clinical enterprise; what counts as a good health care system; and what ought to be the doctor-patient relationship? We focus first on goals.

The *goals of medicine* are important in themselves, and as a matter for public consensus, if on both the research and clinical side those goals are to serve human welfare and the pursuit of health. The market, with no mind of its own, is in no position to lead medicine in a good direction. By its profit-driven bias toward satisfying individual preferences, whatever they might be, market thinking can and has often led medicine in a bad direction. At the clinical level, the dividing line between therapies directed at health improvement and those styled as "lifestyle" therapies has almost disappeared. What's good for people, it increasingly seems, is whatever they want and are willing to pay for—and it is not the task of the market to pass judgments on their preferences.

The almost transcendental status of the profit principle in the pharmaceutical industry, its implicit defense of the crudest supply-and-demand calculations, can hardly promote appropriate research priorities. What sells is not now, and never has been, a good guide to a good society, much less a good medicine. The National Institutes of Health, by contrast—government financed and managed, with salaried researchers—remains a superior model of a research organization, even though subject to strong political pressures. It goes to great trouble to determine health needs and priorities, guided by considerations beyond those of individual interests (though they are not ignored).

Seen from the perspective of history and practice, the goals of medicine can be stated in fairly simple terms, though there is surely cultural and individual variation in interpreting them: the prevention of disease and illness among those who are otherwise healthy, the relief of pain and suffering brought about by diseases and accidents, the avoidance of premature death and the provision of palliative care for the critically ill and dying, and the rehabilitation and care of those who cannot be cured of their malady.[5] The fundamental question concerning these goals in the context of this book is whether the market or government is most likely to advance them. The market has no internal guidance mechanisms for grappling with the nature of health, the meaning of the goals of medicine, and the place of health in human life. But there can be no good medicine unless those most basic of issues are confronted and debated—and a serious effort made to reach at least a rough consensus on them. Can government do better? It can if it sees its role as one of seeking consensus, of stimulating reflection, and of using politics and the legislative process as a means of embodying the best ethical and social values.

Every American and every person from the developing countries ought to envy the Europeans for their commitment to solidarity, a value that grasps the need for human interdependence and mutual support in the struggle against disease, illness, and death. No market system could have created that potent a force for the common welfare. It was Adam Smith's genius to acknowledge that the market lacked a moral core, and that it was the underlying society and culture that had to compensate for that lack. Notably missing from the rhetoric of the more ardent market proponents is the need for a societal moral core to keep a market in health care functioning in a civilized way; and the promotion of consumer choice cannot constitute such a core.

Health Care. We have already suggested above why we believe that the kinds of health care systems that have been a mark of European societies seem to us ideal. But let us put the matter in a slightly different way now. It is the task of a health care system to organize the provision of health care in a way that embodies the goals of medicine, in both its research and delivery agendas. Yet to function properly it needs two important features. One of them is that it must aim for the health of all citizens, regardless of their ability to pay for health care. It is intrinsic to the historical values of medicine, which underlie health care systems, that they make no distinctions among persons. Only one thing counts: that our finite bodies are ever at risk, whether we be young or old, rich or poor, educated or uneducated; that's the point of solidarity as a core value. A good health care system is one that puts that fact at the very center of its efforts to provide people, all the people, with what they need to deal with that finiteness.

In a curious way, pre-modern medicine and pre-modern health care could more easily take that value seriously. Little could be done for the sick other than some diagnosis followed by sympathetic care and concern. The finiteness of the body was an inescapable and unchangeable reality. All of that changed with medical progress, which took as its main target precisely that finiteness. The message became one of all-out warfare: something can and should be done about our finitude, which no longer need be passively accepted as the human fate. That medical progress has brought with it great health progress, great health care system complexity, and great costs.

People in earlier times feared illness, not simply because of the pain and suffering it brought, but also because it could rob them of the capacity to make a living. Thus the earliest forms of health insurance in the nineteenth century were aimed not at paying for medical care, which was in any case cheap, but to provide an income for those who could no longer work; that was a fear almost as great as the fear of death in societies that had no welfare safety net.

The other important feature of good health care systems is that they provide affordable and efficient care of a high quality. When it was reported in 2003 in the United States that 47 percent of the uninsured postponed medical care because of cost, and 37 percent did not fill a prescription for the same reason, and 35 percent skipped recommended treatment, it should not be hard to imagine the fear and anxiety that such situations invoked in those who could not pay for what they needed. The market value of choice was not their concern; their need was more fundamental than that: help me.

The Doctor-Patient Relationship. At the heart of traditional medicine was the doctor-patient relationship, and it remains to this day of great importance to patients. Since no one has ever proved, or rarely even studied, the actual impact of that relationship on health outcomes, there must be something more than health at stake. Our surmise is that, when in need, the sick seek someone who cares about their illness—and, more specifically, cares about them as persons, not merely as the carriers of disease. To be sure, a great deal of health care is impersonal, and some doctors show little interest in the patient as a person; for them the sick body is a machine that needs repair, and for desperately ill persons that can be enough. It is not sufficient, however, to satisfy the ethical ideals of good medicine.

While choice, we have suggested, is hardly the highest value in health care as a general rule, it does seem of considerable importance in the doctor-patient relationship. For all of their regulatory clout and the need to control costs, the governments behind universal health care systems have been wise enough to allow patients to choose their own doctors and for doctors to practice medicine more or less as they see fit. It is, in other words, crucial that both patients and doctors enter and sustain their relationship as free people. And even if it is a peculiar kind of relationship—where one of the partners needs what the other has to give and may not be able to make any other choice in the actual context of illness, and where the other partner, to maintain professional integrity and freedom of medical judgment, is under no obligation to automatically do what the patient wants—it is a very special one.

What the history of medicine seems to show is that the doctor-patient relationship can succeed, even flourish, within all kinds of health care systems, all the way from fee-for-service medicine to a salaried employee role for the physician. What might well be agreed to by proponents or opponents of market health care is that neither the market nor government should get in the way of the doctor-patient relationship. To the extent that either direction creates obstacles to that relationship, to that extent it should count as a black mark against it. One of the early aims of our research on medicine and the market was to assess the impact of market practices on the doctor-patient relationship. Surprisingly, we could find little information on that point. It remains an important area for research, at least for one reason: to what extent is a good doctor-patient relationship compatible with the efficient delivery of high-quality care?

We suspect, but cannot prove, that there may be some dissonance between these two values. American health maintenance organizations (HMOs) failed to control costs for more than a few years, or to gain the efficiency that for a time looked possible, not because they were badly managed but because many of their practices interfered with patient and physician freedom. Freedom of choice, it turns out, can be expensive and can get in the way of cost control. The necessary price of an affordable universal health care system is that both doctors and patients have to give up some degree of freedom; and the trick seems to be to walk a fine line between a limitation on freedom and the provision of enough good services to keep everyone reasonably satisfied with the tradeoff.

Prevention and Avoidable Mortality

Since the time of Hippocrates, medicine and health care have had two basic aims: keeping people well and caring for them when they are sick. The emergence of effective medical treatments and cures, and the organization of modern health care systems, complex and expensive, shifted the balance of interest heavily in the therapeutic direction, and that opened the way for market initiatives. Most market debates have focused on the care of the sick in those systems; they are not much to be found in the field of public health, which even in the United States remains heavily in the hands of government, state or federal. Yet two regularly slighted issues in the context of dramatic developments in medical technology have a bearing on market debates. One of them is the potential place of market practices in preventive medicine, by which we here mean primary prevention, aiming to keep people well. The other is the comparative role of health care and socioeconomic influences in the maintenance and promotion of health.

It is hardly a secret that neither market proponents nor observable market practices in any part of the world have given much attention to prevention. Instead, when market practices catch public and media attention, it is almost always because of technological developments, most of which come out of the private, commercial sector, that are enthusiastically publicized. Not only do those developments seem most to capture attention, visible manifestations of medical progress, but they tend also to put in the shade other health knowledge of great importance, and especially in the area of prevention.

In 1993, two distinguished public health researchers, J. M. McGinnis and W. H. Foege, published an important study showing that close to 50 percent of deaths in the United States could be traced to modifiable behaviors.[6] In 2004, Mokdad and his colleagues closely replicated that study.[7] They came up with similar results, which they and the earlier researchers called "actual causes of death." Diabetes, for example, is increased in prevalence by obesity, just as lung cancer and heart disease are increased by smoking. Among the leading actual causes of death are tobacco, poor diet and physical inactivity, alcohol consumption, toxic substances, firearm incidents, sexual behavior, and illicit use of drugs.

Mokdad and colleagues concluded—in the kind of understatement not at all displayed in, say, the announcement of the mapping of the human genome or the discovery of the potential benefits of stem cell research—that "the findings in this study argue persuasively for the need to establish a more preventive orientation in health care and public health systems in the United States."[8] No media or Hollywood celebrities have come forward to endorse and promote that conclusion, nor have any of the large pharmaceutical, biotechnology, or device companies jumped at the chance to be counted on that issue. To say this is not to deny that efforts are afoot in the United States and elsewhere to develop research and educational programs to encourage health promotion and disease prevention. But they are not coming from market proponents or those who make great profits from what has been called "sick care" as distinguished from "health care."

While it is beyond the scope of this book to note the many ways in which the American way of life promotes unhealthy lifestyles, many of them market-driven, we need to underscore the failure of the market debate to make unhealthy behaviors a central topic worthy of attention. It has been said many times that the for-profit health care industries show little interest in prevention because there is little possibility of great profit in that direction; and that is no doubt true. But more than a failure by omission is at stake here. By focusing market energies, money, publicity, and political clout on providing goods, technologies, and services for sickness care and cure—where the money is to be made—it helps promote a relative indifference to, and distraction from, modifying bad health behavior and attending as well to the background socioeconomic conditions that enhance health status. Attention is focused instead on the provision of health care as the key to healthy lives.

Yet it has been well known for some decades now that most of the improvement in individual and population health comes, not from health care, but from the social and economic conditions under which people live. Thomas McKeown did important work in the 1960s and 1970s showing that health care contributed little to population health.[9] Tracing the decline in mortality in England and Wales between 1848/54 and 1971, he showed that the decline began long before effective health care became available (mainly because of better nutrition, he believed). Most of the decline in deaths from tuberculosis, for instance, came prior to the introduction of immunization and effective chemotherapy, dropping from almost 4,000 deaths per million population in 1838 to 500 by 1940, just prior to effective treatment and vaccination. Later researchers amended his research by noting that effective treatment increased the rate of decline, but his research has stood the test of time. J. P. Mackenbach and colleagues, in a study of infectious disease in the Netherlands over approximately the same time period, found that antibiotics were introduced after mortality had already declined to a significant degree, though, there also, they accelerated the decline. They concluded from their analysis that only somewhere between 5 and 18 percent of the total decline in deaths between 1875 and 1970 could be attributed to health care.[10]

McKeown was one of the pioneers in studies of what are now called "avoidable deaths," or "mortality amenable to health care."[11] An important recent study of the question "does health care save lives?" was sponsored by the English Nuffield Foundation. It made a point of arguing that recent technological advances in medicine and better-organized health care systems in recent decades may show greater improvements in mortality resulting from health care than was earlier true, and they present some recent data to make their case (such as a decline in deaths from heart disease). Even so (though with many methodological qualifications), they acknowledge that there is "the lack of a demonstrable association [of mortality rate] with health care resources."[12] It is the socioeconomic conditions that are most important, something that can be observed in developing countries as well, where in most places there has been a decline in mortality even in the presence of very poor health services. At present, the estimates of the contribution of health care to mortality reduction range in developed countries from 20 to 40 percent. Much less is known about morbidity and disability rates, and it may be that health care makes a greater contribution there.

The Infinity Problem: Unlimited Desires, Finite Resources

The importance of prevention and avoidable mortality is that they reveal how limited the range of market potentialities are, even in principle. And it is evident, despite the wealth of literature and discussion on medicine and the market, how absent those two topics are. The clue in a Sherlock Holmes mystery story is "the dog that did not bark," and that applies here. Now, to that characterization it might well be objected that no one has claimed that market theory and practice have any likely significance beyond formal health care systems—that is, in those contexts where there are various ways of organizing such systems, and influencing the behavior and medical practices of those who take part in them. Moreover, if the data on amenable mortality show that only a minority portion of population health comes from health care, they no less show that, within that portion directly pertinent to market practices, there are many possibilities for improvement, and probably more so now than in the past.

With those qualifications in mind, we want to return finally to what we believe the greatest threats of the market are: first, in creating and then feeding an ultimately harmful appetite for a constant, and intrinsically insatiable, technological progress and innovation centered on individual preference satisfaction; and, second, in promoting the false view that the source of real medical progress and good health lies with clinically oriented health care systems and the technological access they make possible. Prevention strategies and good social and economic conditions are by any statistical calculation the most likely source of improved future human health. But market thinking, most notably of the political and entrepreneurial kind, helps to fertilize the medicine- and sick-care-oriented way of thinking by constantly seeking new and expanded markets for health care products, the more expensive and profitable the better, and by a radical relativizing of any and all health needs and desires. If people will buy medical products and services of whatever kind, and there is no direct individual physical harm, then no one, and particularly the government, should stand in their way. Who is to say, and who is to judge, just what is good and bad for people anyway? That, in essence, seems to be the market argument.

The great advantage of the European health care systems is that, by invoking the value of solidarity, they posit goods of a community kind that are superior to indiscriminately satisfying individual preferences. The great disadvantage of the American health care way of life is that it has ingested far too much of that latter point of view. For both political American liberals and conservatives, any notion of limiting technological innovation, of rationing health care for a societal benefit, is considered anathema. The American pharmaceutical industry gives market politicals the industry they like and technologically enthusiastic liberals the industry they deserve.

The third greatest market threat is the infinity model of medicine and health, in essence the unlimited, boundless drive for better health, for progress without end in overcoming the limits and decay of the human body. The success of medical research in extending life expectancies, still going on, is the source of one problem in the provision of health care, that of aging societies filled with people who still die (as in the old days, but no longer seen as the good old days), but more slowly and expensively. Innovative technologies, together with higher standards of living, are still another sign of research and clinical success. If they typically do not cure us in middle or old age, they can keep us going, but rarely in some cheap, simple way; they prop up our bodies for some additional years, with ever-new drugs and ever more sophisticated diagnostic and surgical procedures. And then, along the way, we are encouraged to hope for more from research, to expect more from our doctors and hospitals with their dazzling array of machines and tubes, with this year's versions marginally better than last year's, and sometimes even better than that. The market alone is hardly responsible for this drive, but it is a major stimulant and particularly hazardous because it has nothing of use to offer in determining either its value or its limits.

We may know in our more lucid moments that there is a likely down side to this endless hope and endless progress—our earlier death from cancer averted, transformed into a later death from Alzheimer's, or our grandfather's death from a sudden heart attack replaced by our own drawn-out death from congestive heart failure. But the whole point of progress is to move on, even when it is not clear that we will necessarily be better off; that is taken for granted. Yet the Harvard psychiatrist Arthur Barsky some years ago showed, with solid historical and survey data, that the actual improvement of health over recent decades has not been matched by a subjective sense of better health. Not only do people "report more frequent and longer-lasting episodes of serious, acute illness than they did 60 years ago . . . [there is also] a progressive decline in our threshold of tolerance for minor disorders and isolated symptoms, along with a greater inclination to view uncomfortable symptoms as pathologic—as signs of disease."[13] The aggressive merchandising of drugs aimed at those "minor disorders" and the relief of "uncomfortable symptoms" is surely part of the situation Barsky describes. In short, he showed, the baseline of what counts as good health and the baseline of patient demand are constantly rising. Wherever we are is not good enough; there is always better health, less pain, a delayed aging, and a later death to be sought; and then some more after that.

AFFORDABLE, SUSTAINABLE MEDICINE AND HEALTH CARE

We come then to a final question: what strategies for the provision of health care will prove most effective for the development of affordable and sustainable medicine and health care in the face of the triple threat of aging societies, technological innovation, and always rising public demand? We mean by *affordable* what most people will be able to access and by *sustainable* what will be financially viable over the long run (as distinguished from ad hoc coping, in a management fashion, with financial pressures). This challenge will be difficult both for a market-oriented or a government-oriented perspective and, for that matter, probably some combination of both as well.

No government, whatever its regulatory power, is likely to be able to finance endless progress in aging societies. Infinite desires and possibilities cannot be paid for with the finite budgets of governments, even in the most affluent societies. At some point or other, already reached in many high-taxation societies, other social and economic needs will begin to get slighted and, even if that does not happen in any damaging way, taxpayers will revolt, even when they are the direct beneficiaries of that taxation. In Europe, the beginning of resistance to an unlimited welfare state is already underway, stimulated by a weak economy. But even in better economic times, future aging societies will mean greater health care needs than in the past, and with more effective, albeit more expensive, technologies potentially available to deal with them. That potentiality will be harder and harder to pay for.

The demand-side tactics that did not work well in the past (but rarely were abandoned) will have to be far more draconian in the future, as evidenced by the sharp increase in deductibles and copayments in the United States, both in business health care coverage and in the federal Medicare program. That development will clash with the higher baseline of what counts as good health care, instilled in modern societies by the constant progress of medicine. Limits tolerated earlier may not be tolerated later—but the economic pressures to put them in place will be far stronger than before. Even if the role of government is seen as providing just a safety net for the poor, the expense of modern medicine will put more people in that category even if, by ordinary historical standards, they are not by any means destitute.

There is a market solution, many would say: let the market have its sway, not only giving people more choice than they now have, but also forcing choice upon them. They will have to decide whether they are willing to pay the high cost of contemporary medicine and the increased cost of new technologies or do without; it will be up to them. This may appeal to some people, particularly the affluent (as with medical savings accounts), but when the pinch of high costs comes to the middle class and those otherwise well off, they are likely to balk. They are then likely to turn to government for relief, as is happening with pharmaceuticals in the United States. Even if, technically, many people can afford the drugs, that would only be possible by sacrificing other things in their lives that are of importance also; at some point, the tension would be intolerable, and choice would be a tyranny not a liberation.

The Weakness of the Market Case

Alternatively, market proponents might well argue that, if the market is given its head, serious competition and suitable market incentives could control costs at least as effectively as government can. That has been said, but never anywhere demonstrated on a national scale. There has been considerable experience in recent decades with government-controlled health care policies; that is far less true with market practices, much less market theory (too much of which is based on hypothetical possibilities, not empirically grounded practices). Will an unregulated pharmaceutical industry, with its shareholders as the main claimants on its economic benefits, be likely to do its bit to help control costs? Will the various for-profit institutions in some countries, such as hospitals, be willing to help out as well—help out, that is, by reducing their profit margins?

There is, in the end, a fundamental incoherence, even a contradictory impulse, in a market-oriented health care, at least one that is not systematically indifferent to a decent public access to necessary health care. How can it be that a profit-oriented health care, aiming to please and reward those who put up the investment money to make it work, will turn out to be the engine of full coverage for all, much less the engine for the control of costs? One person's costs is someone else's profits. Other than public outrage and opprobrium, what incentive is there for those selling health care products to hold down their prices in the name of health?

Shareholders are a notably self-interested group, investing their money where it looks like a good bet. Few people (we surmise) invest in the drug industry to save lives and reduce suffering, the reason given by the industry in its public relations effort for its very existence. Of course, some might invoke Adam Smith's invisible hand at this point, that of the collective benefit of self-interested market decisions. And if the industry could put aside its high-minded public relations rhetoric, it might effectively argue that, yes, its aim is (really) profit, not improved health, but that the actual outcome turns out to be better health for everyone. That result, they could say, is a good result for everyone, and a perfect example of Smith's point about the real meaning of the invisible hand—that there is no necessary connection between the motives for various actions and their actual benefits. But that case might be hard to make with any effectiveness: too many people, particularly in developing countries, get to see the disastrous shortcomings of the invisible hand; it is a hand with a few fingers missing.

Let us finish up by returning to our original question: what strategies for the provision of medicine and health care will be most effective in the face of the growing cost and other pressures on health care systems? Various ingredients can be proposed.

The Case for Government

One such ingredient is that only universal health care systems, government run and financed, or at least governmentally managed and monitored, will be able to cope with those pressures. The market is too much of a wild card to be depended upon to control costs, and is congenitally prone to introduce unfettered efforts to expand choice beyond affordable boundaries and to let individual preferences, regardless of their social or economic implications, rule the day. There are several things that government, and only government, can do. The first is to keep a central eye on the entire health care system and to manage it in a way aiming at the public interest. A good federal government system will decentralize as much as possible, giving regions or states considerable control over their local and regional policy, but it will work to coordinate all of them toward a common end: equitable and high-quality care. A second role of government is that, through its political system, it can find ways to gain the contribution of all citizens in defining the goals of the system; argument and debate will be the rule, but that is as it should be in democratic societies. This will be all the more important if we are correct in projecting cost pressures that will, for earlier specified reasons, just get worse and worse, with little chance of turning back. Those pressures will necessitate rationing and priority-setting, sometimes in ways that will deny people the kind and quality of health care they desire, and even on occasion need. It is well understood that unlimited space travel is not possible with limited budgets, and so finite goals are set. It is far less understood that unlimited medical goals will not be possible with finite budgets. But such budgets are necessary and, in the future, will probably allow far less managerial maneuvering than is now possible. The necessity for citizens' active role in setting priorities and determining limits—their informed consent to being denied treatments they want—will be all the more imperative. But that is only possible with integrated national systems, not fragmented mixtures of public and private health care with no guiding—and visible—hand, which is government's role.[14]

Prevention

Another ingredient is a much expanded role for prevention to promote good health, and a recognition of the limited role that organized health care systems play in advancing health. Efforts are already underway to improve prevention efforts, but far more needs to be done. Research efforts to understand how to help people improve their health-related behavior are imperative, but they need to be complemented by a research effort that has the same status and money lavished on the $3 billion Human Genome Project. We are as ignorant about how to promote good health-related behavior as we are about the role of genetics in making us what we are.

Exhortations not to smoke, to put our seat belts on, to get more exercise, obviously have limited effectiveness. A full exploration of all the social and economic forces inducing us to unhealthy behavior needs to be made. Education programs, moreover, need to bring a tough message to the public: in the future you are not likely to have available at affordable prices all the expensive rescue technologies you might like or need. In short, get smart, start living right—or be prepared to accept the consequences. That message has been delivered in the United States to the baby boomers about their Social Security benefits: you had better start saving some money because the Social Security supports in the future will not be adequate for a good retirement. So too with health care: take care of yourself, you will not get lavish government-provided health care in the future. Hardly less important will be to educate people about the limited role that organized health care, "sick care," plays in our lives. In short, where people now tend to think of health care as available care when they are sick, they will have to think of it as a limited factor in their health, and, for policy purposes, as being limited as a government obligation.

Introducing Market Practices

Yet another ingredient, and a third contribution of a government role, will be to see if some agreement can be reached on where and how to bring in market practices. While we have seen no evidence that widespread market practices in health care systems have more than, at best, a marginal contribution to make to efficiency, cost control, or quality—and sometimes do harm— it would be wise to continue market experiments, but under a number of conditions. We have already suggested some criteria for the use of market practices, but more needs to be said. Just as we have proposed a research investment in disease prevention, market practices might well be seen as an area for more systematic research and experimentation.

At the same time, the interest in the market stems in part from a desire of most people to have considerable freedom in the health care they choose; freedom counts in health care as much as many other places (though with its own nuances). But that desire must be respected, and market ideas cannot simply be rejected out of hand. A viable role must be found for respecting patients' preferences, and the market offers some ways of doing that. It would be foolish to dismiss them, as market opponents usually do. We would like to as well, but prudence and common sense say: let's see them as experiments, maybe useful and maybe not. The point would be to let the evidence decide, not ideological and political commitments to the market.

We have cast a skeptical eye on the market as a health care panacea, in great part as a reaction to the politicals, whose zeal and faith rests on little discernible evidence, not to mention systematically ignoring the evidence that is available, on both market mechanisms and the role of government. They seem to see the market as *the* great solution, the savior, to health care problems. That is neither plausible nor helpful. To put a fine point on it: the need is to find ways to test market practices, but outside the penumbra of market ideologues and true believers. No market failures seem likely to make any difference to them. The instrumentalists, whose approach is not without its problems, are the best placed to help organize and then assess market practices. Their contribution could be all the greater if, together with others, they found a way to encompass prevention and avoidable mortality in their calculations.

Beyond that, the organization of health care systems ends in the hands of administrators and legislators and, ultimately, the general public. However health care systems are organized in the future, the existing economic trends and improvements in most parts of the world—many of them attributable to the adoption of market theory and practice in national economies outside of health care—will bring an improvement to population health. But people will still get sick and be threatened with death, even if later in life than in earlier times; and people tend to worry more about what will happen to them when they get sick than how to keep well in the first place. If that bias will have to change, they will still worry about getting sick. The market is not the way to go as a general panacea for health care, even if it works well in other sectors of society. But possibly it can contribute something. We want to leave that door open, looking carefully before entering.

Notes

INTRODUCTION: OF MONEY, THE MARKET, AND MEDICINE

1. Christopher Pass et al., eds., *The Harper Collins Dictionary of Economics* (New York: Harper Perennial, 1991), 321.

2. Richard B. Saltman and Josep Figueras, *European Health Care Reform: Analysis of Current Strategies* (Copenhagen: World Health Organization, 1997), 40.

3. Stuart M. Butler, "A New Policy Framework for Health Care Market," *Health Affairs* 23, no. 2 (2004): 22.

4. Joseph P. Newhouse, "Medical Care Costs: How Much Welfare Loss?" *Journal of Economic Perspectives* 6 (1992): 3–21. See also Albert A. Okunade and Vasudeva N. R. Murhty, "Technology as a 'Major Driver' of Health Care Costs: A Cointegration Analysis of the Newhouse Conjecture," *Journal of Health Economics* 21 (2002): 147–59; Thomas Bodenheimer, "Rising Health Care Costs. Part 2: Technological Innovation," *Annals of Internal Medicine* 142, no. 11 (2005): 932–97.

5. Richard Wilkinson and Michael Marmot, eds., *The Solid Facts: The Social Determinants of Health,* 2nd ed. (Copenhagen: World Health Organization, 2003), 80.

6. William Haseltine quoted in Lawrence M. Fisher, "The Race to Cash in on the Genetic Code," *New York Times,* 29 August 1999, C-1.

7. Eva Topinkova and Daniel Callahan, "Culture, Economics, and Alzheimer's Disease," *Journal of Applied Gerontology* 18, no. 4 (1999): 411–22.

8. See Timothy Evans et al., eds., *Challenging Inequities in Health: From Ethics to Action* (New York: Oxford University Press, 2001).

CHAPTER 1: FROM ADAM SMITH TO HMOS

1. Plato, *Republic,* 342d, 346a–c.

2. Adam Smith, *An Inquiry into the Nature and Causes of the Wealth of Nations,* Glasgow Edition, ed. R. H. Campbell and A. S. Skinner, 2 vols. (Oxford: Oxford University Press, 1976), 1.ii.27.

3. Bo Petersson, "Health, Doctors and the Good Life," in *Dimensions of Health and Health Promotion,* ed. Lennart Nordenfeldt and Per-Erik Liss (Amsterdam: Editions Rodopi, 2003), 13.

4. Jerry Z. Muller, *The Mind and the Market: Capitalism in Modern European Thought* (New York: Alfred A. Knopf, 2002), 62.

5. Ibid.

6. Adam Smith, *Lectures on Jurisprudence,* Glasgow Edition, ed. R. L. Meek, D. D. Raphael, and P. G. Stein (Oxford: Oxford University Press, 1978), 239.

7. Smith, *Wealth of Nations,* 5.i.f.50, 782.

8. Ibid., 4.vii.c.91, 91–108, 631–41.

9. Ibid., 1.viii, 36, 96.

10. Emma Rothschild, "Commerce and the State: Turgot, Condorcet and Smith," *Economic Journal* 102 (September 1992): 88–89.

11. E. G. Hundert, *The Enlightenment Fable: Bernard Mandeville and the Discovery of Society* (Cambridge: Cambridge University Press, 1994).

12. Stephen Darwall, "Sympathetic Liberalism: Recent Work on Adam Smith," *Philosophy and Public Affairs* 28, no. 2 (1999): 139–65.

13. Benjamin Franklin, "Letter to Joseph Priestly, Passy, France, February 8, 1780," in *The Private Correspondence of Benjamin Franklin,* ed. William Temple Franklin (London: Henry Colborn, 1817), 52.

14. Benjamin Rush, "Observations on the Duty of a Physician," *Medical Inquiries and Observations* 1 (1815); quoted in Dorothy Porter, Robert Baker, and Roy Porter, eds., *The Codification of Medical Morality* (Dordrecht: Kluwer Academic, 1993), 2:16.

15. Henry Pritchett, "The Medical School and the State," *Journal of the American Medical Association* 63 (1914): 28.

16. James C. Riley, *Rising Life Expectancy: A Global History* (Cambridge: Cambridge University Press, 2001), 7.

17. United Nations, *The Determinants and Consequences of Population Trends* (New York: United Nations, 1953).

18. Thomas McKeown, *The Rise of Population* (London: Edward Arnold, 1976); Riley, *Rising Life Expectancy,* 9.

19. Abdel Omran, "The Epidemiological Transition Theory: A Preliminary Update," *Journal of Tropical Pediatrics* 29 (1983): 305–16.

20. Riley, *Rising Life Expectancy,* 21–24.

21. Daniel Callahan, *What Price Better Health? Hazards of the Research Imperative* (Berkeley: University of California Press, 2003), chap. 1.

22. Frederick T. Gates, *Chapters in My Life* (New York: Free Press, 1977), 188.

23. Paul Starr, *The Social Transformation of American Medicine* (New York: Basic Books, 1982), 219.

24. Callahan, *What Price Better Health?* chap. 8.

25. Wilhelm Hennis, *Max Weber: Essays in Reconstruction* (London: Allen and Unwin, 1988).

26. Muller, *Mind and the Market,* 86.

27. Ibid., 87.

28. Quoted in ibid., 87.

29. Muller, *Mind and the Market,* 136.

30. Ibid., 131, 141.

31. Jay Katz, *The Silent World of Doctor and Patient* (New York: Free Press, 1984).

32. Muller, *Mind and the Market,* 395–96.

33. Daniel Bell, *The Cultural Contradictions of Capitalism* (New York: Basic Books, 1976), 33.

34. Daniel Yergin and Joseph Stanislaw, *The Commanding Heights: The Battle of the World Economy* (New York: Touchstone Books, 1998), xii.

35. Friedrich A. Hayek, *The Road to Serfdom,* 5th ed. (Chicago: University of Chicago Press, 1992), 6, 18.

36. Ibid., 65.

37. Ibid.

38. Ibid, 133.

39. Milton Friedman, "How to Cure Health Care," *Public Interest* 142 (winter 2001): 194–95.

40. Regina Herzlinger, *Market-Driven Health Care* (Reading, MA: Addison-Wesley, 1997), 283, 4.

41. Michael Moran, "Explaining the Rise of the Market in Health Care," in *Markets and Health Care: A Comparative Perspective,* ed. Wendy Ranade (London: Longmans, 1998), 30.

42. Muller, *Mind and the Market,* 386–87.

43. Amartya Sen, *Development as Freedom* (New York: Anchor Books, 1999), 112.

44. Richard B. Saltman and Josep Figueras, *European Health Care Reform: Analysis of Current Strategies* (Copenhagen: World Health Organization, 1997), 40–41.

45. Maurizio Ferrera, "The Rise and Fall of Democratic Universalism: Health Care Reform in Italy," *Journal of Health Politics, Policy and Law* 20, no. 2 (1995): 275–302.

46. Julian Le Grand, "Markets and Quasi-Markets in Health Care," *Eurohealth* 1 (1995): 3.

47. Victor R. Fuchs, "Economics, Values, and Health Care Reform," *American Economic Review* 86, no. 1 (1996): 1–24. See also Roger Feldman and Michael Morrissey, "Health Economics: A Report on the Field," *Journal of Health Politics, Policy and Law* 15, no. 3 (1990): 627–46.

48. Kenneth J. Arrow, "Uncertainty and the Welfare Economics of Medical Care," *American Economic Review* 53 (1963): 941–73; Peter J. Hammer et al., eds., *Uncertain Times: Kenneth Arrow and the Changing Economics of Health Care* (Durham: Duke University Press, 2003).

49. James C. Robinson, *The Corporate Practice of Medicine* (Berkeley: University of California Press, 1999).

50. Fuchs, "Economics, Values, and Health Care Reform," 1.

51. Ibid., 6, 10.

52. Ibid., 10

53. Robert G. Evans, "Going for the Gold: Redistributive Agenda behind Market-Based Health Care Reform," *Journal of Health Politics, Policy and Law* 22, no. 2 (1997): 456.

54. Evan M. Melhado, "Economists, Public Provision, and the Market: Changing Values in Policy Debate," *Journal of Health Politics, Policy and Law* 23, no. 2 (1998): 251.

55. Evans, "Going for the Gold," 456.

56. Regina Herzlinger, "Prix Fixe Rip-Offs," *Wall Street Journal,* 13 June 2003, A6; Clark C. Havighurst, *Health Care Choices: Private Contracts as Instruments of Health Reform* (Washington, DC: American Enterprise Institute, 1995); Richard A. Epstein, *Mortal Peril: Our Inalienable Right to Health Care* (Reading, MA: Addison-Wesley, 1997).

57. Wendy Ranade, ed., *Markets and Health Care: A Comparative Perspective* (London: Longmans, 1998), 2.

58. John Appleby, "Economic Perspectives on Markets and Health Care: Introduction," in Ranade, *Markets and Health Care,* 41.

59. Alain Enthoven and Richard Kronick, "A Consumer Health Plan for the 1990s," *New England Journal of Medicine* 320, no. 1 (1989): 29–37; Mark V. Pauly et al., "A Plan for 'Responsible National Health Insurance,'" *Health Affairs* 10, no. 1 (1991): 5–25.

60. Thomas Rice, "Can Markets Give Us the Health System We Want?" *Journal of Health Politics, Policy and Law* 22, no. 2 (1997): 422–23.

61. Mark Pauly, "Who Was That Straw Man Anyway? A Comment on Evans and Rice," *Journal of Health Politics, Policy and Law* 22 (1997): 470.

62. Thomas Rice, *The Economics of Health Care Reconsidered,* 2nd ed. (Chicago: Health Administration Press, 2002).

63. Richard B. Saltman, "Balancing State and Market in Health System Reform," *European Journal of Public Health* 7 (1997): 119–20.

64. Kevin M. Murphy and Robert H. Topel, eds., *Measuring the Gains from Medical Research* (Chicago: University of Chicago Press, 2003).

65. Irving Kristol, *Two Cheers for Capitalism* (New York: Basic Books, 1978).

66. Robert Baker et al., "Crisis, Ethics, and the American Medical Association," *Journal of the American Medical Association* 278, no. 2 (1997): 164.

67. Ezekiel J. Emanuel and Nancy Dubler, "Preserving the Physician Patient Relationship in an Era of Managed Care," *Journal of the American Medical Association* 273, no. 4 (1995): 324–25.

68. Karen I. Titlow, Jonathan E. Rackoff, and Ezekiel J. Emanuel, "What Will It Take to Restore Physician Trust?" *Business and Health* 17, no. 6 (1999): 14–18; Steffie Woolhandler and David U. Himmelstein, "When Money Is the Mission: The High Costs of Investor-Owned Care," *New England Journal of Medicine* 341, no. 6 (1999): 441–46; Leon Eisenberg, "Health Care for Patients or for Profit?" *American Journal of Psychiatry* 143, no. 8 (1986): 1015–19.

69. Steffie Woolhandler and David U. Himmelstein, "Extreme Risk—The New Corporate Proposition for Physicians," *New England Journal of Medicine* 333, no. 25 (1995): 446.

70. Milton Friedman, *Capitalism and Freedom* (Chicago: University of Chicago Press, 2002), 46.

71. Arnold S. Relman, "What Market Values Are Doing to Medicine," *Atlantic Monthly* 269, no. 30 (1992): 99, 102.

72. Jerome P. Kassirer, "Our Endangered Integrity: It Can Only Get Worse," *New England Journal of Medicine* 336, no. 23 (1997): 1666–67.

73. Arnold S. Relman and Uwe Reinhardt, "An Exchange on For-Profit Health Care," in *For-Profit Enterprise in Health Care* (Washington, DC: National Academy Press, 1986).

74. Ibid., 209.

75. Linda Emanuel, "Bringing Market Medicine to Professional Account," *Journal of the American Medical Association* 277, no. 12 (1997): 1004–5.

76. Marsha R. Gold et al., "A National Survey of the Arrangements Managed-Care Plans Make with Physicians," *New England Journal of Medicine* 333, no. 25 (1995): 1678–83.

CHAPTER 2: A TALE OF TWO CULTURES

1. Carolyn Hughes Tuohy, *Accidental Logics: The Dynamics of Change in the Health Care Arena in the United States, Britain, and Canada* (New York: Oxford University Press, 1999).

2. Seymour Martin Lipset, *Continental Divide: The Values and Institutions of the United States and Canada* (New York: Routledge, 1990), 8.

3. Frank Underhill, *In Search of Canadian Liberalism* (Toronto: Macmillan of Canada, 1960), 222.

4. E. A. Tollefson, *Bitter Medicine: The Saskatchewan Medical Feud* (Saskatoon: Modern Press, 1963); David C. Naylor, *Private Practice, Public Payment: Canadian Medicine and the Politics of Health Insurance* (Montreal: McGill-Queen's University Press, 1986), chap. 7.

5. Nuala P. Kenny, *What Good Is Health Care? Reflections on the Canadian Experience* (Ottawa: CHA Press, 2002), 46–47.

6. Tollefson, *Bitter Medicine,* 17–20.

7. R. Bothwell and J. English quoted in Kenny, *What Good Is Health Care?* 48. See also Jacelyn Duffin, "The Guru and the Godfather: Henry Sigerist, Hugh Maclean, and the Politics of Reform in 1940s Canada," *Canadian Bulletin of Medical History* 9, no. 2 (1952): 191–218.

8. Joyce Appleby quoted in Gordon S. Wood, "Early American Get up and Go," *New York Review of Books* 47, no. 11 (2000): 52. See also Joyce Appleby, *Inheriting the Revolution: The First Generation of Americans* (Cambridge: Harvard University Press, 2000).

9. Alexis de Tocqueville, *Democracy in America,* trans. George Lawrence (Garden City, NY: Doubleday, 1969), 621.

10. George Rosen, *The Structure of American Medical Practice: 1875–1941* (Philadelphia: University of Pennsylvania Press, 1983), 19.

11. Paul Starr, *The Social Transformation of American Medicine* (New York: Basic Books, 1982), 21–22.

12. Rosen, *Structure of American Medical Practice,* 31.

13. Ibid., 4.

14. Starr, *Social Transformation of American Medicine,* 61.

15. Charles D. Weller, " 'Free Choice' as a Restraint of Trade in American Health Care Delivery and Insurance," *Iowa Law Review* 69, no. 5 (1984): 1351–78.

16. Nancy Tomes, "Merchants of Health: Medicine and Consumer Culture in the United States, 1900–1940," *Journal of American History* 88, no. 2 (2001): 540.

17. Ibid., 541.

18. Adapted from Kenny, *What Good Is Health Care?* 250. See also "Health-Reform Cycle," in *Getting Health Reform Right*, ed. Mark S. Roberts et al. (New York: Oxford University Press, 2004), 21–39.

19. D. Bricker and E. Greenspon, *Searching for Certainty: Inside the New Canadian Mindset* (Toronto: Doubleday Canada, 2001), 181.

20. Ibid., 183.

21. Robert S. Bothwell and John R. English, *Pragmatic Physicians: Canadian Medicine and Health Care Insurance, 1910–1940* (Montreal: McGill-Queens University Press, 1992).

22. Tuohy, *Accidental Logics*, 46; for an interesting comparison with the United States, see Miriam K. Laugesen and Thomas Rice, "Is the Doctor In? The Evolving Role of Organized Medicine in Health Policy," *Journal of Health Politics, Policy and Law* 28, no. 2–3 (2003): 289–316.

23. Naylor, *Private Practice, Public Payment*, chaps. 6 and 8.

24. Tuohy, *Accidental Logics*, 51.

25. Colin D. Howell, "Medical Science and Social Criticism: Alexander Peter Reid and the Ideological Origins of the Welfare State in Canada," in *Canadian Healthcare and the State: A Century of Evolution*, ed. C. David Naylor (Montreal: McGill-Queen's University Press, 1992), 16–37.

26. Malcolm Taylor, *Health Insurance and Canadian Public Policy: The Seven Decisions That Created the Canadian Health Insurance System* (Montreal: McGill-Queen's University Press, 1979), 164–66.

27. Ibid., 163.

28. Tuohy, *Accidental Logics*, 44.

29. Starr, *Social Transformation of American Medicine*, 287.

30. Theda Skocpol, *Boomerang: Health Care Reform and the Turn against Government* (New York: W. W. Norton, 1997).

31. Terence Sullivan and Patricia M. Baranak, *First Do No Harm: Making Sense of Canadian Health Care* (Vancouver: University of British Columbia Press, 2002), 28–29.

32. Ibid., 1–2.

33. Bricker and Greenspon, *Searching for Certainty*, 189.

34. T. J. Murray, "Balancing Values, Funding and Americanization of Expectations in the Canadian Health System," in *Proceedings of the 37th International Congress on the History of Medicine* (Galveston: University of Texas Medical Branch, 2002), 89–98.

35. Robert Evans and Noralo P. Roos, "What Is Right about the Canadian Health Care System?" *Milbank Quarterly* 77, no. 3 (1999): 393.

36. Michael Adams, *Fire and Ice: The United States, Canada, and the Myth of Converging Values* (Toronto: Penguin Canada, 2003), 141.

37. C. David Naylor, "Health Care in Canada: Incrementalism under Fiscal Duress," *Health Affairs* 18, no. 3 (1999): 9–26.

38. Clifford Krauss, "Long Lines Mar Canada's Low-Cost Health Care," *New York Times*, 13 February 2003, A3.

39. Monique Begin, "Renewing Medicare," *Canadian Medical Association Journal* 167, no. 1 (2002): 46–47; Stephen Lewis et al., "Ending Waiting-List Mismanagement: Principles and Practices," *Canadian Medical Association Journal* 162 (2000): 1297–1300; Shafer Parker, "The Symptoms Get Worse: No Governments in Canada Will Admit Healthcare Is Becoming Inadequate," *The Report*, 5 February 2001.

40. Conference Board of Canada, *Defining the Canadian Advantage* (Ottawa: Conference Board of Canada, 2003), 32–36.

41. Premier's Advisory Council on Health, *A Framework for Reform* (Edmonton: Premier's Advisory Council on Health, 2001), 5.

42. Ibid., 43. Regina Herzlinger's "don't call them patients" is in *Market-Driven Health Care* (Reading, MA: Addison-Wesley, 1997), 283.

43. Standing Committee on Social Affairs, Science and Technology, *The Health of Canadians—the Federal Role* (Toronto: Standing Senate Committee on Social Affairs, Science and Technology, October 2002).

44. Premier's Advisory Council, *Framework for Reform*.

45. Ibid., 9.

46. Stephen Harper quoted in Ken Warn, "Massive Federal Cash Injection Urged for Canadian Healthcare," *Financial Times* (London), 29 November 2002, 11.

47. Allan S. Detsky and C. David Naylor, "Canada's Health Care System: Reform Delayed," *New England Journal of Medicine* 345, no. 8 (2003): 804–10; John K. Iglehart, "Revisiting the Canadian Health Care System," *New England Journal of Medicine* 342, no. 26 (2000): 2007–12.

48. Detsky and Naylor, "Canada's Health Care System," 810.

49. Janice MacKinnon, "The Arithmetic of Health Care," *Enjeux Publics* 5, no. 3 (2004): 16.

50. Conference Board of Canada, *Understanding Health Care Costs and Escalators* (Ottawa: Conference Board of Canada, March 2004), i–ii.

51. Mark Heinzl and Christopher J. Chipello, "Shock Treatment for Canadian Health Care," *Wall Street Journal*, 13 June 2005, B3; Supreme Court of Canada, *Chaoulli v. Quebec (Attorney General)*, 2005 SCC 35.

52. Will Lester, "Public Supports Health Care for All," *Los Angeles Times*, 20 October 2003.

53. Michael M. Chernew, Richard A. Hirt, and David M. Cutler, "Increased Spending on Health Care: How Much Can the United States Afford?" *Health Affairs* 22, no. 4 (2003): 15–24; Gerald F. Anderson et al. "It's the Prices Stupid: Why the United States Is Different from Other Countries," *Health Affairs* 22, no. 3 (2003): 89–105.

54. Tuohy, *Accidental Logics*, 161.

55. Laugesen and Rice, "Is the Doctor In?"

56. John K. Iglehart, "Changing Health Insurance Trends," *New England Journal of Medicine* 347, no. 12 (2002): 956–62.

57. James C. Robinson, "The End of Managed Care," *Journal of the American Medical Association* 285, no. 20 (2001): 2622.

58. Gerald Burke, "And Now the Good News," *Health Systems Review* 26 (1996): 21.

59. Alain C. Enthoven and Sarah J. Singer, "Markets and Collective Action in the Regulation of Managed Care" (ms., 1997).

60. Alain C. Enthoven, "Employment-Based Health Insurance Is Failing: Now What?" *Health Affairs,* Web Exclusive, 2003, W3–338.

61. David Mechanic, "Managed Care as a Target of Distrust," *Journal of the American Medical Association* 277, no. 22 (1997): 1810–11. See also James C. Robinson, "From Managed Care to Consumer Health Insurance: The Fall and Rise of Aetna," *Health Affairs* 23, no. 2 (2004): 43–55.

62. Robert M. Crane and Laura A. Tollen, "Out of the Frying Pan and into the Fire?" *Health Affairs,* Web Exclusive, 2003, W139–54.

63. Uwe W. Reinhardt, "Employer-Based Health Insurance: A Balance Sheet," *Health Affairs* 18, no. 6 (1999): 124.

64. Robert Galvin and Arnold Milstein, "Large Employers' New Strategies in Health Care," *New England Journal of Medicine* 347, no. 12 (2002): 939–42.

65. Regina E. Herzlinger, ed., *Consumer-Driven Health Care* (New York: Jossey-Bass, 2004).

66. John A. Gabel, Anthony T. L. Sassao, and Thomas Rice, "Consumer-Driven Health Plans: Are They More Than Talk Now?" *Health Affairs,* Web Exclusive, 2002, W395–407.

67. Karen Davis, "Consumer-Driven Health Care: Will It Improve Health System Performance?" *Health Services Research* 39, no. 4, pt. 2 (2004): 1230.

68. James C. Robinson, *The Corporate Practice of Medicine: Competition and Innovation in Health Care* (Berkeley: University of California Press, 1999), 2, 5.

69. Ibid., 14–15, 235.

70. Sidney Lutz and E. Preston Gee, *The For-Profit Healthcare Revolution: The Growing Impact of Investor-Owned Health Systems* (Chicago: Irwin Professional Publishing, 1996), ix.

71. Ibid., 177.

72. David Shactman et al., "The Outlook for Health Spending," *Health Affairs* 22, no. 6 (2003): 12–26.

73. Victor Fuchs, "Managed Care and Merger Mania," *Journal of the American Medical Association* 277, no. 11 (1997): 921.

74. David M. Cutler and Jill R. Horowitz, "Community Hospitals from Not-for-Profit to For-Profit Status" (Working Paper 6672, National Bureau of Economic Research, Washington, DC, 1998).

75. L. K. Nichols, "Are Market Forces Strong Enough to Deliver Efficient Health Care Systems? Confidence Is Waning," *Health Affairs* 23, no. 2 (2004): 8–21.

76. Physicians' Working Group for Single-Payer Health Insurance, "Proposal of the Physicians' Working Group for Single-Payer National Health Insurance," *Journal of the American Medical Association* 290, no. 6 (2003): 799.

77. John Conyers, "A Fresh Approach to Health Care in the United States: Improved and Expanded Medicare for All," *American Journal of Public Health* 93, no. 2 (2003): 193.

78. D. J. Palmisano, D. W. Emmons, and G. D. Wozniak, "Expanding Insurance Cover-

age through Tax Credits, Consumer Choice, and Market Enhancements: The American Medical Association Proposal for Health Insurance Reform," *Journal of the American Medical Association* 291, no. 18 (2004): 2238.

79. Enthoven, "Employment-Based Health Insurance Is Failing," W243–47.

80. Alain C. Enthoven, "Market Forces and Efficient Health Care Systems," *Health Affairs* 23, no. 2 (2004): 26–27.

81. Ezekiel J. Emanuel and Victor R. Fuchs, "The Universal Cure," *New York Times,* 18 November 2003, A25.

82. Stuart M. Butler, "A New Policy Framework for Health Care Markets," *Health Affairs* 23, no. 2 (2004): 22–23.

83. David M. Cutler, *Your Money or Your Life* (New York: Oxford University Press, 2004), 116. Notably absent from Cutler's scheme is any significant role for the market. See also Leif Wellington Haase, *A New Deal for Health: How to Cover Everyone and Get Medical Costs under Control* (New York: Century Foundation Press, 2005). His plan blends mandatory individual purchasing of health insurance, government subsidies for those who cannot afford it, and a combination of payroll and compound taxes and general revenue to pay for it, aided by assorted market practices.

84. See, e.g., John E. Wennberg, "Variations in the Use of Medicare Services among Regions and Selected Academic Medical Centers" (Duncan W. Clark Lecture, ms., New York Academy of Medicine, 24 January 2005); and a collection of essays on Wennberg's findings over the years: "Variations Revisited," *Health Affairs,* Web Exclusive Collection, 2004.

85. Jonathan Oberlander, *The Political Life of Medicare* (Chicago: University of Chicago Press, 2003).

86. Cited in ibid., 179.

87. Laurie McGinley et al., "A Guide to Who Wins and Who Loses in Medicare Bill," *Wall Street Journal,* 18 November 2003, B1.

88. Dick Armey, "Say 'No' to the Medicare Bill," *Wall Street Journal,* 21 November 2003, A12.

89. John K. Iglehart, "The New Medicare Prescription-Drug Benefit—A Pure Power Play," *New England Journal of Medicine* 350, no. 8 (2004): 826–33.

90. "Review and Outlook: Bad Political Medicine," editorial, *Wall Street Journal,* 21 November 2003, A12.

CHAPTER 3: THE ENDURANCE OF SOLIDARITY

1. Richard B. Saltman and Hans F. W. Dubois, "The Historical and Social Base of Social Health Insurance Systems," in *Social Health Insurance Systems in Western Europe,* ed. Richard B. Saltman, Reinhard Busse, and Josep Figueras (Maidenhead, UK: Open University Press, 2004), 21–32.

2. United Nations, *International Covenant on Economic, Social and Cultural Rights,* art. 12 (New York: United Nations, 3 January 1976).

3. Daniel Callahan, "The WHO Definition of Health," *Hastings Center Studies* 1, no. 3 (1973): 77–87.

4. Alan Jacobs, "Seeing Difference: Market Health Reform in Europe," *Journal of Health Politics, Policy and Law* 23, no. 1 (1998): 1–53. For an illuminating examination of the diversity of European health care systems and the institutional influences on them, see "Special Issue: Legacies and Latitude in European Health Policy," *Journal of Health Politics, Policy and Law* 30, no. 1–2 (2005).

5. This section draws heavily on a report commissioned for this book from Alan Cribb, "Markets and Healthcare in the UK" (ms., 2003); all citations of Cribb in the text refer to this report. See also Donald Light, "Universal Health Care: Lessons from the British Experience," *American Journal of Public Health* 93, no. 1 (2003): 125–30; Rudolf Klein, "Big Bang Health Care Reform—Does It Work? The Case of Britain's 1991 National Health Service Reforms," *Milbank Quarterly* 73, no. 3 (1995): 299–337; Michael Calnan, "The NHS and Private Health Care," *Matrix* 10, no. 3 (2000): 3–19; Ray Robinson and Ann Dixon, "United Kingdom," in *Health Care Systems in Transition* (Copenhagen: European Observatory on Health Care Systems, 1999); Clive Snee, "United Kingdom," *Journal of Health Politics, Policy and Law* 25, no. 5 (2000): 945–51; Alain C. Enthoven, *Reflections on the Management of the National Health Service* (London: Nuffield Provincial Hospitals Trust, 1985).

6. Henry Aaron and William B. Schwartz, *The Painful Prescription: Rationing Health Care* (Washington, DC: Brookings Institution, 1984).

7. Robinson and Dixon, "United Kingdom," 104.

8. Klein, "Big Bang Health Care Reform," 333.

9. We draw here on another paper commissioned for this book: Ruud ter Meulen and Christi Nierse, "Medicine and the Market: Sweden" (ms., 2003). See also Catharine Hjortsberg and Ola Ghatnekar, *Health Care Systems in Transition: Sweden* (Copenhagen: European Observatory on Health Care Systems, 2001); Finn Diderichsen, "Sweden," *Journal of Health Politics, Policy and Law* 25, no. 5 (2000): 930–35.

10. Hjortsberg and Ghatnekar, *Health Care Systems in Transition: Sweden*, 91.

11. This section on Italy draws heavily on a paper commissioned for the book: N. Pasini and L. Fasano, "The Impact of Market Thinking and Italian Culture on the National Health Service" (ms., 2003). Citations of Pasini and Fasano in the text refer to this report.

12. Signal Vallarta et al., "Denmark," in *Health Care Systems in Eight Countries: Trends and Challenges*, ed. Anna Dixon and Elias Mossialos (Copenhagen: European Observatory on Health Care Systems, 2002), 17–30.

13. Simone Sandier et al., "France," in Dixon and Mossialos, *Health Care Systems in Eight Countries*, 31–46; Jean Pierre Poullier and Simone Sandier, "France," *Journal of Health Politics, Policy and Law* 25, no. 2 (2000), 899–905.

14. This section on Germany draws heavily on a report prepared for this book by Kurt Fleischauer, "Medicine and the Market: Germany" (ms., 2003). See also Christa Altensetter, "Insights from Health Care in Germany," *American Journal of Public Health* 93, no. 1 (2003): 38–43; Richard Busse and Annette Riesberg, *Health Care Systems in Transition: Germany* (Copenhagen: European Observatory on Health Care Systems, 2000); Martin Pfaff and Dietmar Wassener, "Germany," *Journal of Health Politics, Policy and Law* 25, no. 5 (2000): 907–14.

15. This section on the Netherlands draws heavily on a paper commissioned for this book from Christi Nierse and Ruud ter Meulen, "Medicine and the Market: The Netherlands" (ms., 2003). See also Andre den Exter et al., *Health Care Systems in Transition: The Netherlands* (Copenhagen: European Observatory on Health Care Systems, 2002); Reinhard Busse, "The Netherlands," in Dixon and Mossialos, *Health Care Systems in Eight Countries,* 61–74; Jan-Kees Helderman et al., "Market-Oriented Health Care Reforms and Policy Learning in the Netherlands," *Journal of Health Politics, Policy and Law* 30, no. 1–2 (2005): 197–209.

16. This section on Switzerland is heavily indebted to a report prepared for this book by Hanspeter Kuhn, "Medicine and the Market—Country Study: Switzerland" (ms., 2003). See also an interesting exchange: Regina E. Herzlinger and Ramin Parsa-Parsi, "Consumer-Driven Health Care: Lessons from Switzerland," *Journal of the American Medical Association* 292, no. 10 (2004): 1213–20; and Uwe E. Reinhardt, "Consumer-Driven Health Care: Lessons from Switzerland," *Journal of the American Medical Association,* 292, no. 10 (2004): 1213–20.

17. Judith Healy, "Australia," in Dixon and Mossialos, *Health Care Systems in Eight Countries,* 3–16.

18. Bruce Rosen, *Health Systems in Transition: Israel* (Copenhagen: European Observatory on Health Care Systems, 2003); Bruce Rosen, "Script—Israel: A Case Study of Equitable Health Care," *EIU Healthcare International,* 2nd quarter (1999): 15–21. This section on Israel has also profited from a conference that Callahan organized in Tel Aviv in 1999, a fractious but interesting collection of Israeli economists, political scientists, and government officials.

19. We draw here on a study commissioned for this book from Eva Krizova, "Medicine and the Market in the Czech Republic" (ms., 2003); citations of Krizova in the text refer to this report. See also Martin Bojar (former Health Minister for the Czech Republic), "Transformation of Health Care System—Czech Republic 1990–1994" (paper presented at Hastings Center Conference, Prague, 1999).

20. Document quoted by Krizova, "Medicine and the Market in the Czech Republic."

21. Robin Gauld, "Revolving Doors: New Zealand's Health Reforms," *Social Policy Journal of New Zealand* 18 (2002): 202–4, 815–44; Commonwealth Fund, "The New Zealand System: Views and Experiences of Adults with Health Problems" (Commonwealth Fund, New York, 2003).

22. Robin Gauld, "Big Bang and the Policy Prescription: Health Care Meets the Market in New Zealand," *Journal of Health Politics, Policy and Law* 25, no. 5 (2002): 826.

23. Organization for Economic Cooperation and Development (OECD), *Health at a Glance 2003: OECD Countries Struggle with Rising Demand for Health Spending* (Paris: Organization for Economic Cooperation and Development, 2003), 1.

24. Charles Fleming, "Europeans Face Health Costs," *Wall Street Journal,* 17 November 2003, A18.

25. Calum R. Paton, "Analysis of Market Reforms in Europe," *Eurohealth* 6, no. 4 (2000): 30.

26. Michael Moran, "Explaining the Rise of the Market in Health Care," in *Markets and Health Care,* ed. Wendy Ranade (London: Longmans, 1998), 18.

27. Ranade, *Markets and Health Care,* 1, 6.

28. Reinhard Busse, "Impact of Market Forces: Six Hypotheses and Limited Evidence," *Eurohealth* 6, no. 3 (2000): 31–34.

29. Ibid.

30. Ibid.

31. Though published in 1997, a study by Richard B. Saltman and Josep Figueras points to cost-escalating forces that have not changed since then: *European Health Care Reform: Analysis of Current Strategies* (Copenhagen: World Health Organization, 1997).

32. James Morone, "Citizens as Shoppers? Solidarity under Siege," *Journal of Health Politics, Policy and Law* 25, no. 5 (2000): 958–68.

33. Ruud ter Meulen, Wil Arts, and Ruud Muffels, eds., *Solidarity in Health and Social Care in Europe* (Dordrecht: Kluwer Academic, 2001), 1.

34. Ibid.

35. Saltman and Dubois, "Historical and Social Base of Social Health Insurance Systems," 27.

36. Richard B. Saltman, "Social Health Insurance in Perspective," in Saltman, Busse, and Figueras, *Social Health Insurance Systems in Western Europe,* 5.

37. Hans Maarse and Aggie Paulus, "Has Solidarity Survived? A Comparative Analysis of the Effect of Social Health Insurance Reform in Four European Countries," *Journal of Health Politics, Policy and Law* 28, no. 4 (2003): 589–614; Colleen M. Flood, Mark Stabile, and Carolyn Hughes Tuohy, "The Borders of Solidarity: How Countries Determine the Public/Private Mix in Spending and the Impact on Health Care," *Matrix* 12 (2000): 297–355; Wil Arts and Rudi Verburg, "Modernisation, Solidarity and Care in Europe: The Sociologist's Tale," in ter Meulen, *Solidarity in Health and Social Care in Europe,* 15–40.

38. Vivienne Kendall, *The Prospects for Private Health Care in Europe* (London: Economist Intelligence Unit, 1999).

39. Ibid., vii.

40. Richard B. Saltman, "The Western European Experience with Health Care Reform" (Secretariat, World Health Organization Regional Office for Europe, Copenhagen, 2003), 3.

CHAPTER 4: THE MARKET IN DEVELOPING COUNTRIES

1. United Nations Development Programme (UNDP), *Human Development Report 2003: Millennium Development Goals: A Compact among Nations to End Human Poverty* (Oxford: Oxford University Press, 2003).

2. World Health Organization (WHO), *The World Health Report* (Geneva: World Health Organization, 2003).

3. Basil Davidson, *African Civilization Revisited* (Trenton, NJ: Africa World Press, 1991).

4. G. Mashaba, "Culturally-Based Health-Illness Patterns in South Africa and Humanistic Nursing Care Practices," in *Transcultural Nursing: Concepts, Theories, Re-*

search, and Practices, ed. M. M. Leininger, College Custom Series USA (New York: McGraw Hill, 1995), 591–602.

5. Meredeth Turshen, *Privatizing Health Services in Africa* (New Brunswick, NJ: Rutgers University Press, 1999), 15–18.

6. Stephen Owoahene-Acheampong, *Inculturation and African Religion: Indigenous and Western Approaches to Medical Practice* (New York: Peter Lang, 1998).

7. Turshen, *Privatizing Health Service in Africa,* 25–28.

8. Ibid., 28.

9. Ibid.

10. Zambian Ministry of Health, *National Health Care Financing Policy* (Lusaka: Government Printer, 1998).

11. Government of Kenya, *Sessional Paper No. 10 on African Socialism and Its Applications to Planning in Kenya* (Nairobi: Government Printer, 1965).

12. Wasunna Owino, *Delivery and Financing of Health Care Services in Kenya: Critical Issues and Research Gaps,* IPAR Discussion Papers Series DP no. 002 (Nairobi: Institute of Policy Analysis and Research, 1997), 2.

13. Government of Kenya, *Sessional Paper No. 10,* 2.

14. Owino, *Delivery and Financing of Health Care Services in Kenya,* 3.

15. S. E. Chambua, "The Development Debates and Crisis of Development Theories: The Case of Tanzania with Special Emphasis on Peasants, State and Capital," in *African Perspectives on Development,* ed. U. Himmelstrand, K. Kinyanjui, and E. Mburugu (London: James Currey, 1994), 37–50.

16. K. J. Havnevik, *Tanzania—the Limits to Development from Above* (Motala: Nordisk Afrikainstitutet, in cooperation with Mkuki na Nyota, 1993).

17. Alice Shiner, "Shaping Health Care in Tanzania: Who's Pulling the Strings?" *Lancet* 362 (2003): 829–30.

18. A. Tripp and M. L. Swantz, *What Went Right in Tanzania: People's Response to Directed Development* (Dar-es-Salaam: Dar Es Salaam University Press, 1996).

19. Ministry of Health, Tanzania, *National Health Policy* (Dar-es-Salaam: Ministry of Health, 1990).

20. Ministry of Health, Tanzania, *Population and Development in Tanzania* (Dar-es-Salaam: Ministry of Health, 1985).

21. World Bank, *Adjustment in Africa: Reforms, Results, and the Road Ahead* (New York: Oxford University Press, 1994).

22. Ibid.

23. Ibid.

24. Audrey R. Chapman and Leonard S. Rubenstein, eds., *Human Rights and Health: The Legacy of Apartheid* (Washington, DC: American Association for the Advancement of Science, 1998).

25. Ibid.

26. Ibid.

27. Solomon R. Benatar, "Health Care Reform in the New South Africa," *New England Journal of Medicine* 336, no. 12 (1997): 891–95.

28. Ibid.

29. J. P. H. Rossouw and B. E. Hofmeyr, "Infant and Child Mortality in South Africa: Levels, Differentials and Determinants," in *South Africa's Demographic Future*, ed. W. P. Mostert and J. M. Lötter (Pretoria: Human Sciences Research Council, 1995), 33–44.

30. See S. Tang et al., *Financing Rural Health Services in China: Adapting to Economic Reform*, Institute of Development Studies Research Report no. 26 (Brighton, UK: Institute of Development Studies, University of Sussex, 1994).

31. Ibid.; Gerald Bloom, "Financing Rural Health Services in China," in *Marketizing Education and Health in Developing Countries: Miracle or Mirage*, ed. Christopher Colclough (Oxford: Clarendon Press, 1997), 222–42.

32. Bloom, "Financing Rural Health Services in China," 223.

33. William Hsiao and Yuanli Liu, "Economic Reform and Health Lessons from China," *New England Journal of Medicine* 335, no. 6 (1996): 430–31.

34. Bloom, "Financing Rural Health Services in China," 224.

35. Gerald Bloom, *Primary Health Care Meets the Market: Lessons from China and Vietnam*, Institute of Development Studies Working Paper 53 (Brighton, UK: University of Sussex, 1997).

36. Ibid.

37. R. J. Cima, *Vietnam: A Country Study* (Washington, DC: Library of Congress, 1987).

38. N. T. Hien et al., "The Pursuit of Equity: A Health Sector Case Study from Vietnam," *Health Policy* 33 (1995): 191–204.

39. Ibid.

40. Bloom, *Primary Health Care Meets the Market*, 5.

41. Swedish International Development Cooperation Agency, "Economic Reform in Vietnam: Achievements and Prospects" (series of reports for the International Seminar, Jakarta, Indonesia, 1994).

42. Lincoln Chen and Linda G. Hiebert, "From Socialism to Private Markets: Vietnam's Health in Rapid Transition" (Harvard Center for Population and Development Studies, Working Paper Series no. 94, Harvard School of Public Health, Cambridge, October 1994), 11.

43. Ibid.

44. Socialist Republic of Vietnam, *Tong Diea Dan So Viet Nam—1989: Statistical Data of the Socialist Republic of Vietnam* (Hanoi: General Statistical Office, 1986–1991).

45. Chen and Hiebert, "From Socialism to Private Markets," 11.

46. Government of India, *Report of the Health Survey and Development Committee* (New Delhi: Manager of Publications, 1946).

47. Siddhartha Gupta, "Fifty-three Years of 'Independence' and Our Health," *People's March, Voice of the Indian Revolution* 1, no. 9 (2000), www.peoplesmarch.com/archives/2000/nov2k/fifty.htm.

48. Sonia Fleury, Susana Belmartino, and Enis Baris, eds., *Reshaping Health Care in Latin America: A Comparative Analysis of Health Care Reform in Argentina, Brazil, and Mexico* (Singapore: International Development Research Centre, 2000).

49. Cristian Baeza, "A Script: Taking Stock of Healthcare Reform in Latin America," *EIU Healthcare International,* 2nd quarter (1998): 1–12.

50. Ibid.

51. This discussion on Chile draws heavily from a paper commissioned for this book: Miguel Kottow, "Medicine and Market in Chile, with a Brief Report on Argentina and Brazil" (ms., 2003).

52. Armando Barrientos and Peter Lloyd-Sherlock, "Reforming Health Insurance in Argentina and Chile," *Health Policy and Planning* 15, no. 4 (2000): 417–23.

53. Varun Gauri, "Are Incentives Everything? Payment Mechanisms for Health Care Providers in Developing Countries?" (World Bank Development Research Group Working Paper 2624, Washington, DC, 2001), 3.

54. World Bank, *World Bank Development Report: From Plan to Market* (Oxford: Oxford University Press, 1996).

55. Bloom, *Primary Health Care Meets the Market,* 6–8.

56. M. Madeo and S. Spinaci, "Health Sector Reforms in Developing Countries," *Giornale Italiano di Medicina Tropical* 5 (2000): 1–2.

57. Kim Reiseman, "The World Bank and the IMF: At the Forefront of the World Transformation," *Fordham Law Review* 60 (1992): 349–51.

58. Rajesh Swaminathan, "Regulating Development: Structural Adjustment and the Case for National Enforcement of Economic and Social Rights," *Columbia. Journal of Transnational Law* 37 (1998): 161.

59. Reiseman, "World Bank and the IMF," 349–51.

60. World Bank, *Q & A, Facts and Figures about the World Bank Group* (Washington DC: World Bank, 1998), 1. See also Adam Wagstaff, "Economics, Health and Development: Some Ethical Dilemmas Facing the World Bank and the International Community," *Journal of Medical Ethics* 27 (2001): 262–67.

61. Kamran Abbasi, "The World Bank and World Health: Health Care Strategy," *British Medical Journal* 318, no. 7188 (1999): 3–6.

62. This section on reform prescriptions (and the next, on increasing the role of the market) draws heavily on a paper commissioned from Migai Akech, "Medicine and the Market in Developing Countries" (ms., 2003).

63. Vittorio Corbo and Stanley Fischer, "Adjustment Programs and Bank Support: Rationale and Main Results," in *Adjustment Lending Revisited: Policies to Restore Growth,* ed. Vittorio Corbo et al. (Washington, DC: World Bank, 1992).

64. Swaminathan, "Regulating Development," 161.

65. World Bank, *Better Health in Africa: Lessons Learned* (Washington, DC: World Bank, 1994).

66. Sue McGregor, "Neoliberalism and Health Care," *International Journal of Consumer Studies* 25, no. 2 (2001): 83–86.

67. Akech, "Medicine and the Market in Developing Countries."

68. The Structural Adjustment Participatory Review International Network (SAPRIN), *Structural Adjustment: The SAPRI Report—The Policy Roots of Economic Crisis, Poverty, and Inequality* (Washington, DC: Zed Books, 2004).

69. Akech, "Medicine and the Market in Developing Countries."

70. McGregor, "Neoliberalism and Health Care," 83, 86.

71. Melitta Jakab et al., "The Introduction of Market Forces in the Public Hospital Sector: From New Public Sector Management to Organizational Reform" (World Bank HNP Discussion Paper, World Bank, Washington, DC, 2002), 6.

72. Madeo and Spinaci, "Health Sector Reforms in Developing Countries," 1–2.

73. Ann Mills, "To Contract or Not to Contract? Issues for Low and Middle Income Countries," *Health Policy and Planning* 13 (1998): 191.

74. Ibid.

75. World Health Organization/UNICEF, *International Conference on Primary Health Care* (Alma-Ata, USSR: World Health Organization, 1978).

76. G. C. Griffin, "User Charges for Health Care in Principle and Practice," in *Health Care Financing,* Proceedings of Regional Seminar on Health Care Financing, Asian Development Bank, Philippines, 27 August 1987 (Manila: Asian Development Bank, 1987).

77. Joseph Stiglitz, *Globalization and Its Discontents* (New York: W. W. Norton, 2003): xiii, xiv.

78. Carol Welch, Friends of the Earth, and Jason Oringer, "In Focus: Structural Adjustment Programs," *Economic Justice Now* 3, no. 3 (1998): 3.

79. Stiglitz, *Globalization and Its Discontents,* 40.

80. David Ellerman, "Mixing Truth and Power: Implications for a Knowledgeable Organization," *SA Newsletter* (World Bank Group), 2001, 3.

81. Charlotte Denny, "Don't Bank on It: Factions at the World Bank Argue," *Guardian* (London), 4 July 2000.

82. Günther Taube, "Social Dimensions of Adjustment: Conceptual Issues and Empirical Evidence from Afrika," *Spectrum* 28, no. 2 (1993): 165–83.

83. Mills, "To Contract or Not to Contract?" 196–210.

84. Turshen, *Privatizing Health Services in Africa,* 33.

85. Griffin, "User Charges for Health Care."

86. See L. A. Biljmakers, M. T. Basset, and D. M. Sanders, "Health and Structural Adjustment in Rural and Urban Zimbabwe," *Scandinavian Institute of African Studies Research Report* 101 (1996).

87. G. Mwabu, J. Mwanzia, and W. Liambila, "User Charges in Government Health Facilities in Kenya: Effect on Attendance and Revenue," *Health Policy and Planning* 10, no. 2 (1995): 64–170.

88. Erik Blas and M. E. Limbambala, "User-Payment, Decentralization and Health Service Utilization in Zambia," *Health Policy and Planning* 16, no. 2 (2001): 19–28.

89. A. K. Hussein and P. G. Mujinja, "Impact of User Charges on Government Health Facilities in Tanzania," *East Africa Medical Journal* 74, no. 12 (1997): 751–57.

90. Lucy Gilson, "The Lessons of User Fee Experience in Africa," *Health Policy and Planning* 12, no. 4 (1997): 273–85.

91. World Bank, *World Development Report: The State in a Changing World* (Oxford: Oxford University Press, 1997).

92. Turshen, *Privatizing Health Services in Africa,* 33.

93. Sara Bennet and Elias Ngalande-Banda, *Public and Private Roles in Health: A*

Review and Analysis of Experience in Sub-Saharan Africa (Geneva: World Health Organization, Division of Strengthening of Health Services, 1994).

94. Arhin-Tenkorang, "Mobilizing Resources for Health: The Case for User Fees Revisited" (WHO Commission on Macroeconomics and Health Working Paper WG3:6, World Health Organization, Geneva, 2000), 5.

95. SAPRIN, *Structural Adjustment.*

96. Ibid.

97. World Health Organization, "Global AIDS Epidemic Shows No Sign of Abating," www.who.int/mediacentre/releases/2003/prunaids/en/print.html (accessed 3 December 2003).

98. Amar A. Hamoudi and Jeffrey D. Sachs, "The Economics of AIDS in Africa," in *AIDS in Africa,* ed. M. Essex et al. (New York: Kluwer Academic, 2002).

99. Madeo and Spinaci, "Health Sector Reforms in Developing Countries," 2.

100. World Bank, *World Development Report 1993: Investing in Health* (New York: Oxford University Press, 1994).

101. Ann-Louise Colgan, "Africa Action Position Paper: Hazardous to Health: The World Bank and IMF in Africa," *Africa Policy E-Journal* 0204 (2002): 1.

102. Phillip Musgrove, "Economic Crisis and Health Policy Response," in *Demographic Responses to Economic Adjustment in Latin America,* ed. Georges Tapinos, Andrew Mason, and Jorge Bravo (Lille, France: International Union for the Scientific Study of Population, 1997).

103. Anna Breman and Carolyn Shelton, "Structural Adjustment and Health: A Literature Review of the Debate, Its Role Players and Presented Empirical Evidence" (WHO Commission on Macroeconomics and Health, Working Paper WG6:6, World Health Organization, Geneva, 2001).

104. Michel Garenne and Eneas Gakusi, "Health Effects of Structural Adjustment Programs in Sub-Saharan Africa" (working paper, French Center for Population and Development Studies, Paris, 2000).

105. International Monetary Fund, International Development Association, Gobind Nankani, and Masood Ahmed, *Review of the Poverty Reduction Strategy Paper (PSRP) Approach: Early Experience with Interim PRSPs and Full PRSPs* (Washington, DC: International Monetary Fund and International Development Association, 2002).

106. Charles Abugre, "Still SAPping the Poor: A Critique of IMF Poverty Reduction Strategies," *World Development Movement Report* (2000), www.wdm.org.uk/campaigns/cambriefs/debt/sappoor.pdf.

107. Jeff Ruster, Chiaki Yamamoto, and Khama Rogo, "Franchising in Health: Emerging Models, Experiences and Challenges in Primary Care" (World Bank Group, Private Sector and Infrastructure Network, Washington, DC, 2003).

108. Colgan, "Africa Action Position Paper."

109. William Hsiao, "What Should Macroeconomists Know about Health Care Policy? A Primer" (International Monetary Fund, Working Paper WP/00/136, Washington, DC, 2000).

110. Ibid.

111. WHO, *World Health Report* (2003).

112. Hsiao, "What Should Macroeconomists Know?" 18.

113. Government of Kenya, "Sessional Paper on National Social Health Insurance: The National Social Health Insurance Fund Bill" (Government of Kenya, Nairobi, 2004); "Free Care on the Way," *Daily Nation* (Nairobi), 8 January 2003.

114. Ministry of Health, Tanzania, *Proposals for Health Sector Reform* (Dar-es-Salaam: Government Printer, 1994).

115. David Dollar and Jakob Svennson, "What Explains the Success and Failure of Structural Adjustment Programs?" (Policy Research Working Paper 1938, World Bank Macroeconomics and Growth Group, Washington, DC, 1998).

116. Welch et al., "In Focus: Structural Adjustment Programs," 3.

117. Natasha Palmer et al., "A New Face for Private Providers in Developing Countries: What Implications for Public Health?" *Bulletin of the World Health Organization* 81 (2003): 4.

118. Ernst & Young, "Health Care Systems and Health Market Reform in the G20 Countries" (report presented at the World Economic Forum, Davos, Switzerland, January 2003).

119. Joint United Nations Program on AIDS/World Health Organization, *Epidemiological Fact Sheet—South Africa* (Geneva: U.N. Program on AIDS/World Health Organization, 2002).

120. Bloom, *Primary Health Care Meets the Market,* 12–13.

121. Ibid.

122. Yanrui Wu, "China's Health Care Sector in Transition: Resources, Demand and Reforms," *Health Policy* 39, no. 2 (1997): 137–52.

123. Jun Gao et al., "Changing Access to Health Services in Urban China: Implications for Equity," *Health Policy and Planning* 16, no. 3 (2001): 302–12.

124. State Council, "Decision of the Central Committee of the Chinese Communist Party and the State Council on Health Reform and Development" (Beijing, 15 January 1997).

125. Deborah Davis and Nancy E. Chapman, "Turning Points in Chinese Health Care: Crisis or Opportunity?" *Yale-China Health Journal* 1 (2002): 3–9.

126. Ernst & Young, "Health Care Systems and Health Market Reform."

127. Zhizheng Du, "Health Care and the Market in China" (ms., 2003).

128. Bloom, *Primary Health Care Meets the Market,* 12–13.

129. Peter Wonacott, "Ailing Patient: In Rural China, Health Care Grows Expensive, Elusive," *Wall Street Journal,* 19 May 2003, A1.

130. Jun Gao et al., "Changing Access to Health Services in Urban China," 302–12.

131. Davis and Chapman, "Turning Points in Chinese Health Care."

132. Meng-Kin Lim et al., "Public Perceptions of Private Health Care in Socialist China," *Health Affairs* 23, no. 6 (2004): 222–34.

133. Francis Markus, "China's Ailing Health Care," *British Broadcasting Corporation,* Shanghai (8 December 2004).

134. Ernst & Young, "Health Care Systems and Health Market Reform."

135. Brijesh Purohit, "Private Initiatives and Policy Options: Recent Health System Experience in India," *Health Policy and Planning* 16, no. 1 (2001): 88–89.

136. Ramesh Bhat, "The Private/Public Mix in Health Care in India," *Health Policy and Planning* 8, no. 1 (1993): 43–56.

137. See C. David Naylor et al., "A Fine Balance: Some Options for Private and Public Health Care in Urban India," in *Human Development Network* (Washington, DC: World Bank, 1999).

138. Chen and Hiebert, "From Socialism to Private Markets," 11.

139. Paul Gertler and Jennie Litvack, "Access to Health Care during Transition: The Role of the Private Sector in Vietnam," in *Household Welfare and Vietnam's Transition* (Washington, DC: World Bank Group, 1998).

140. Brian Abel-Smith, "Recent Developments in Health Insurance" (paper presented at a Conference in Hanoi, Vietnam, 1992).

141. Nguyen Thi Hong Ha, Peter Berman, and Ulla Larsen, "Household Utilization and Expenditure on Private and Public Health Services in Vietnam," *Health Policy and Planning* 17, no. 1 (2002): 61–70.

142. Peter Berman, "Rethinking Health Care Systems: Private Health Care Provision in India," *World Development* 26, no. 8 (2000): 1463–79.

143. Paul Smithson, *Health Financing and Sustainability in Vietnam,* Report for Save the Children Fund, UK, Sustainability in the Health Sector Project (London: Save the Children UK, 1993).

144. Bloom, *Primary Health Care Meets the Market,* 12–18.

145. Figure presented by Vietnam Health Insurance at Vietnam Health Week, Hanoi, 22–23 June 1999.

146. T. Ensor and P. San, "Health Sector Reform in Asian Transition Countries" (Study on Social Sector Issues in Asian Transition Economies, Asian Development Bank, 1996).

147. G. Dahlgren, "Some Key Issues Related to the Regulatory Role of the Government in the Health Sector" (presented at Vietnam Health Week, Hanoi, 22–23 June 1999).

148. WHO, *World Health Report* (2003).

149. Pham Huy Dung, "The Political Process to Increase the Private Health Sector's Role in Vietnam," in *Private Health Sector Growth in Asia: Issues and Implications,* ed. William Newbrander (Chichester: John Wiley, 1997).

150. Bloom, *Primary Health Care Meets the Market,* 18–25.

151. Gertler and Litvack, "Access to Health Care during Transition."

152. Baeza, "Script: Taking Stock of Healthcare Reform," 1–12.

153. Fleury et al., *Reshaping Health Care in Latin America,* 12.

154. Baeza, "Script: Taking Stock of Healthcare Reform," 1–12.

155. E. Medina, "Descentralización y Privatización del Sistema de Salud," *Estudios Publicos* 39 (1990): 5–66.

156. Kottow, "Medicine and Market in Chile."

157. Ibid.

158. A. Barrientos, "Health Policy in Chile: Is the Public Sector Dominant Again?" (ID21 Health, Manchester, UK, 2002), www.id21.org/health/h1ab1g3.html (accessed 12 February 2005).

159. A. Barrientos, "Private Wealth, Private Health: Challenging Healthcare Inequal-

ities in Chile" (ID21 Health, Manchester, U.K., 2001), www.id21.org/health/h2ab1g2 .html (accessed 12 February 2005).

160. Ibid., 21.

161. Ernst & Young, "Health Care Systems and Health Market Reform."

162. Ibid.

163. Ibid.

164. Armando Barrientos and Peter Lloyd-Sherlock, "Reforming Health Insurance in Argentina and Chile," *Health Policy and Planning* 15, no. 4 (2000): 422–23.

165. Peter Berman and Thomas Bossert, "A Decade of Health Sector Reform in Developing Countries: What Have We Learned?" in *DDM Report no. 81* (Cambridge: Harvard School of Public Health, 2000), 1–21.

166. WHO, *World Health Report* (2003).

167. UNDP, *Human Development Report 2003*.

168. Peter Bourne, "Asking the Right Questions: Lessons from the Cuban Health Care System" (inaugural U.K. Health Equity Network annual lecture, London School of Economics, London, March 2003).

169. Alexander S. Preker, "Global Development Challenges and Health Care Reform" (Health, Nutrition and Population Series, World Bank, Washington, DC, 2001).

170. Rene Loewenson, "Structural Adjustment and Health Policy in Africa," *International Journal of Health Services* 23, no. 4 (1993): 717–30.

171. Yuanli Liu et al., "Transformation of China's Rural Health Care Financing," *Social Science and Medicine* 8 (1995): 1085–93.

172. Ricardo Britrán and Fernando Xavier Almarza, *Las Instituciones de Salud Previsional (ISAPRE) en Chile* (Santiago: Comisión Económico para América Latina y el Caribe, 1997).

173. Bona Chita et al., *Decentralization of Health Systems in Zambia,* Partnerships for Health Reform Technical Report (Bethesda, MD: Partnerships for Health Reform, 2000).

174. Lucy Gilson and Ann Mills, "Health Sector Reforms in Sub-Saharan Africa: Lessons of the Last 10 Years," *Health Policy* 32, no. 1–3 (1995): 215–43.

175. W. C. Newbrander, I. W. Aitken, and R. L. Kolehmainen-Aitken, "Performance of the Health System under Decentralization," in *Decentralization in a Developing Country: The Experience of Papua New Guinea and Its Health Service,* ed. J. Thomason, W. C. Newbrander, and R. L. Kolehmainen-Aitken (Canberra: Australian National University, 1991), 64–75.

176. Berman and Bossert, "Decade of Health Sector Reform," 14.

177. V. Brijal and L. Gilson, "Understanding Capacity: Financial Management within the District Health System" (Center for Health Policy Monograph, Johannesburg, 1997); J. A. Cooksey and R. M. Krieg, "Metropolitan Health Policy Development: Barriers to Implementation," *Journal of Public Health Policy* 17, no. 3 (1996): 261–74.

178. Berman and Bossert, "Decade of Health Sector Reform," 10.

179. M. W. Kroneman and J. Van der Zee, "Health Policy as a Fuzzy Concept: Methodological Problems Encountered when Evaluating Health Policy Reforms in an International Perspective," *Health Policy* 40 (1996): 139–155; William C. Hsiao, "Comparing

Health Care Systems: What Nations Can Learn from One Another," *Journal of Health Politics, Policy and Law* 17, no. 4 (1992): 613–36; R. A. Carr-Hill, "Efficiency and Equity Implications of the Health Care Reforms," *Social Science and Medicine* 39, no. 9 (1994): 1189–201.

180. C. Pollitt, "Justification by Works or by Faith? Evaluating the New Public Management," *Evaluation* 1, no. 2 (1995): 133–54.

181. Andrea Giovanni Cornia, "Investing in Human Resources: Health, Nutrition and Development for the 1990s," in *Human Development and the International Development Strategies for the 1990s,* ed. Keith Griffin and John Knight (London: Macmillan, 1990).

182. World Bank, *World Bank Development Report: From Plan to Market* (Oxford: Oxford University Press, 1996).

183. Thomas Rice, *The Economics of Health Reconsidered,* 2nd ed. (Chicago: Health Administration Press, 2003); Preker, "Global Development Challenges."

184. A. S. Preker et al., "Health Care Financing for Rural and Low-Income Populations: The Role of Communities in Resource Mobilization and Risk Sharing—a Synthesis of the Community Financing Experience" (submitted to the WHO Commission on Macro-Economics and Health, Geneva, 2001).

185. Preker, "Global Development Challenges."

CHAPTER 5: THE MARKET WILD CARD

1. In light of the important role Smith gave to government in alleviating human suffering and deprivation, it is remarkable that this feature of his work is so often overlooked.

2. Christine Kinealy, *A Death-Dealing Famine: The Great Hunger in Ireland* (Ann Arbor: University of Michigan Press, 1997).

3. IMS World Review, "IMS Reports a 9 Percent Constant Dollar Growth in '03 Global Pharma Sales," *IMS Insights,* 2004, 1.

4. Ibid.

5. John Harwood, "Despite Rx Benefit, White House Faces a Medicare Problem," *Wall Street Journal,* 3 March 2004, A4.

6. Quoted in ibid.

7. Robert Dubois et al., "Explaining Drug Spending Trends: Does Perception Match Reality?" *Health Affairs* 19, no. 2 (2000): 231–39.

8. Cynthia Smith, "Retail Prescription Drug Spending in the National Health Accounts," *Health Affairs* 23, no. 1 (2004): 160–67.

9. Henry J. Kaiser Family Foundation, *California Seniors and Prescription Drugs* (Menlo Park: Henry J. Kaiser Family Foundation, 2002).

10. Arnold S. Relman and Marcia Angell, "America's Other Drug Problem," *New Republic* 4, no. 587 (2002): 27–41; Marcia Angell, *The Truth about Drug Companies: How They Deceive Us and What to Do about It* (New York: Random House, 2004); Jerry Avorn, *Powerful Medicines: The Benefits, Risks, and Costs of Prescription Drugs* (New York: Knopf, 2004).

11. David Blumenthal and E. G. Cambell, "Academic Industry Relationships in Biotechnology: A Primer on Policy and Practice," *Cloning* 2, no. 3 (2000): 129–36. See also Hamilton Moses III and Joseph B. Martin, "Academic Relationships with Industry: A New Model for Biomedical Research," *Journal of the American Medical Association* 285, no. 7 (2001): 933–35.

12. Robert Pear, "Drug Companies Increase Spending on Efforts to Lobby Congress and Governments," *New York Times,* 1 June 2003, A33.

13. Ibid.

14. Martin T. Garhart et al., "Examining the FDA's Oversight of Direct-to-Consumer Advertising," *Health Affairs,* Web Exclusive, February 2003, W3-120–23.

15. Joel S. Weissman et al., "Consumers' Reports on the Health Effects of Direct-to-Consumer Drug Advertising," *Health Affairs,* Web Exclusive, 2003, W3-82–95.

16. Robert W. Dubois, "Pharmaceutical Promotion: Don't Throw the Baby Out with the Bath Water," *Health Affairs,* Web Exclusive, 2003, W96–103.

17. T. E. Henney, "Challenges in Regulating Direct-to-Consumer Advertising," *Journal of the American Medical Association* 284, no. 17 (2000): 2242.

18. Weissman et al., "Consumers' Reports on Health Effects."

19. Gardiner Harris, "Novartis to Give Consumer Ads a Big Role in Selling Drugs," *New York Times,* 20 November 2003, C1.

20. Garhart et al., "Examining the FDA's Oversight."

21. Pharmaceutical Research and Manufacturers of America, "PhRMA Adopts New Marketing Code" (Washington, DC, 19 April 2002), www.phrma.org/mediaroom/press/releases/19.04.2002.390.cfm.

22. J. D. Kleinke, "Just What the HMO Ordered: The Paradox of Increasing Drug Costs," *Health Affairs* 19, no. 2 (2000): 78–91.

23. Michael Dickson, Jeremy Hurst, and Stéphane Jacopzone, *Survey of Pharmacoeconomic Assessment Activity in Eleven Countries,* OECD Working Papers (Paris: Organization for Economic Cooperation and Development, 2003), 3.

24. Ibid., 31.

25. Peter J. Neumann et al., "Are Pharmaceuticals Cost-Effective? A Review of the Evidence," *Health Affairs* 18, no. 2 (2000): 104.

26. Uwe E. Reinhardt, "An Information Infrastructure for the Pharmaceutical Market," *Health Affairs* 23, no. 1 (2004): 107–12. See also John F. Hoadley, "The Continued Need for Independent Research on Prescription Drugs" *Health Affairs* 23, no. 1 (2004): 244–49.

27. Dickson, Hurst, and Jacopzone, *Survey of Pharmacoeconomic Assessment Activity,* 42.

28. Bruce E. Landon, James D. Reschovsky, and David Blumenthal, "Physicians' Views of Formularies: Implications for Medicare Drug Benefit Design," *Health Affairs* 23, no. 1 (2004): 224–25.

29. Peter J. Neumann, "Evidence-Based and Value-Based Formulary Guidelines," *Health Affairs* 23, no. 1 (2003): 124–34.

30. Bob Tedeschi, "As the Debate Continues, Opinions Are Divided over the Merits of Allowing Online Drug Purchasing from Canada," *New York Times,* 8 March 2004, C4.

31. Jillian Clare Cohen, "The Moral Dilemma of International Internet Pharmacies," *Hastings Center Report* 34, no. 2 (2004): 5.

32. Wayne Guglielmo, "Rx Price Control: Maine Gets a Go-Ahead," *Medical Economics* 78, no. 13 (2001): 23.

33. Leila Abboud, "Texas Health Plan Curbs Lilly Drug," *Wall Street Journal,* 1 March 2004, B3.

34. Robert Pear, "U.S. Limiting Costs of Drugs for Medicare," *New York Times,* 21 April 2003, A1.

35. Melody Petersen, "U.S. to Back Heart Device in More Cases," *New York Times,* 7 June 2003, C1.

36. Richard G. Frank, "Government Commitment and Regulation of Prescription Drugs," *Health Affairs* 22, no. 3 (2003): 48.

37. J. D. Kleinke, "Access versus Excess: Value-Based Cost Sharing for Prescription Drugs," *Health Affairs* 23, no. 1 (2004): 43.

38. Ibid.

39. Canadian Institute for Health Information, *Health Care in Canada* (Ottawa: Canadian Institute of Health Information, 2002), 84.

40. Ibid., 88.

41. Patricia M. Danzon and Michael E. Furukawa, "Price and Availability of Pharmaceuticals: Evidence from Nine Countries," *Health Affairs,* Web Exclusive, 2003, W3-520–21.

42. Steven G. Morgan, Morris L. Borer, and Jonathan D. Agrew, "Whither Seniors' Pharmacare: Lesson from (and for) Canada." *Health Affairs* 22, no. 3 (2003): 52.

43. Aslam H. Anis, "Pharmaceutical Policies in Canada: Another Example of Federal-Provincial Discord," *Canadian Medical Association Journal* 62, no. 4 (2000): 523.

44. Morgan, Borer, and Agrew, "Whither Seniors' Pharmacare," 54; see also Minority Staff, Committee on Government Reform, "Response to Drug Industry Claims on Prescription Drug Differences between the United States and Other Countries" (U.S. House of Representatives, Washington, DC, 2002).

45. "We Need Romanow's National Drug Industry," editorial, *Canadian Medical Association Journal* 168, no. 3 (2003): 253.

46. Standing Committee on Social Affairs, Science and Technology, *The Health of Canadians—the Federal Role,* vol. 6: *Recommendations for Reform* (Toronto: Standing Senate Committee on Social Affairs, Science and Technology, October 2002), 12.

47. Vanessa Fuhrmans and Gautan Naik, "Drug Makers Fight to Fend Off Cuts in European Prices," *Wall Street Journal,* 7 June 2002, A1.

48. Ibid.

49. Ian Cowell, "European Union Expansion Has Drug Makers Worried," *New York Times,* 20 November 2003, W7.

50. Ibid.

51. The CEO is quoted in Fuhrmans and Naik, "Drug Makers Fight to Fend Off Cuts," A1.

52. Ibid., A7.

53. Gavin Permanand and Elias Mossialos, "Theorizing the Development of the

European Union Framework for Pharmaceutical Regulation" (LSE Health and Social Care Discussion Paper no. 13, London School of Economics and Political Science, London, 2004), 4.

54. Ibid., 7.

55. Michael Vandergrift and Panos Kanavos, "Health Policy versus Industrial Policy in the Pharmaceutical Sector: The Case of Canada," *Health Policy* 41, no. 3 (1997): 255.

56. Daniel Callahan, *False Hopes* (New York: Simon and Schuster, 1998).

57. Richard B. Saltman and Josep Figueras, *European Health Care Reform: Analysis of Current Strategies* (Copenhagen: World Health Organization, 1997), 177.

58. Dickson, Hurst, and Jacopzone, *Survey of Pharmacoeconomic Assessment Activity,* 25.

59. Katharine Levit et al., the Health Accounts Team, "Health Spending Rebound Continues in 2002," *Health Affairs* 23, no. 1 (2004): 149.

60. Dickson, Hurst, and Jacopzone, *Survey of Pharmacoeconomic Assessment Activity,* 25–29.

61. Saltman and Figueras, *European Health Care Reform,* 177ff.; Elias Mossialos, Monique Mrazek, and Tom Walley, *Regulating Pharmaceuticals in Europe: Striving for Efficiency, Equity, and Quality* (Maidenhead, UK: Open University Press, 2004).

62. European Court of Justice, "The Competition Rules of the EC Do Not Preclude German Sickness Fund Associations from Determining Ceilings for Payments in Respect of Certain Medicinal Products" (European Court of Justice, Luxembourg, 16 March 2004), cases C-264/01, C-306/01, C-351/01, C-355/01.

63. "Drug Bill Upheld," *BBC News,* 5 June 2004.

64. Associated Press, "European Court Backs Discount Medical Imports" (1 April 2004).

65. Panos Kanavos and Uwe Reinhardt, "Reference Pricing for Drugs: Is It Compatible with U.S. Health Care?" *Health Affairs* 22, no. 3 (2003): 16–30.

66. Alan Maynard and Karen Bloor, "Dilemmas in Regulation of the Market for Pharmaceuticals," *Health Affairs* 22, no. 3 (2003): 38, 39.

67. World Bank, *World Development Report 1993: Investing in Health* (New York: Oxford University Press, 1994).

68. R. Hartog, "Essential and Non-Essential Drugs Marketed by 20 Largest European Pharmaceutical Companies in Developing Countries," *Social Science and Medicine* 37, no. 7 (1993): 897–904.

69. World Health Organization, *The Use of Essential Drug,* 6th Report of the Expert Committee, WHO Technical Report Series no. 850 (Geneva: World Health Organization, 1995).

70. Turshen, *Privatizing Health Services in Africa,* 108–10.

71. World Health Organization, *Framework for Action in Essential Drugs and Medicines Policy* (Geneva: World Health Organization, 2000), 2.

72. Y. Liu et al., "Transformation of China's Rural Health Care Financing," *Social Science and Medicine* 41, no. 8 (1995): 1085–93; Alexandra Wyke, ed., "HealthCare International: China's Pharmaceutical Industry—in Difficulties," *EIU HealthCare International,* 2nd quarter (1997): 46–58.

73. Wyke, "HealthCare International."

74. Ramesh Govindaraj, G. Chellaraj, and C. J. L. Murray, "Health Expenditures in Latin America and the Caribbean," *Social Science and Medicine* 44, no. 2 (1997): 157–69; World Bank, *World Development Report 1993.*

75. K. Diarra and S. Coulibaly, "Financing of Recurrent Health Costs in Mali," *Health Policy* 5 (1990): 126–38; World Health Organization, "Framework for Containing Resistance to Antimicrobial Drugs" (WHO Presentation at Infectious Diseases Partners Initial Meeting, U.S. Agency for International Development, Washington, DC, 16–17 December 1997).

76. Ramesh Govindaraj, Michael R. Reich, and Jillian C. Cohen, *World Bank Pharmaceuticals,* HNP Discussion Paper (Washington, DC: World Bank, September 2000), 8.

77. World Bank, *Better Health in Africa: Experiences and Lessons Learned* (Washington, DC: World Bank, 1994), 77.

78. William Newbrander, "Equity and Coverage of Health Care Provision in Kenya" (report prepared for the BASICS Project, Partnership for Child Health Care, Arlington, VA, 1995).

79. Sjaak Van der Geest, "The Efficiency of Inefficiency: Medicine Distribution in South Cameroon," *Social Science and Medicine* 25, no. 3 (1982): 293–305.

80. A. Alland, Jr., *Adaptation in Cultural Evolution: An Approach to Medical Anthropology* (New York: Columbia University Press, 1970), 170. Also quoted in Sjaak Van der Geest et al., "User Fees and Drugs: What Did the Health Reforms in Zambia Achieve?" *Health Policy and Planning* 15, no. 1 (2000): 62.

81. Mission for Essential Drugs and Supplies, "Report of an Annual Conference" (Mission for Essential Drugs and Supplies, Nairobi, Kenya, 1993).

82. A. Ron, B. Abel-Smith, and G. Tamburi, *Health Insurance in Developing Countries: A Social Security Approach* (Geneva: International Labor Office, 1990); C. Normand and A. Weber, *Social Health Insurance: A Guidebook for Planning,* WHO/SHS/94.3 (Geneva: World Health Organization, 1994); J. Kutzin and H. Barnum, *How Health Insurance Affects the Delivery of Health Care in Developing Countries* (Washington, DC: World Bank; 1992), 1–20.

83. World Health Organization/Drug Action Programme (WHO/DAP), *Global Comparative Pharmaceutical Expenditure: Health Economics and Drugs,* DAP Series no. 3 (Geneva: World Health Organization, 1997).

84. World Bank, *Better Health in Africa,* 75.

85. World Health Organization, *Public-Private Roles in the Pharmaceutical Sector: Implications for Equitable Access and Rational Drug Use,* WHO/DAP/97.12 (Geneva: World Health Organization, 1997), 15.

86. Harvey Bale, "WHO Should Build Partnerships with the Pharmaceutical Industry to Improve Public Health," *Lancet* 361, no. 9351 (2003): 4.

87. World Health Organization, *Counterfeit Drugs Guidelines for the Development of Measures to Combat Counterfeit Drugs* (Geneva: World Health Organization, 1999), 11–12.

88. Van der Geest, "Efficiency of Inefficiency."

89. World Bank, *Better Health in Africa,* 77.

90. H. V. Hogerzeil et al., "Field Test for Rational Drug Use in Twelve Developing Countries," *Lancet* 342, no. 8884 (1993): 1408–10; World Bank, *Better Health in Africa.*

91. F. M. Haaijer-Ruskamp and P. Denig, "New Approaches to Influencing Physicians' Drug Choices: The Practice-Based Strategy," in *Contested Ground,* ed. P. Davis (Oxford: Oxford University Press, 1996).

92. Turshen, *Privatizing Health Services in Africa,* 108–10.

93. WHO/DAP, *Global Comparative Pharmaceutical Expenditure*; B. McPake and E. Ngalande-Bande, "Contracting out Health Services in Developing Countries," *Health Policy and Planning* 9, no. 1 (1994): 25–30; Ann Mills, "Contractual Relations between Government and the Commercial Private Sector in Developing Countries: Are They a Good Idea in Health?" in *Private Health Providers in Developing Countries: Serving the Public Interest?* ed. S. Bennet, B. McPake, and A. Mills (London: Zed Press, 1997).

94. Macroeconomics and Health Strategy/World Health Organization/Drug Action Programme, *Managing Drug Supply,* 2nd ed. (Hartford, CT: Kumarian Press, 1997).

95. Ibid.

96. "Ranbaxy in R&D Tie-up with Glaxo," editorial, *Hindu* (Chennai, Madras) 24 October 2003.

97. S. C. Benjamin, Obinna E. Omujekwe Uzochukwu, and Cyril O Akpala, "Effect of the Bamako-Initiative Drug Revolving Fund on Availability and Rational Use of Essential Drugs in Primary Health Care Facilities in South-East Nigeria," *Health Policy and Planning* 17, no. 4 (2002): 378–83.

98. WHO/DAP, *Global Comparative Pharmaceutical Expenditure.*

99. Ibid.

100. G. Bevan, *Equity in the Use of Health Care Resources: Current Concern,* Social and Human Science Paper no. 3, WHO/SHS/CC/91.1 (Geneva: World Health Organization, 1991).

101. K. Walsh, *Public Services and Market Mechanisms: Competition, Contracting, and the New Public Management* (Basingstoke, UK: Macmillan, 1996).

102. Govindaraj, Reich, and Cohen, *World Bank Pharmaceuticals.*

103. Bernard Pecaoul et al., "Access to Essential Drugs in Poor Countries: A Lost Battle?" *Journal of the American Medical Association* 281, no. 4 (1999): 361–67; H. David Banta, "Worldwide Interest in Global Access to Drugs," *Journal of the American Medical Association* 285, no. 22 (2001): 2844–46; P. Boulet et al., *Pharmaceuticals and the WTO TRIPS Agreement: Questions and Answers* (Geneva: World Health Organization, 2000).

104. Kristen K. Jensen, "Thompson May Seek to Void Cipro Patent If Talks Fail," *Bloomberg,* 23 October 2001.

105. *The Pharmaceutical Manufacturers' Association of South Africa et al., vs. the President of the Republic of South Africa, the Honorable Mr. N. R. Mandela N.O. et al.,* High Court of South Africa, case no. 4183/98.

106. David Henry and Joel Lexchin, "The Pharmaceutical Industry as a Medicines Provider," *Lancet* 360, no. 9345 (2002): 1590–95; "Patent Protection versus Public Health," editorial, *Lancet* 358, no. 9293 (2001): 1563.

107. Doha World Trade Organization Ministerial, "Declaration on the TRIPS Agreement and Public Health" (World Trade Organization, Geneva, 14 November 2001).

108. World Health Organization and World Trade Organization Secretariats, "Workshop on Differential Pricing and Financing of Essential Drugs," Norwegian Foreign Affairs Ministry, Global Health Council, 8–11 April 2001, Hosbjor, Norway (World Health Organization, Geneva, 2001).

109. Frederick M. Abbott, *Compulsory Licensing for Public Health Needs: The TRIPS Agenda at the WTO after the Doha Declaration on Public Health,* Occasional Paper 9 (Geneva: United Nations Office, February 2002), 17.

110. A. Barrett, "Fifty Ways to Keep Your Patent," *Business Week,* 12 July 2001.

111. Patrice Trouiller et al., "Drug Development for Neglected Diseases: A Deficient Market and a Public-Health Policy Failure," *Lancet* 359, no. 9324 *(2002):* 2188–94.

112. Global Forum for Health Research, *The 10/90 Report on Health Research 2000* (Geneva: Global Forum for Health Research, 2000).

113. Leena Menghaney quoted in Reuters, "Patent Bill in India Could Raise AIDS Drug Prices," *New York Times,* 23 March 2005, A1.

114. Rachel Cohen, spokeswoman for Doctors Without Borders, in an interview with Rachel Zimmerman-See, "Merck Still Draws Fire for HIV Drug for Poor Nations," *Wall Street Journal,* 3 March 2004, D3.

115. Ibid.

116. Donald G. McNeil, Jr., "Patents or Poverty? A New Debate over Poor AIDS Care in Africa," *New York Times,* 5 November 2001, A1–6.

117. Gordon Perkin quoted in DELIVER, "The Importance of Logistics in HIV/AIDS Programs, No Product? No Program!" 2003, www.deliver.jsi.com.

118. William G. Rothstein, "Pharmaceuticals and Public Policy in America: A History," in *American Health Care: Current Issues in Socio-Historical Perspective,* ed. William G. Rothstein (Madison: University of Wisconsin Press, 1995), 381.

119. Frank R. Lichtenberg, "Pharmaceutical Development, Mortality Reduction, and Economic Growth," in *Measuring the Gain from Medical Research: An Economic Approach,* ed. Kevin M. Murphy and Robert H. Topel (Chicago: University of Chicago Press, 2002).

120. Rothstein, "Pharmaceuticals and Public Policy in America," 388.

121. M. N. Graham Dukes, "Accountability of the Pharmaceutical Company," *Lancet* 360, no. 9346 (2002): 1682–84.

122. Dean Baker, "Financing Drug Research: What Are the Issues?" (issue brief, Center for Economic and Policy Research, Washington, DC, 22 September 2004).

123. Pharmaceutical Research and Manufacturers of America, *Annual Report: 2003–2004* (Washington, DC: Pharmaceutical Research and Manufacturers of America, 2004), 2.

124. Dickson, Hurst, and Jacopzone, *Survey of Pharmacoeconomic Assessment Activity.*

125. Merrill Goszner, *The $800 Million Pill* (Berkeley: University of California Press, 2004), 230–46.

126. Donald Light and Joel Lexchin, "Will Lower Drug Prices Jeopardize Drug Research? A Fact Sheet," *American Journal of Bioethics* 4, no. 1 (2004): W1-4.

127. James Love, "Evidence Regarding Research and Development Investments in Innovative and Non-Innovative Medicines" (Consumer Project on Technology, Washington, DC, 23 September 2003).

128. Alan Seger and Deborah Socolar, "Do Drug Makers Lose Money on Canadian Imports?" (Data Brief no. 6, Boston University School of Public Health, Boston, 15 April 2004).

CHAPTER 6: THE VALUE OF THE MARKET

1. Mark V. Pauly et al., "A Plan for 'Responsible National Health Insurance,' " *Health Affairs* 10, no. 1 (1991): 5-25.

2. William James, *The Principles of Psychology* (Cambridge: Harvard University Press, 1981), 462.

3. Thomas Rice, *The Economics of Health Reconsidered,* 2nd ed. (Chicago: Health Administration Press, 2003), 272.

4. Alain Enthoven, "Introducing Market Forces in Health Care: A Tale of Two Countries" (ms., July 2002).

5. See the discussion of "guild free choice" in the section "The Early American Background" in chapter 2.

6. Alain Enthoven, "Consumer-Choice Health Plan," *New England Journal of Medicine* 298, no. 12, pt. 1 (1978): 650-98.

7. Ronald C. Lippincott and James W. Begun, "Competition in the Health Sector: A Historical Perspective," *Journal of Health Politics, Policy and Law* 7, no. 2 (1982): 463.

8. Alain Enthoven, "Employment-Based Health Insurance Is Failing: Now What?" *Health Affairs,* Web Exclusive, suppl. 2003, W3-237-49.

9. Robert H. Miller, "Competition in the Health System: Good News and Bad News," *Health Affairs* 15, no. 2 (1996): 2.

10. Ibid., 7; Robert H. Miller and Harold S. Luft, "Does Managed Care Lead to Better or Worse Quality of Care?" *Health Affairs* 16, no. 5 (1997): 7-25.

11. Eli Ginzburg, "Managed Care and the Competitive Market in Health Care," *Journal of the American Medical Association* 277, no. 22 (1997): 1813.

12. Anil Bamezai et al., "Price Competition and Hospital Cost Growth in the United States (1989-1994)," *Health Economics* 8, no. 3 (1999): 233-43.

13. James C. Robinson, "Consolidation and the Transformation of Competition in Health Insurance," *Health Affairs* 23, no. 6 (2004): 11-24.

14. Susan Marquis, Jeannette A. Rogowski, and Jose J. Escarce, "The Managed Care Backlash: Did Consumers Vote with Their Feet?" *Inquiry* 41, no. 41 (winter 2004/2005): 376-90.

15. Mitchell P. V. Glavin et al., "An Examination of Factors in the Withdrawal of Managed Care Plans for the Medicare and Choice Program," *Inquiry* 39, no. 4 (2002/2003): 341-54.

16. Thomas Scully quoted in Uwe W. Reinhardt, "The Medicare World from Both Sides: A Conversation with Tom Scully," *Health Affairs* 22, no. 6 (2003): 168.

17. Bryan Dowd, Robert Coulan, and Roger Feldman, "A Tale of Four Cities: Medicare Reform and Competitive Pricing," *Health Affairs* 19, no. 3 (2000): 9–29.

18. D. Farley, "Competition among Hospitals: Market Structure and Its Relationship to Utilization, Costs, and Financial Position" (Research Note 7, National Center for Health Services Research, Washington, DC, 1985); Zack Zwanziger and Glenn A. Melnick, "The Effects of Competition and the Medicare PPS Program on Hospital Cost Behavior in California," *Journal of Health Economics* 7 (1988): 301–20; James C. Robinson and Harold S. Luft, "Competition and the Cost of Hospital Care, 1972 to 1982," *Journal of the American Medical Association* 257, no. 23 (1987): 3241–45.

19. James Robinson and Harold S. Luft, "Competition, Regulation, and Hospital Costs, 1982–1986," *Journal of the American Medical Association* 260, no. 18 (1988): 2678.

20. A. Bamezai et al., "Price Competition and Hospital Cost Growth in the United States (1989–1994)," *Health Economics* 81 (1999): 233.

21. Robinson and Luft, "Competition, Regulation, and Hospital Costs," 2676.

22. Emmett Keeler, Glen Melnick, and Jack Zwanziger, "The Changing Effects of Competition on Non-Profit Hospital Pricing Behavior," *Journal of Health Economics* 18, no. 1 (1999): 69.

23. Bamezai et al., "Price Competition and Hospital Cost Growth," 233–34.

24. P. A. Rivers, S. Glover, and G. Munchus, "Hospital Competition in Major U.S. Metropolitan Areas: Empirical Evidence," *Journal of Health and Human Services Administration* 23, no. 1 (2000): 47–48.

25. J. Zwanziger, G. A. Melnick, and A. Bamezai, "The Effect of Selective Contracting on Hospital Costs and Revenues," *Health Services Research* 35, no. 4 (2000): 849–67.

26. Richard Freeman, "Competition in Context: The Politics of Health Care Reform in Europe," *International Journal for Quality in Health Care* 10, no. 5 (1998): 400.

27. Richard B. Saltman and Josep Figueras, "On Solidarity and Competition: An Evidence-Based Perspective," *Eurohealth* 2, no. 4 (1996): 20; Rice, *Economics of Health Reconsidered,* 273.

28. Rice, *Economics of Health Reconsidered,* 272.

29. Enthoven, "Introducing Market Forces in Health Care," 11, 12.

30. See the section "The United States: Postwar Years, Postwar Frustrations" in chapter 2.

31. Burton A. Weisbrod, "Competition in Health Care: A Cautionary View," repr. in Jack Myers, ed., *Market Reforms in Health Care: Current Issues, New Directions, Strategic Decisions* (Washington DC: American Enterprise Institute for Public Policy Research, 1993), 71.

32. James C. Robinson, "Consolidation and Competition in Health Insurance," *Health Affairs* 23, no. 6 (2004): 11–24.

33. Paul T. Menzel, "Economic Competition in Health Care: A Moral Assessment," *Journal of Medicine and Philosophy* 12, no. 1 (1987): 63–84; John K. Iglehart, "The

Emergence of Physician-Owned Specialty Hospitals," *New England Journal of Medicine* 352, no. 1 (2005): 78–84.

34. J. Akin, "Fees for Health Services and Concern for Equity for the Poor," *World Bank PHN Technical Note Series* 86 (1986): 10.

35. Richard B. Saltman and Josep Figueras, *European Health Care Reform: Analysis of Current Strategies* (Copenhagen: World Health Organization 1997), 115–39.

36. Ibid.

37. Robert Evans et al., "It's Not the Money, It's the Principle: Why User Charges for Some Services and Not Others" (Discussion Paper no. 94-06, Centre for Research on Economic and Social Policy, University of British Columbia, January 1994).

38. D. Griffin, "Welfare Gains from User Charges for Government Health Services," *Health Policy and Planning* 7 (1992): 177–80; International Bank for Reconstruction and Development, *Financing Education in Developing Countries: An Exploration of Policy Options* (Washington, DC: World Bank, 1986); E. Jiminez, *Pricing Policy in Social Sectors: Cost Recovery for Education and Health in Developing Countries* (Baltimore: Johns Hopkins University Press, for the World Bank, 1987).

39. Lucy Gilson, *Government Health Care Charges: Is Equity Being Abandoned?* EPC Publication no. 15 (London: European Policy Centre, 1988).

40. James C. Robinson, "Renewed Emphasis on Consumer Cost Sharing in Health Insurance Benefit Design." *Health Affairs,* Web Exclusive, suppl. 2002, W139–54.

41. Barbara Martinez, "Shifting Burden: With Medical Costs Climbing Workers Are Asked to Pay More," *Wall Street Journal,* 16 June 2003, A1.

42. Geoffrey F. Joyce et al., "Employer Drug Benefit Plans and Spending on Prescription Drugs," *Journal of the American Medical Association* 288, no. 14 (2002): 1733–39.

43. Robinson, "Renewed Emphasis on Consumer Cost Sharing."

44. Joseph P. Newhouse, "Consumer-Directed Health Plans and the RAND Health Insurance Experiment," *Health Affairs* 23, no. 6 (2004): 107–13.

45. Jay M. Gellert, "The Role of the Consumer in Managed Care's Future," *Health Affairs,* Web Exclusive, suppl. 2002, W160–61.

46. Saltman and Figueras, *European Health Care Reform,* 83–100.

47. Ibid.

48. B. Abel-Smith and P. Rawall, "Can the Poor Afford 'Free' Health Care? A Case Study of Tanzania," *Health Policy and Planning* 7, no. 4 (1992): 329–41.

49. See B. Abel-Smith et al., *Choices in Health Policy: An Agenda for the European Union* (Luxembourg/Aldershot: Office of Official Publications of the European Communities/Dartmouth Publishing, 1995).

50. Organization for Economic Cooperation and Development, "The Reform of Health Care Systems: A Review of Seventeen OECD Countries," *Health Policy Studies* 5 (1994): 45.

51. Victor G. Rodwin and Simone Sander, "Health Care under French National Health Insurance," *Health Affairs* 12, no. 3 (1993): 111–31.

52. R. J. Rubin and D. N. Mendelson, *A Framework for Cost-Sharing Policy Analysis* (Basle: Pharmaceutical Partners for Better Health Care, 1995); Saltman and Figueras, *European Health Care Reform,* 83–100.

53. Organization for Economic Cooperation and Development, *Health at a Glance: OECD Indicators 2003* (Paris: Organization for Economic Cooperation and Development, 2003), 45.

54. Saltman and Figueras, *European Health Care Reform,* 83–100.

55. Joseph P. Newhouse, *Free for All: Lessons from the RAND Health Insurance Experiment* (Cambridge: Harvard University Press, 1993).

56. A. Adams and T. Harnett, "The Poor and Cost Sharing in the Social Sectors of Sub-Saharan Africa" (World Bank, Human Resources and Poverty Division, Africa, Technical Department, Washington, DC, 1995); Lucy Gilson, "The Political Economy of User Fees with Targeting: Developing Equitable Health Financing Policy," *Journal of International Development* 7, no. 3 (1995): 369–401.

57. B. Nolan and V. Turbat, *Cost Recovery in Public Health Services in Sub-Saharan Africa* (Washington, DC: Economic Development Institute, Human Resources Division, 1993).

58. D. Booth et al., "Coping with Cost Recovery" (report to Swedish International Development Cooperation Agency, Commissioned through the Development Studies Unit, Department of Social Anthropology, Stockholm University, 1995); S. J. Fabricant, C. W. Kamara, and A. Mills, "Why the Poor Pay More: Household Curative Expenditures in Rural Sierra Leone," *Journal of International Health Planning and Management* 14, no. 3 (1999): 179–99; J. K. Mbugua, G. H. Bloom, and M. M. Segall, "Impact of User Charges on Vulnerable Groups: The Case of the Kibwezi in Rural Kenya," *Social Science and Medicine* 41, no. 6 (1995): 829–35; R. Sauerborn, A. Adams, and N. Hien, "Household Strategies to Cope with the Economic Costs of Illness," *Social Science and Medicine* 43, no. 3 (1996): 291–301.

59. C. Leighton, *22 Policy Questions about Health Care Financing in Africa* (Washington, DC: Health and Human Resources Analysis for Africa/Health Financing and Sustainability Projects, U.S. Agency for International Development, 1995); J. Litvack and C. Bodart, "User Fees Plus Quality Equals Improved Access to Health Care: Results of a Field Experiment in Cameroon," *Social Science and Medicine* 37, no. 3 (1993): 369–83.

60. Abel-Smith and Rawall, "Can the Poor Afford 'Free' Health Care?" 329–41.

61. J. Kutzin, "Experience with Organizational and Financing Reform of the Health Sector: Current Concerns" (SHS Paper no. 8, WHO/SHS/CC94.3, World Health Organization, Geneva, 1995).

62. Booth et al., "Coping with Cost Recovery." See also T. Ensor and San Phan Bich, "Access and Payment for Health Care: The Poor of Vietnam," *International Journal of Health Planning and Management* 11, no. 1 (1996): 69–83.

63. F. Diop, A. Yazbeck, and R. Bitran, "The Impact of Alternative Cost Recovery Schemes on Access and Equity in Niger," *Health Policy and Planning* 10, no. 3 (1995): 223–40.

64. A. Creese and J. Kutzin, "Lessons from Cost Recovery in Health" (paper prepared for workshop on Social and Economic Effects of Alternative Methods of Financing Education and Health Services in Developing Countries, Institute of Development Studies, University of Sussex, Brighton, 28 February–2 March 1994); J. Thomason, N. Mulou, and

C. Bass, "User Charges for Rural Health Services in Papua New Guinea," *Social Science and Medicine* 39, no. 8 (1994): 1105–15.

65. Gilson, "Political Economy of User Fees," 369–401.

66. Lucy Gilson, "The Lessons of User Fee Experience in Africa," *Health Policy and Planning* 12, no. 4 (1997): 273–85.

67. Brian Nolan and Vincent Turbat, *Cost Recovery in Public Health Services in Sub-Saharan Africa* (Washington, DC: Economic Development Institute, World Bank, 1993).

68. Elias Mossialos and Ann Dixon, "Funding Health Care: An Introduction," in *Funding Health Care Options for Europe,* ed. Elias Mossialos et al. (Buckingham, UK: Open University Press, 2002), 4–6.

69. Stephen Young, "The Nature of Privatization in Britain 1979–1985," *Western European Politics* 9 (1986): 235–52.

70. Alan Maynard and Ann Dixon, "Private Health Insurance and Medical Savings Accounts: Theory and Experience" in Mossialos et al., *Funding Health Care Options for Europe,* 109–26; D. J. Chollet and M. Lewis, "Private Insurance Principles and Practice," in *Innovations in Health Care Financing: Proceedings of a World Bank Conference, 10–11 March 1997,* ed. G. J. Schieber (Washington, DC: World Bank, 1997).

71. Chollet and Lewis, "Private Insurance Principles and Practice."

72. Rice, *Economics of Health Reconsidered,* 216–19.

73. E. van Doorslaer et al., "The Redistributive Effect of Health Care Finance in Twelve OECD countries," *Journal of Health Economics* 7, no. 4 (1999): 281–89; A. Wagstaff et al., "Equity in the Finance of Health Care: Some Further International Comparisons," *Journal of Health Economics* 18, no. 3 (1999): 263–90.

74. K. Stocker, H. Waitzkin, and C. Iriart, "The Exportation of Managed Care to Latin America," *New England Journal of Medicine* 340, no. 14 (1999): 1131–35.

75. Allen Buchanan, "Privatization and Just Health Care," *Bioethics* 9, no. 3/4 (1995): 220–39.

76. Ha T. Tu and James D. Reschovsky, "Assessments of Medical Care by Enrollees in For-Profit and Nonprofit Health Maintenance Organizations," *New England Journal of Medicine* 346, no. 17 (2002): 1288.

77. B. M. Kinzbrunner, "For Profits vs. Not-for-Profit Hospice: It Is the Quality That Counts," *Journal of Palliative Care Medicine* 5, no. 4 (2002): 483.

78. Donald H. Taylor, "What Price For-Profit Hospitals?" *Canadian Medical Association Journal* 166, no. 11 (2002): 1418.

79. Elaine M. Silverman, Jonathan S. Skinner, and Elliot S. Fisher, "The Association between For-Profit Hospital Ownership and Increased Medical Spending," *New England Journal of Medicine* 341, no. 6 (1999): 420.

80. Bradford H. Gray, *The Profit Motive and Patient Care: The Changing Accountability of Doctors and Hospitals* (Cambridge: Harvard University Press, 1991); Dan W. Brock and Allen Buchanan, "Ethical Issues in For-Profit Health Care," in *For-Profit Enterprise in Health Care,* ed. Bradford Gray (Washington, DC: National Academy Press, 1986), 224–49.

81. Steffie Woolhandler and David Himmelstein, "Cost of Care and Administration

at For-Profit and Other Hospitals in the United States," *New England Journal of Medicine* 336, no. 11 (1997): 769.

82. Ibid., 774.

83. Silverman, Skinner, and Fisher, "Association between For-Profit Hospital Ownership and Increased Medical Spending."

84. Glenn Melnick, Emmett Keeler, and Jack Zwanziger, "Market Power and Hospital Pricing: Are Nonprofits Different?" *Health Affairs* 18, no. 3 (1999): 173.

85. Cristina Boccuti and Marilyn Moon, "Comparing Medicare and Private Insurers: Growth Rates in Spending over Three Decades," *Health Affairs* 22, no. 2 (2003): 236.

86. Public Citizen' Research Group, "Large Differences among Medical HMOs in Enrollees Appeals," *Public Citizen's Health Research Group Health Letter* 11 (1995): 1–4.

87. Himmelstein and Woolhandler, "Cost of Care and Administration," 769; P. Born and C. Geckler, "HMO Quality and Financial Performance," *Journal of Health Care Finance* 24 (1998): 65–67; Tu and Reschovsky, "Assessments of Medical Care," 1288; Peter J. Devereaux et al., "A Systematic Review and Meta-Analysis of Studies Comparing Mortality Rates of Private For-Profit and Private Not-for-Profit Hospitals," *Canadian Medical Association Journal* 166, no. 11 (2002): 1399–1406; P. J. Devereaux et al., "Comparison of Mortality between Private For-Profit and Private Not-for-Profit Hemodialysis Centers," *Journal of the American Medical Association* 288, no. 19 (2002): 2449–57.

88. Eric C. Schneider, Alan M. Zaslavsky, and Arnold M. Epstein, "Use of High-Cost Operative Procedures by Medical Beneficiaries Enrolled in For-Profit and Not-for-Profit Health Plans," *New England Journal of Medicine* 350, no. 2 (2004): 143–50.

89. Patrick Romano et al., "A National Profile of Patient Safety in U.S. Hospitals," *Health Affairs* 21, no. 2 (2002): 163.

90. Anne Elixhauser, Claudia Steiner, and Irene Fraser, "Volume Thresholds and Hospital Characteristics in the United States," *Health Affairs* 22, no. 2 (2003): 175.

91. Kaiser Family Foundation, *For-Profit Health Care Companies: Trends and Issues* (Menlo Park: Kaiser Family Foundation, 1998), 21.

92. Mark Schlesinger, Shannon Mitchell, and Bradford Gray, "Measuring Community Benefits Provided by Nonprofit and For-profit HMOs," *Inquiry* 40, no. 2 (2003): 126, 127.

93. Ibid., 129.

94. William Baldwin, "Unsocializing Medicine," *Forbes* 169, no. 11 (2002): 24.

95. Martin Feldstein, "Health and Taxes," *Wall Street Journal,* 19 January 2004, 13A.

96. Ron Lieber, "Getting Uncle Sam to Cover Your Massage: Rush to Use up Medical Savings Accounts Prompts Creative Reading of Rules; a Tax Break for Dieters," *Wall Street Journal*, 5 November 2002, D1.

97. Baldwin, "Unsocializing Medicine," 24; Samuel E. D. Shortt, "Medical Savings Accounts in Publicly Funded Health Care Systems: Enthusiasm versus Evidence," *Canadian Medical Association Journal* 167, no. 2 (2002): 160.

98. S. Matisonn, "Medical Savings Accounts in South Africa" (study 234, National Center for Policy Analysis, Dallas, 2000).

99. Michael Barr, "Medical Savings Accounts in Singapore: A Critical Inquiry," *Journal of Health Politics, Policy and Law* 26, no. 4 (2001): 709. See also Jeremiah Hurley, "Medical Savings Accounts in Publicly Financed Health Care Systems: What Do We Know?" (McMaster University Centre for Health Economics and Policy Analysis, Research Working Paper 01-12, Hamilton, Ontario, December 2001).

100. Barr, "Medical Savings Accounts in Singapore," 712, 713.

101. Ibid., 716. See also Chris Ham, "Values and Health Policy: The Case of Singapore," *Journal of Health Politics, Policy and Law* 26, no. 4 (2001): 742.

102. Barr, "Medical Savings Accounts in Singapore," 716.

103. Ibid., 717.

104. Mark Pauly, "Medical Savings Accounts in Singapore: What Can We Know?" *Journal of Health Politics, Policy and Law* 26, no. 4 (2001): 730.

105. Shortt, "Medical Savings Accounts in Publicly Funded Health Care Systems," 161.

106. David Gratzer, "It's Time to Consider Medical Savings Accounts," *Canadian Medical Association Journal* 167, no. 2 (2002): 151.

107. Evelyn L. Forget, Raisa Deber, and Leslie L. Roos, "Medical Savings Accounts: Will They Reduce Costs?" *Canadian Medical Association Journal* 167, no. 2 (2002): 143–47.

108. Malcolm Gladwell, "The Moral Hazard Myth," *New Yorker,* 20 August 2005, 49.

109. Kate Christensen, "Ethically Important Distinctions among Managed Care Organizations," *Journal of Law Medicine and Ethics* 23 (1995): 223–29. See also David Orentlicher, "Paying Physicians More to Do Less: Financial Incentives to Limit Care," *University of Richmond Law Review* 30 (1996): 155–97; Managed Health Care Improvement Task Force, "Financial Incentives for Providers in Managed Care Plans" (background paper, National Advisory Council on Professional and Organizational Ethics Conference, Oakland, CA, 26 May 1999).

110. Managed Health Care Improvement Task Force, "Financial Incentives for Providers," 74.

111. Ibid., 82–85; Orentlicher, "Paying Physicians More to Do Less," 162.

112. Douglas A. Conrad et al., "The Impact of Financial Incentives on Physician Productivity in Medical Groups," *Health Services Research* 37, no. 4 (2002): 885–906.

113. M. Gaynor and M. V. Pauly, "Compensation and Productive Efficiency in Partnerships: Evidence from Medical Group Practice," *Journal of Political Economy* 98, no. 3 (1990): 544–73; M. Gaynor and P. Gertler, "Moral Hazard and Risk Spreading in Partnerships," *Rand Journal of Economics* 26, no. 4 (1995): 591–613.

114. Douglas Conrad et al., "Primary Care Physician Compensation Method in Medical Groups," *Journal of the American Medical Association* 279, no. 11 (1998): 853–58; 856.

115. Dolores Clement et al., "Access and Outcomes for Elderly Patients Enrolled in Managed Care," *Journal of the American Medical Association* 271, no. 19 (1994): 1487–92.

116. Council on Ethical and Judicial Affairs, American Medical Association, "Ethi-

cal Issues in Managed Care," *Journal of the American Medical Association* 273 (1995): 330–35; David Sulmasy, "Managed Care and Managed Death," *Archives of Internal Medicine* 155, no. 2 (1995): 133–36.

117. Managed Health Care Improvement Task Force, "Financial Incentives for Providers," 78–79.

118. Orentlicher, "Paying Physicians More to Do Less," 161–62.

119. Ibid.

120. Managed Health Care Improvement Task Force, "Financial Incentives for Providers," 82–87.

121. Varun Gauri, "Are Incentives Everything? Payment Mechanism for Health Care Providers in Developing Countries" (World Bank Development Research Group, Working Paper 2624, World Bank, Washington, DC, 2001), 13.

122. Richard B. Saltman, Reinhard Busse, and Josep Figueras, *Social Health Insurance Systems in Western Europe* (Maidenhead, UK: Open University Press, 2004); further citations of this source (SHI study) are in the text.

123. OECD, *Health at a Glance,* 45.

124. Elizabeth A. McGlynn, "There Is No Perfect Health Care System," *Health Affairs* 23, no. 3 (2004): 100–102.

125. John Cogan, Glenn Hubbard, and Daniel Kessler, "Healthy, Wealthy and Wise," *Wall Street Journal,* 4 May 2004, A1. Cogan is a former deputy director of the Office of Management and Budget; Hubbard, former chairman of George W. Bush's Council of Economic Advisors; and Kessler, a professor at Stanford University. For similar ideas, see also Newt Gingrich, *Saving Money and Saving Lives: Transforming Health and Healthcare* (Washington, DC: Alexis de Tocqueville Foundation, 2003).

126. Cogan, Hubbard, and Kessler, "Healthy, Wealthy and Wise."

127. Peter S. Hussey et al., "How Does the Quality of Care Compare in Five Countries?" *Health Affairs* 23, no. 3 (2004): 90.

128. Ibid., 91–92.

129. Cogan, Hubbard, and Kessler, "Healthy, Wealthy and Wise."

130. Karen Davis, "Taking a Walk on the Supply Side: Ten Steps to Control Health Care Costs" (Commonwealth Fund, New York, 9 March 2005).

131. John C. Goodman et al., *Lives at Risk: Single-Payer National Health Insurance around the World* (Lanham, MD: Rowan and Littlefield, 2004), 909.

132. J. Hurst and L. Siciliani, "Tackling Excessive Waiting Times for Elective Surgery: A Comparison of Policies in Twelve OECD Countries" (OECD working paper, Organization for Economic Cooperation and Development, Paris, July 2003); cited in Gerard F. Anderson et al., "Health Spending in the United States and the Rest of the Industrialized World," *Health Affairs* 24, no. 4 (2005).

133. Anderson et al., "Health Spending in the United States."

134. Roger D. Feldman, ed., *American Health Care: Government, Market Processes, and the Public Interest* (New Brunswick, NJ: Transaction Publishers, 2000); further citations of this source are in the text.

135. Richard A. Epstein, "Antidiscrimination Principle in Health Care: Community Rating and Preexisting Conditions," in Feldman, *American Health Care,* 224.

136. Alain Enthoven, "Market Forces and Efficient Health Care Systems," *Health Affairs* 23, no. 2 (2004): 26.

CHAPTER 7: THE FUTURE OF THE MARKET IN HEALTH CARE

1. Health Insurance Association of America, *The Impact of Medical Technology on Future Health Care Costs* (Bethesda, MD: Health Insurance Association of America, 2001); David Cutler, "Technology, Health Costs, and the NIH" (ms., 1995); for a more complex story of American health care costs, see also Uwe Reinhardt, Peter S. Hussey, and Gerald F. Anderson, "U.S. Health Care Spending in an International Context," *Health Affairs* 23, no. 3 (2004): 10–25.

2. Uwe E. Reinhardt, "Does the Aging of the Population Really Drive the Demand for Health Care?" *Health Affairs* 22, no. 6 (2003): 27–39.

3. Thomas Rice, *The Economics of Health Reconsidered,* 2nd ed. (Chicago: Health Administration Press, 2003), 73 ff.

4. Ibid., 273.

5. Hastings Center, "The Goals of Medicine: Setting New Priorities," *Hastings Center Report* 26, no. 6 (1996): S1–S27.

6. J. M. McGinnis and W. H. Foege, "Actual Causes of Death in the U.S.," *Journal of the American Medical Association* 270, no. 18 (1993): 2207–12.

7. Ali H. Mokdad et al., "Actual Causes of Death in the United States, 2000," *Journal of the American Medical Association* 291, no. 10 (2004): 1238–45.

8. Ibid., 1243.

9. Thomas McKeown, *The Role of Medicine: Dream, Mirage, or Nemesis?* (Oxford: Blackwell, 1979).

10. J. P. Mackenbach et al., "Regional Differences in Mortality from Conditions Amenable to Medical Interventions in the Netherlands: A Comparison of Four Time Periods," *Journal of Epidemiology and Community Health* 42 (1998): 325–32.

11. Ellen Nolte and Martin McKee, *Does Health Care Save Lives? Avoidable Mortality Revisited* (London: Nuffield Trust, 2004).

12. Ibid., 43.

13. Arthur J. Barsky, *Worried Sick: Our Troubled Quest for Wellness* (Boston: Little, Brown, 1988), 187.

14. Norman Daniels and James E. Sabin, *Setting Limits Fairly: Can We Learn to Share Medical Resources?* (New York: Oxford University Press, 2002).

Index

Daniel Callahan is Director, International Program, The Hastings Center. He was a cofounder of the center and for many years its president. He has a B.A. from Yale and a Ph.D. in philosophy from Harvard. He is an elected member of the Institute of Medicine, National Academy of Sciences, and a fellow of the American Association for the Advancement of Science. He is also a senior scholar at the Institute for Politics and Policy at Yale University and an honorary faculty member of the Charles University Medical School, Prague, the Czech Republic. He is the author or editor of many books, most recently *What Price Better Health: Hazards of the Research Imperative.*

Angela Wasunna is Associate, International Program, The Hastings Center. She is an Advocate of the High Court of Kenya and has a Bachelor of Laws (LL.B.) degree from the University of Nairobi, Kenya , a Master of Laws (LL.M.) degree with a bioethics specialization from McGill University, Canada, and an LL.M. from Harvard Law School. Her research interests include health and human rights, intellectual property law, financing of health care in developing countries, legal and ethical issues raised by international research, and HIV/AIDS law and policy. She is an elected board member of the International Association of Bioethics and a member of the International Bar Association, the Pan African Bioethics Initiative, and the Law Society of Kenya.